The
Medical Interview:
A Primer
for Students of
the Art

The Medical Interview:
A Primer for Students of the Art

EDITION 2

JOHN L. COULEHAN, M.D., F.A.C.P.
Professor of Medicine
State University of New York at Stony Brook
Stony Brook, New York

MARIAN R. BLOCK, M.D., A.B.F.P.
Chairman, Department of Family Medicine
The Western Pennsylvania Hospital
Pittsburgh, Pennsylvania

 F. A. DAVIS COMPANY • Philadelphia

F. A. Davis Company
1915 Arch Street
Philadelphia, PA 19103

Printed in the United States of America

Last digit indicates print number: 10 9 8 7 6 5 4

NOTE: As new scientific information becomes available through basic and clinical research, recommended treatments and drug therapies undergo changes. The author(s) and publisher have done everything possible to make this book accurate, up-to-date, and in accord with accepted standards at the time of publication. The authors, editors, and publisher are not responsible for errors or omissions or for consequences from application of the book, and make no warranty, expressed or implied, in regard to the contents of the book. Any practice described in this book should be applied by the reader in accordance with professional standards of care used in regard to the unique circumstances that may apply in each situation. The reader is advised always to check product information (package inserts) for changes and new information regarding dose and contraindications before administering any drug. Caution is especially urged when using new or infrequently ordered drugs.

Library of Congress Cataloging-in-Publication Data

Coulehan, John L., 1943–
    The medical interview : a primer for students of the art / John L. Coulehan, Marian R. Block. — Ed. 2.
        p.   cm. — (Essentials of medical education series)
    Includes bibliographical references and index.
    ISBN 0-8036-1996-0 (softbound : alk. paper) : $20.00 (est.)
    1. Medical history taking.   I. Block, Marian R., 1947–
II. Title.   III. Series.
    [DNLM: 1. Medical History Taking.   2. Physician-Patient Relations. WB 290 C855m)
RC65.C68   1991
616.07′51 — dc20
DNLM/DLC
for Library of Congress   91-25137
                                                                                CIP

To Our Families

Foreword
From the Patient's Perspective

This splendid book is both interesting and important because it is concerned with real patients in the natural setting of clinical medicine. Given that the work of medicine is about the care of real patients, it is strange but true that this book is one of the few of its kind.

The fact of this volume's distinctiveness requires some comment. Solid grounds exist for considering the 20th century as the period when science entered medicine in full force. The contributions of science to medicine pervade every dimension of clinical medicine, from understandings of basic mechanisms of disease, to the discernment of diagnostic technology, to the power of current therapeutics.

Another trend characteristic of 20th century medicine is the emphasis on the sick person—the subject of medical care. How the illness interferes with the patient's function claims our attention not only for its diagnostic information but also because of our genuine concern for the interference in the patient's life caused by the disease. Treatment choices are commonly made with the patient's viewpoint in mind.

Another aspect of the pre-eminence of the person in medicine is the current understanding that how a disease presents itself, what course it runs, and what its outcome will be depends in part on *who* the patient is. We see diseases as confined to organ systems or parts of the body, whereas the cumulative effects of disease on the person extend, we know, to the person's relationships with others, to the family, and even, on occasion, to the community.

From the late 19th century and well into the early decades of this century, physicians were not directly concerned with patients' perspectives. They were almost solely interested in finding what disease a patient had. That attitude is natural enough considering the fact that diseases as they are presently known had just been "invented" in the early years of the 19th century and were *the* exciting advance of the times. The two fundamental tenets of classical disease theory are that each disease is characterized by a unique pathologic abnormality and that every disease has a unique cause. Little wonder that physicians spent their time trying to ferret out the pathologic abnormality that was the seat of the patient's illness, as well as hunting for its particular cause. In the light of these beliefs, it is not surprising that there was not much room in medicine for the sick person *as sick person.*

On March 19, 1927, Francis Peabody published in the *Journal of the American Medical Association* a now-famous paper called "The Care of the Patient," in which he pointed out the detrimental effect on patient care that is produced by the single-minded pursuit of disease. He showed the problems raised when a patient is dismissed as having nothing wrong just because no disease can be found to account for the symptoms. The startling feature of his essay, and what makes it a landmark, is that it discusses these issues *from the point of view of the patient.* Peabody was not alone, however, in promoting the importance of the sick person in medicine. The blossoming of the modern discipline of psychology and the work of Freud and his followers were also of great importance in promoting an appreciation of the effect of emotions in the production and amelioration of illness. Since the Second World War, the place of the subject in medicine—the importance of the sick person—has become an established part of the medical scene.

Or has it? A multitude of external evidence supports the idea of the central position of the sick person. Entering medical students are imbued with the importance of the patient. Virtually every medical school curriculum has courses devoted to humanities in medicine, ethics, or similar person-oriented subjects. In sharp contrast, however, is the perspective one gets from within a modern teaching hospital, where it is clear that the central place of the sick person is more an ephemeral ideal than a reality. In the wards of academic centers, students and house officers are rewarded for their command of science and technology rather than their understanding of the perspective of the patient. How can it be that something as characteristic of the medicine of this era as the centrality of the sick person is so *informally* accepted and so formally problematic? The answer lies in the almost paradoxical fact that *both* the importance of the sick person *and* science are what characterize modern medicine. It is in exploring the contest and friction between science and personal values that we will see what an important book Drs. Coulehan and Block have written.

Acceptable knowledge, from a scientific point of view, is objective, reproducible, and predictable. Numeric data seem best to meet the ideal, but other artifacts such as roentgenograms, electrocardiograms, spirometric tracings, and slides of tissue are also acceptable. In medicine, we call such information "hard" data. On the other hand, information that is subjective, value-laden, or which cannot be measured is considered unscientific and believed to be of lesser value. It is often called "soft." Medical scientists believe that soft data should be replaced by hard data at all times. Unfortunately, the knowledge and information by which we come to know the viewpoint of the sick person—bodily feelings, emotions, needs, desires, fears, beliefs, future concerns, lived past, relationships, and so on—are *always* "soft," subjective (in that they have to do with a subject), value-laden, and unmeasurable. *It has always been so, it will always be so, and it cannot be otherwise.*

The truth of the previous sentence has not been easy for medicine, doctors, or science to accept. Instead, three solutions to the quandary posed by the unscientific nature of personal information have been tries. One has been to banish the person from medicine as practiced. In this view, doctors take care of diseases, and personal factors are thought to be, at best, matters of sentiment and, at worst, contaminants that impede the diagnosis and treatment of disease. This has merely led to bad medicine in which technologic imperatives rule over human needs—we do things because they can be done rather than because they should be done.

A second solution has been to try to *force* personal information into the mold of the scientific ideal by creating questionnaires and scales that can be handled numerically. This may have some uses, but for the care of individual patients it is worse than useless—worse because it fools the doctor and puts off the inevitable recognition that personal information *cannot* meet the scientific ideal.

The third commonly attempted solution is to live by a double standard. On the one hand, formal recognition is given to scientific knowledge and information, while pretending that nothing else is really important in medicine. At the same time, the importance of the perspective of the sick person is given informal acknowledgment by valuing highly such things as caring, humaneness, or compassion, which are thought to be the characteristics of a good doctor. Double standards require people to say one thing but do another. They are inherently unworkable.

Personal information does not meet standards; this cannot be denied. There is another way out of the quandary, however, which is better than the three described. Accept the fact that certain standards of information (scientific) apply to certain types of knowledge—the objective facts of nature. Other standards of information apply to the other type of knowledge—personal information about sick persons. It is not that one is better, the other worse; they are inherently different. A scientist's personal feelings about how RNA transcription occurs, for example, are useless information. Numeric measurements of the patient's feelings are equally useless. The real questions are not whether information is scientific or not, or which type is better; the real questions for doctors are: What is the problem? What kind of information do I need to solve the problem? How do I get the information? How do I ensure maximum reliability of information? How do I think about it? and How do I apply it?

The importance of this book lies in its direct address of these questions. The volume takes the information that patients have to offer about their diseases and themselves to be of fundamental importance in the care of sick persons. The book then offers methods for getting at that information through the relationship between doctor and patient. Then it provides ways to think about and use the information that is developed through the interaction of the doctor with the patient.

The volume's distinctiveness arises from the manner in which its subject is approached. Its teachings are systematic, its system based on theoretic principles, which the authors make perfectly clear. The reader is free to agree or disagree with the theory. But because theoretic underpinnings are provided, readers do not have to model themselves after the authors in order to make effective use of the teachings. This is a refreshing change after all the interviewing cookbooks!

One thing more. I hope that this book will stimulate readers to take part in the development of methods of thinking about the personal information obtained from patients, methods of inquiry that will be as powerful for this type of information as are scientific methods for the objective facts of nature. This book is a wonderful way to begin to learn the ideas and skills that doctors employ throughout their lives—the same ideas and skills that are the first step toward the advances in methods of thought that are necessary to continued progress in medicine.

ERIC J. CASSELL, M.D., F.A.C.P.
New York, New York

Preface

Our course in medical interviewing and ultimately this book originated from our perception of a paradox. We found, on the one hand, that many faculty members at our medical center emphasized the importance of history-taking, both in their lectures to students and house staff, and in their discussion of individual patient cases. On the other hand, medical school and residency curricula put very little emphasis on the systematic teaching of history-taking or medical interviewing. Our students received a "little black book" that outlined a patient's history and presented a long series of suggested questions to ask. The seeming contradiction between the avowed value of history-taking in patient care and its neglect in the curriculum troubled us. There was a sense that students should "pick up" interviewing skills through experience; yet there were few opportunities to monitor or direct that experience. As students and residents discussed clinical problems on rounds, it seemed apparent that they valued historic data considerably less in the decision-making process than they valued other "hard" or "objective" data.

It was our hypothesis that good interviewing skills are not simply something "extra" in health care practice, simply a desirable feature that leads to better rapport with patients or more sensitivity to psychosocial issues. Good interviewing skills also allow health care workers to obtain more complete and more accurate data about illness, data that contribute to better diagnostic and therapeutic decisions. Furthermore, these skills facilitate written communication and cost-effective medical care, and they inhibit dissatisfaction and the proliferation of malpractice claims. Thus, good doctor-patient communication is not simply pleasant or desirable, it lies at the core of the science and logic of clinical medicine.

But just what are the required interviewing skills and how can one teach them? We went to the literature to learn how others had taught medical interviewing, and then went to our own practices, and to those of some of our colleagues and residents, to learn more about the process of interaction between doctor and patient. We did this by audio-taping and videotaping many interviews and carefully studying the tapes. As might be expected, we found both good and bad interviews, and observed a number of patterns. In the best history taking, we found a dynamic balance between an open-ended, non-directive approach that promoted patient acceptance, rapport, and willingness to tell the story; and a clear, task-oriented structure that directed the interview toward accurate and precise information.

The course that we developed for second year medical students was based on these convictions, the taped data we had acquired, and our review of the literature on teaching history-taking and interviewing skills. In particular, we found that a micro-skill approach, developed by Carkhuff, Ivey and Authier, and others for the counseling situation, could be adapted to teaching medical history taking. The first edition of this book was developed over a period of years from materials we prepared for students in that course. Our objective was to provide a step-by-step approach—one that could be useful to students and house officers who simply read the book, tried out its methods, and reflected upon their experience, as well as being useful to those who employed it in the context of organized instruction.

In the years since the first edition was published, we have continued to learn from our students, our patients, and from the burgeoning literature on the analysis of doctor-patient interactions. We have also benefited from thoughtful critiques of our book by a number of colleagues and reviewers. In this second edition, we expand our approach to medical interviewing to include pediatric, ambulatory, and geriatric encounters; and to the assessment of patients' mental status. In addition, we present chapters on recording the medical history, the use of questionnaires and computers in history-taking, and the ethics of doctor-patient interactions.

This book includes numerous examples of doctor-patient interactions. The large majority of these are abstracted from taped interviews, although in every case we have removed any personal references that might serve to identify the physician or patient. In a few cases, we have altered (mostly by shortening) the transcripts in ways that serve to demonstrate specific points more compactly. We wish to thank the patients and physicians who permitted us to tape and study their interviews, thus providing a rich resource for understanding and teaching the skills of history taking.

As in the first edition, we wish to acknowledge our debt to two outstanding physician-educators. Eric J. Cassell, M.D. taught us how to observe the physician-patient interaction *systematically* and supported us throughout this endeavor. Alvan Feinstein, M.D. first taught us that the medical history is a basic source of scientific data about the patient and his or her illness and made us aspire to find the science in the art of history-taking.

We also wish to thank the faculty members of the medical interviewing course at the University of Pittsburgh who, through the years, have provided fruitful ideas, thoughtful discussion, constructive criticism, and unwavering support. In particular, we want to acknowledge Lili Penkower, Noel Poncelet, Laurel Milberg, Donna Nardini, Joel Merenstein, and Larry Pacoe. Finally, we express our thanks to Judy Smith, Marcy Cloherty, and Crystal Latimer, who put up with the administrative nightmare of coordinating students, classrooms, and faculty for several years, and prepared our manuscript through its various revisions.

Although each of us had primary responsibilities for writing certain chapters and for selecting and editing transcripts, this book is a joint product; in a very special sense it is a truly collaborative effort, and we are both responsible for the entire text.

JOHN L. COULEHAN, M.D., M.P.H.
MARIAN R. BLOCK, M.D.

Contents

Time after time I have gone out into my office in the evening feeling as if I couldn't keep my eyes open a moment longer. . . . But once I saw the patient all that would disappear. In a flash the details of the case would begin to formulate themselves into a recognizable outline, the diagnosis would unravel itself, or would refuse to make itself plain, and the hunt was on. Along with that, the patient himself would shape up into something that called for attention, his peculiarities, her reticences or candors. And though I might be attracted or repelled, the professional attitude which every physician must call on would steady me and dictate the terms on which I was to proceed.

William Carlos Williams, from *The Autobiography,* reprinted in W. C. Williams, *The Doctor Stories.* New Directions, New York, 1984.

Introduction:
The Poor Historian

> History-taking, the most clinically sophisticated procedure of
> medicine, is an extraordinary investigative technique: in few other
> forms of scientific research does the observed object talk.
>
> Alvan Feinstein, *Clinical Judgment*

They cluster in the hall on rounds, eight of them—students,
house officers, and attending physician—creating turbulence
and obstructing flow. A medication nurse pushes a cabinet
around them on the way down the hall, while the breakfast lorry
closes in from the other direction. An intern begins the presentation with "Mr. Blank is a 52-year-old man who presents with
abdominal pain . . . the patient is a poor historian. . . ."

The attending physician learns that this sick person claims to
have a number of symptoms and he is apparently taking several
medications. The intern hastens to add that Mr. Blank's compliance is poor, he doesn't seem to understand his illness, and he is,
after all, a "poor historian." Having thus dispensed with prelim-
inaries, the intern moves on to reporting the patient's physical
findings and initial laboratory data. At this point all qualifiers are
dropped: the magnesium level does not *seem* to be 2.2, it *is* 2.2.
Meanwhile, the attending physician reflects on the term "poor
historian," perhaps because of an unconscionable lack of interest
in magnesium. The matrix of numbers vibrating among students
and house officers takes on a life of its own, while the attending
physician wonders about this patient's "poorness." The physician knows what the intern is trying to tell the group with the
phrase "poor historian." The young physician does not intend to
say that the patient is an impoverished professor of history. Nor
does the intern mean that the patient is a failing history student.

1

No, the intern is saying in precise medical shorthand, "I was unable to reconstruct a logical story of the illness in my conversation with this patient. We did not communicate well." Reflecting further, the attending physician finds the term "poor historian" acceptable but wonders if the attribution is correct. Perhaps the intern would be more correct in saying, "The medical history is unclear because *I'm* a poor historian."

This vignette illustrates how data we obtain from speaking with the patient and the therapy we accomplish through the process of doctor-patient interaction are not often topics for discussion during medical rounds. While we consider information about serum magnesium, for which accuracy and precision is assumed, a fit topic for discussion, knowledge of the precise pattern of symptoms or the patient's beliefs about the symptoms appears less scientific and less relevant. The third-year medical student soon learns to spend less time listening to the patient's story and more time among his or her peers at the nurse's station agonizing over the meaning of a magnesium value. The students learn to accept responsibility for how well (or how poorly) they perform a bone marrow aspiration, interpret an x-ray, or insert a proctoscope. As physicians, we rarely blame the patient for an inadequate bone marrow aspirate, yet we believe the hospital is full of patients who perpetrate poor histories.

Stories of sickness and suffering—the kind of human stories that moved us to enter a healing profession in the first place—gradually move to the background as we become "socialized" into the technical culture of medicine. Students and physicians become preoccupied with quite different stories, i.e., technical tales in which organs and instruments rather than people are the protagonists. Sometimes, in fact, the patient's story is entirely forgotten:

> Nowadays it is not rare in hospital practice that investigations bring some unexpected results to light and these lead to more examinations along a side track. After a while the whole staff is interested in, say, the immunoglobulin pattern, and nobody remembers why the patient was admitted. Only on the day the patient is discharged will he say, "But you have not done anything about my backache!"[110]

This illustrates a narrow view of the medical enterprise, one that permeates medical education; the view is that real medicine is solely concerned with objective data, i.e., numbers, graphs, and images. This is associated with the belief that so-called subjective data, for example, the story a patient tells us, is necessarily lacking in quantification and so also must be lacking in clinical value. In other words, what patients feel, the suffering they experience, and the disability that haunts them, all of which they describe only indirectly through the medium of words, are secondary in importance to those physiologic quantities that can be observed directly by physicians. Physicians, so this premise goes, must address what *causes* all this suffering and pain: altered physiology, abnormal biochemical findings, or disease. The real work of medicine requires us to reduce persons and their illnesses to organs and diseases. In this view, if you correct bad numbers, suffering will go away. You don't have to pay much attention to who the patients are or to the fine details of their stories.

In fact, the patient and his or her story often get in the way of "real" medicine. The patient "comes to function as a kind of translucent screen on which the disease is projected . . . (but) the screen has opacities of its own which obscure the accurate perception of the underlying disease."[7] The poor historian, the patient with whom we have difficulty communicating, has many such "opacities." It is difficult to see through the person to the disease.

But should the patient be merely a screen, whether it be translucent or partially opaque? Should we endeavor to subtract the "subjective" from our medical equation? A broader view of medicine holds that the patient's stories—stories of sickness—lie at the center of medical practice. The great clinician and medical educator, William Osler, wrote, "It is a safe rule to have no teaching without a patient for a text, and the best teaching is that taught by the patient himself."[78] In fact, experienced clinicians are aware that, in general, about 70% of diagnoses are made on the basis of patient interviews and over 90% are made on the basis of history and physical examination.[30] Primary physicians spend the largest part of their clinical time talking with patients; the physicians generate most of their diagnostic hypotheses on the basis of the history, and most of the significant bits of information they use arise from this dialogue.

Despite widespread token recognition of this broader view of medicine, until recently medical schools generally did not include interviewing skills in their curricula. Medical educators did not consider history taking and talking with patients appropriate topics for serious study. These educators gave students "little black books" that included lists of questions about symptoms and past diagnoses. If the patient did not answer these questions clearly, concisely, and in a medically acceptable fashion, the patient was labeled a "poor historian." Clinicians told their students, "Talking with patients is important, but you'll pick up how to do it as you go along. The doctor-patient relationship is also important—crucial, in fact—but you'll pick that up as you go along, too. You just need experience."

This attitude toward communication skills in medicine has begun to change for a number of reasons. First, rapid advances in technology have led to a highly specialized and very expensive form of medicine that is missing something. Patients often find themselves doing better but feeling worse. They cannot understand why the "best" medicine—medicine targeted entirely to organ systems or even to specific diseases—does not seem to meet their needs. Academic medicine, in turn, has begun to understand that pain, suffering, and dysfunction must be conceptualized in broad human terms as well as in biochemical terms if we are to be effective healers. Medical practice must be based on a biopsychosocial[43] or holistic[25] model rather than on a purely biological model.

Second, in the past 35 years many investigators have studied the process of interviewing and analyzed its individual components. This work, along with studies in fields as wide ranging as medical anthropology and clinical decision making, has shown that the "art of medicine" can be articulated and taught systematically. It is not simply a matter of intuition and experience.

Third, patient-oriented studies have shown that good patient-doctor communication leads to good outcomes, improved patient satisfaction, and adherence to treatment. On the other hand, poor patient-doctor communication leads to poor outcomes, doctor-shopping, and excessive malpractice suits. Finally, the pressing need to limit the costs of medical care has led to a renewed emphasis on physicians who can use resources more rationally by knowing more about their patients and less about narrow categories of disease.

This book is based on the premise that interviewing and patient-doctor communication are essential to good medical practice. Talking with patients is not a skill reserved for psychiatrists and primary care doctors. It is essential for radiologists as well as internists, ophthalmologists, and pediatricians. Medical interviewing is a basic clinical skill. It is not a matter of common sense nor does it come necessarily with experience. It is a skill that can be broken down into its component parts, and it can be learned. That is the subject of this book.

This book is addressed primarily to students of medicine and other health professions who are about to begin their professional interaction with patients. It is designed to be a guide for those who are just learning to take a medical history as well as a resource for those who are a little farther along in their education and who are beginning to have sustained contact with patients as clinical clerks and postgraduate trainees. Our particular emphasis is on the microskills of the initial patient interview. Although we deal extensively with basic history taking, the same skills serve as building blocks for all types of patient-doctor interactions. They lie at the core of the art and science of medicine.

The book is divided into three major sections. Part 1 presents the basics. It includes chapters on fundamental interviewing skills and a series of chapters on different components of the medical history. It ends with a chapter on the medical write-up. Part 2 deals with more complex or difficult interviewing situations. These might arise because of the setting (e.g., office or clinic practice) or the age or competence of the patient (e.g., pediatrics or geriatrics), or from various other barriers to effective patient-doctor communication that create a "difficult" interview. Part 3 considers some additional topics relevant to the medical interview: screening and case finding through the use of questionnaires (Chap. 12), clinical judgment as manifested in patient-doctor conversations (Chap. 13), and the process of creating a healing connection (Chap. 14). The last chapter summarizes important ethical considerations that apply to medical interviewing and other ordinary patient-doctor interactions.

PART 1

Basic Skills

CHAPTER 1

History Taking
as a Clinical Skill

The means of testing, required to give an inferential element any claim whatsoever to be *knowledge* instead of conjecture, are the data provided by observation—and *only* by observation.

John Dewey, *Propositions, Warranted Assertibility, and Truth*

While modern medicine is based on a group of theoretical sciences, clinical medicine itself is a practical science: it is the science of helping ill people get well, rather than that of understanding disease. As with any other science, clinical medicine has basic units of observation, basic quantities of measurement, and basic instruments for obtaining these measurements. The basic units of observation are signs and symptoms, the quantities of measurement are words and sometimes numbers, and the most important instrument is the medical practitioner.[46] Like any other scientific instrument, the clinician must be objective, precise, sensitive, specific, and reproducible when making observations about the patient's illness (Fig. 1–1).

OBJECTIVITY

What does it mean to be objective when interviewing a patient and taking a medical history? *Objectivity* means removing one's own beliefs, prejudices, and preconceptions before making observations; objectivity involves removing *bias* or systematic distortion from one's observations. Other words for objectivity are accuracy and validity. Your observations should correspond to what the patient really felt and experienced. If, for example, you start out by expecting a typical history of a certain illness and discard or minimize items that do not seem to fit, you are not

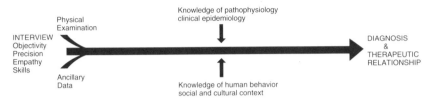

FIGURE 1–1. The medical interview in the context of clinical medicine.

being objective. Consider this interview taken from Platt and McMath[80] in which the physician "knew" that the patient had severe lung disease and so was unable to hear or follow up on the chief complaint:

Dr: Hello, I'm Dr. X; are you Mrs. Y?

Pt: Yes, I'm glad to know you.

Dr: What sorts of troubles have you been having?

Pt: I've been going downhill for 2 years. Nothing seems to be working right.

Dr: What is the worst part?

Pt: My legs. I have constant pain in my legs. It's gotten so bad I can't sleep.

Dr: What about your breathing?

Pt: Oh, that's all right. I can breathe fine. I just hurt so bad in my legs.

Dr: Are you still smoking?

Pt: Yes, with this pain, I've gone back to cigarettes for relief. But I'm down to half a pack or so a day.

Dr: Are you having pains in your chest?

Pt: No.

Dr: How about cough?

Pt: No, I hardly ever cough.

Dr: How much are you actually able to do?

Pt: Well, I was able to do everything until about 2 years ago, but now I can hardly walk half a block.

Dr: Why is that?

Pt: My legs. They hurt.

Dr: Do they swell up?

Pt: Well, they've been a bit swollen the last 2 or 3 weeks, but the pain is there whether they swell or not.

Dr: All right, I want to ask you some things about your medical history now.

The physician in this case seems to ignore the patient's leg pain; when she complains about it, the physician replies with questions about breathing. The physician is undervaluing certain kinds of information—ignoring what is not expected—while overvaluing other data related to a diagnosis that is "known." This not only is unscientific and could lead to a missed diagnosis, it is also likely to make the patient feel ignored. When patients feel ignored, they tend to say less, and data vital to making a diagnosis may be lost.

This is how the same physician might respond on a better day:

Dr: Hello, I'm Dr. X, are you Mrs. Y?
Pt: Yes, I'm glad to know you.
Dr: Thank you, I'm glad to know you too. What sorts of troubles have you been having?
Pt: I've been going downhill for 2 years. Nothing seems to be working right.
Dr: What is the worst part?
Pt: My legs. I have constant pain in my legs. It's gotten so bad I can't sleep.
Dr: Pain in your legs. Tell me more about that.
Pt: Well it's gotten so bad I can hardly walk half a block.
Dr: You mean the pain forces you to stop?
Pt: Yes, that's exactly it. And, well, it gets better when I stop, but never really goes away. Even at night when I'm lying still it wakes me up, it's so bad.

The patient here is giving a history consistent with severe peripheral vascular disease, a story to which the physician is now attending. The patient is now able to volunteer important details about the leg pain that not only aid the diagnostic process but also help her feel understood. The skill in being objective requires, first, effective listening and, then, effective feedback to the patient of what you have heard; in other words, you let the patient know that you hear what is said.

INTERPRETATION VERSUS OBSERVATION

It is easy to confuse *interpretation* with *observation*. When talking with a patient, the observation is what the patient actually says or does; the patient's words are the *primary data* of the symptom. Medical students are sometimes encouraged by preceptors and house officers to use terms that are really interpretations rather than descriptions. One example of such a term is "angina," which means a certain kind of chest pain due to coronary artery disease. This word is an interpretation implying a specific etiology. The primary data of the symptom might be something like: "substernal discomfort of a dull, pressing nature, lasting about 3 minutes, brought on by exertion, and relieved by rest." The use of terms such as angina is a method of shorthand necessary for quick thinking and talking in medicine; such shorthand terms are appropriate to use when the symptom has indeed been shown to be, in this case, secondary to coronary artery disease. *However,* if you interpret the symptom prematurely, you may lose data that point to the correct diagnosis. Once you start using the word angina, you may forget the patient's own story. Premature interpretation compromises objectivity.

Here is an example of a 68-year-old woman who lived for several years with the diagnosis of angina, i.e., coronary artery disease, because her former physician did not listen for the *primary data.* Here is how she described her chest pain:

Dr: Tell me about this chest pain.
Pt: It's a soreness in here, right through here (pointing to midchest) a lot. Some pain in my arm and a feeling in here. And a burning in the middle here and a burning in my throat.
Dr: When does this seem to come on?
Pt: Oh, it can be anytime, doctor. Sometimes I even get it in the middle of the night.
Dr: How about when you walk or are active in any way?
Pt: No, I can just be sitting.

Despite the fact that the patient did not have and had never had exertional chest pain relieved by rest, she had a complete cardiac workup, including coronary angiography. Even though all the test results proved negative, she carried a diagnosis of coronary artery disease. Finally, a new physician heard the complaints of burning and the nocturnal occurrence of pain and ordered an esophagram and upper gastrointestinal series; the physician discovered massive esophageal reflux and spasm. Perhaps it would have been more serious to overlook coronary artery disease, but for the patient much was lost: Frightened that she might die at any moment of a heart attack, she persisted in her belief that she had heart disease and was unable to be rehabilitated to an active life.

Objectivity means not only separating your own interpretations from the data but also separating the patient's interpretations from the data. This is important to remember when a patient tells you "My ulcer is acting up" or "My heart is giving me a lot of trouble" or "I'm here for my Hodgkin's disease." In such instances, the patient is interpreting certain symptoms as indicative of the presence of ulcer disease or heart disease, or is reporting a diagnosis instead of the primary data. For example, here is the statement of a 78-year-old man who called his physician with the following complaint:

> Pt: I don't know what's wrong. Somebody said I must have had the flu but it's lasted so long and I've tried everything and I don't know what to eat, so I just had to call and find out what you thought because it's been going on now 2 weeks and you know me, I don't call unless I really have to. And someone said I must have appendicitis or what's that thing that old people get?

This patient focuses on the etiology of his problem and does not give a story describing his symptoms. All we know is that, whatever has been going on, it has been going on for about 2 weeks. The physician's next response might be:

> Dr: Well, some people who get the flu do feel sick for quite some time.

While this response shows that the physician has heard the patient's theory, the physician still would not know what is going on. A better response might be:

> Dr: Well, some people who get the flu do feel sick for quite a while, but I'm not sure you had the flu. What exactly were your symptoms?
> Pt: Well, I had severe diarrhea—just like water—for a few days and I hurt low down in my belly. And weak, awful weak.

The doctor now has some primary data with which to start putting the diagnostic puzzle together. Although the patient's interpretation should be separated from primary data, the interpretation should not be ignored; it is important to acknowledge his belief about etiology as legitimate whether or not you agree with it. Such a recognition of the patient's point of view is necessary to managing the patient, particularly when explaining the rationale for a particular therapy or course of action.

PRECISION

Precision refers to how widely observations are scattered around the "real" value. Here, we are dealing not with a systematic bias that leads purposefully in one direction or another but rather with the random, unsystematic error induced by vagueness, poor listening, or lack of attention to detail. The basic units of measurement when taking a medical history are words; words are descriptions of sensations perceived by the patient and communicated to the physician. Words are verbal measurements and should be understood precisely; words must, therefore, be as detailed as necessary and as unambiguous as possible. For example, if a patient complains of being tired, does that mean shortness of breath on exertion, muscle weakness, lack of desire for activity, or sleepiness? Although the physician may correctly perceive that the patient says he or she is tired, the physician may have no idea of what is actually being described unless he or she gains enough detail to distinguish among dyspnea on exertion, muscle weakness, lack of motivation, and somnolence. In order to do this, the next question might go something like, "What do you mean by tired?" or "Can you tell me more about this tiredness?" or "How would you describe this feeling without using the word tired?" The good interviewer finds out with as much precision as possible what the patient is actually experiencing. The following is an example of a physician trying to get as much detail as possible about a chief complaint of headache:

Pt: See, I get these migraine headaches.
Dr: What do you mean by migraine headaches?
Pt: The last two headaches—I had two headaches last week, one on Monday and one on Thursday. Now they weren't real, real bad but the ones that I had before that, I threw up. I got real, real cold.

Dr: How often do you get these headaches?

Pt: I had two real bad ones within 2 weeks' time, then I didn't have one for a few weeks. Now the ones that I had last week, I didn't throw up with them, but they were enough that I had to go to bed with them.

Dr: Are the headaches something that occur almost every week, almost every month, or every couple of months?

Pt: I get them all the time. It is just within the last few months that I have been getting them more frequently. But I have averaged maybe one or two a month.

Dr: When you get these headaches, where does it hurt?

Pt: They start here and they just go around. Sometimes they'll go on one side of my face, sometimes on the other side of my face. But they start in the back of my neck here.

Dr: Do you get any kind of problems with your eyes when these headaches are coming on?

Pt: Blurred vision. The light bothers me.

Dr: Both eyes or one eye?

Pt: I have to go—like I go upstairs in my bedroom and like close everything up, and I just lay down with a blanket.

Dr: What kind of problem does the light give you when you have a headache?

Pt: It just bothers me, just the light itself, it's like a glare. The light itself bothers me.

Dr: What do these headaches keep you from doing?

Pt: Everything. I can't do a thing. When I get one, I have to go to bed. That's exactly what I do. Usually I throw up with them. I get real, real cold. It can be 90° outside, I'm freezing. Mostly the throwing up is a light vomiting.

Dr: Is there anything you can think of that triggers these headaches?

Pt: Nothing, it just starts.

Dr: Okay. What kind of person are you?

Pt: Little things will set me off. Like my kids are fighting, that bothers me, or if I feel like I'm overly tired or something like that. Little things bother me, that's all, but I've always been a nervous person.

Dr: When you get upset or you get nervous, is that likely

> to start up your headaches? Is there any kind of con-
> nection between the two?
>
> Pt: I can get up with a headache. If I get up with it, I'm
> done for the whole day. I do nothing at all.
>
> Dr: Do these headaches scare you?
>
> Pt: No, I'm used to them.
>
> Dr: Okay, so they don't frighten you, it's just a matter of
> trying to . . .
>
> Pt: To get rid of them.

There is no unambiguous test for the etiology of headache; only a careful and precise history will distinguish between migraine and muscle contraction headaches. This physician does not accept the patient's or previous doctor's diagnosis of migraine headache ("What do you mean by migraine headache?") and goes on to get many details about frequency, location, visual symptoms, and other associated symptoms.

SENSITIVITY AND SPECIFICITY

Accuracy and precision are two criteria by which we judge medical tests, including the medical history. Two additional criteria are sensitivity and specificity. The sensitivity of a test expresses its ability to "pick up" real cases of the disease in question. The higher the sensitivity, the greater the percentage of cases the test accurately identifies as having a positive test result. Specificity, on the other hand, refers to a test's ability to "rule out" disease in normal people. The higher the specificity, the greater the likelihood that a negative test result actually identifies a person who does not have the disease. Few, if any, tests in medicine approach 100% sensitivity and specificity; certainly the medical interview will not yield such definitive information.

A symptom may be very sensitive (cough, in cases of pneumonia) but not specific at all (dozens of diseases cause cough); it may be relatively specific (nocturnal midepigastric pain relieved by eating, in cases of duodenal ulcer) but not very sensitive (most persons with duodenal ulcer do not have that symptom). This relative lack of sensitivity and specificity for individual symptoms is one reason why physicians often minimize the value of their history taking and rush into more "scientific" tests. However, an individual symptom is not the appropriate unit on which to base decisions; we deal, rather, in symptom complexes, patterns, or pictures. We consider a detailed reconstruction of the illness, rather than isolated statements about symptoms.

A complete symptom complex may well be quite sensitive and specific; it may be adequate, in fact, to serve as the basis for diagnosis and therapeutic decisions. For example, Schmitt and his coworkers found that, among patients admitted to the hospital with a chief complaint of shortness of breath, clinicians could have made the correct diagnosis on the basis of history alone in 74% of cases.[91] Even when the "complete history" is not enough information for a correct diagnosis, the history usually contains *most* of the needed information. The history narrows the range of possible problems dramatically and yields a very small number of hypotheses to be supported, ruled out, or confirmed by physical examination and further studies. Thus, Rich and associates[87] found that—even in a high-technology setting such as a university's internal medicine training program—residents regarded the medical history as having much higher diagnostic value than either a physical examination or information from laboratory or radiographic tests. The well-conducted patient interview will yield a firm (and large) database on which to design an efficient (and small) diagnostic plan. In order to achieve this result, however, the physician must approach the task objectively and precisely. The *real* sensitivity and specificity of a symptom complex are irrelevant in a given situation if the instrument through which the data are obtained, the clinician, lacks accuracy and precision.

REPRODUCIBILITY

Reproducibility is another important characteristic of scientific tests, including medical interviewing. However, reproducibility of the medical history must be tempered by several considerations about human nature and the interactive process. In caring for a patient in the hospital, three or four observers often obtain three or four different versions of the patient's history. Much of the time, the differences may not be of great significance, but sometimes they will be crucial. Only one of four observers, for example, may note that the patient has had bright red rectal bleeding intermittently for the last 3 months. This fact might be lost in the review of systems and was only elicited by a direct question because the patient actually came into the hospital for chest pain and was either too embarrassed to mention the bleeding or, perhaps, too concerned about his heart to mention a seemingly unrelated problem. It suddenly becomes an important issue when you find the patient has a stool test that demonstrates occult blood or a hematocrit of 32%. The whole medical team might have to shift gears from ischemic heart disease workup to lower gastrointestinal (GI) bleeding workup. Of course, just as in the laboratory, data that change from one "experiment" to the next are always suspect. Reproducibility is a characteristic highly valued in testing; the apparent lack of reproducibility makes many physicians question the value of medical history taking.

Of course, one problem is that different history-taking instruments (physicians) manifest different levels of accuracy and precision. There are, however, several other reasons why various observers may get varying stories at different times.

First, patients come to the hospital or to the doctor with a personal story that includes a series of symptoms but often with no index of which symptoms are more or less important in explaining their underlying disease. A severe headache may cause the patient more pain than a sudden swelling of the left leg; but the latter could be secondary to lymphatic obstruction by metastatic cancer, while the former may have no pathologic significance at all. Each time a person is interviewed and constructs his or her story, the person learns, by virtue of what questions are asked and what seems to hold the interviewer's attention, what is of most importance to the interviewer. The patient will, in a sense, learn to "package" the story and make it more efficient or relevant or interesting to the clinician. Therefore, it is likely that later observers will get a more clearly connected and flowing— or at least different—history than the first interviewer.

Second, a corollary to this "educational" process is that patients may learn to consider important some things that they had not bothered to mention originally. The person may have forgotten the first episode of syncope or may have considered an illness occurring 3 years ago as something entirely unrelated to the present one. Repetition and focusing on symptoms will not only make the story more coherent but will also refresh the patient's memory or, perhaps, set the stage for some new insight. Therefore, it is reasonable that later observers may pick up entirely new information that the patient neglected to mention earlier. For example, here is how a first interview might go with a patient complaining of headaches. Knowing the importance to the diagnosis of differentiating new headaches from chronic ones, the clinician, a student, proceeds:

Dr: Tell me about your headaches. When did they start?
Pt: Well, I started getting them about 3 months ago.
Dr: Is that the first time you ever had this headache?
Pt: Well, yes.
Dr: So headaches are really new for you.
Pt: Well, now that I think about it, I can remember one something like it about 2 years ago. I remember, we were on vacation and I had to stay in the hotel. I thought I had the flu or something.
Dr: That's interesting. When did you get the next one?

For the next clinician, the attending physician, who interviews this patient, the story may be revealed as follows:

Dr: Tell me when these headaches started.
Pt: Well, I guess the first time I ever had one was about 2 years ago. But then I only had one every few months or so; they weren't frequent, until about 3 months ago when I started getting them every week.

Although both interviewers ask similar questions, notice how the patient's story is more organized and straightforward on the second telling.

Third, sick people may have already "organized" their illness in some way that makes sense to them, even before they see the doctor.[4] They may have tried getting rid of the symptoms on their own and perhaps may have asked for advice from family or friends. They may have read health columns in newspapers or seen a "TV doctor" discussing a problem similar to theirs. In addition, some patients may have religious or cultural beliefs that "frame" their understanding of illness in general. In these ways, patients usually develop some hypotheses about the kind of problems they have and what can or should be done about them. Consequently, they are likely to tell their tales in ways consistent with these hypotheses; they will emphasize symptoms that support their theories and minimize or forget symptoms that do not. The primary data are filtered through the patient's own hypotheses and beliefs. In the process of being interviewed by several different people trying to direct the flow of data toward medical hypotheses, a patient's own hypotheses may change. And when the story is filtered through a different set of beliefs, the story's elements, that is, perceptions, symptoms, and attributions, appear to change.

Fourth, different histories may be obtained at different times because the patient simply and consciously changes the story. Medical students or doctors often invoke this reason when they dislike the patient or are unable to account for the symptoms. The more the symptoms seem to be unrelated to "objective" findings or diagnostic tests, the more likely they are to be considered imaginary and susceptible to change from one history-taking session to another. Although some patients, of course, do change their story, the so-called unreliable patient is actually a much less frequent explanation for "changing" symptoms than the other factors we are considering.

Fifth, it is clear that interviewing skills play a part as well: An empathic physician who lets the patient tell his or her story is much more likely to obtain an accurate picture than a physician who asks a list of questions by rote. Skill in interviewing probably bears a general relationship to the person's experience level (medical student, intern, resident, attending physician); but when one considers an individual interview of an individual patient, all bets are off. The inexperienced medical student who can spend time with a patient in a nonthreatening atmosphere may learn a lot more than a hurried attending physician. In general, interviewing skills that maximize objectivity and precision reduce the rate of false-positive and false-negative histories.

THE SCIENCE AND THE ART OF HISTORY TAKING

As you develop clinical skills, you learn techniques to achieve objectivity and precision in gathering primary data from patients (see Fig. 1–1). This is good science and, what is more, it allows the patient to tell his or her story without fear of being prejudged. Objectivity demands removing your own beliefs and those of the patient to get at the primary data; objectivity involves suspending critical judgment and accepting the patient's story as his or her unique experience. Objectivity and precision involve understanding or knowing as though you were having the same symptom that the patient is describing. It is interesting to note that Carl Rogers defined empathy as "understanding exactly." This suggests that the skills required to be objective and precise are the same skills as those required to be a compassionate and empathic observer.

Thus, a *scientific* approach to history taking permits and reinforces an *artful* approach to the patient. Is there a contradiction between a "just get the facts" interview and an empathic interview? We would argue that there is no such contradiction, that you cannot get the facts without understanding exactly and without suspending judgment. Otherwise, the facts that you get may not be the relevant facts. With such an approach, you will embark on a vicious cycle that will lead you to undervalue history taking and rely more and more on a "shotgun" approach to diagnostic tests. To get the facts, you must understand and not judge; if you do otherwise, you will lose primary data essential to making the correct diagnosis. And when you understand and are nonjudgmental, your interview will build rapport—often the start of a therapeutic relationship—and will gather the data that tell not only *what* the diagnosis is but *who* the patient is.

A patient says this best. The following is part of an interview in which the patient describes how it feels to be understood and not judged:

Pt: Aw, I'm not usually this able to talk to people like this. I don't really know you . . .

Dr: That's true. I'm a total stranger.

Pt: And all of a sudden I have gone completely down the line and told you everything I could possibly think of to tell you. I've never been able to do that. I have very few people that I talk to personally or talk to about the way I feel . . . um . . . I talk to my family but there are only certain things that you can talk to your family about, and I have never had anyone I could talk to. I have always kept everything to myself. And now, all of a sudden, I've just flowed over like a broken toilet.

Dr: Was it helpful?

Pt: Yes, because I just learned something else about myself. The funny thing is, I have said all these things to you, and most times talking to people, I always think

> before I talk. I have said everything I have said to you
> without thinking about it first, and without wondering
> what you are going to think about what I am saying to
> you. And I can honestly say that I have never done that
> with anyone.
>
> Dr: Uh huh.
>
> Pt: I . . . um . . . have, maybe, I have a lot of friends but I
> mean, people you can really sit down and tell every lit-
> tle thing that happens in your life. There are very few
> of those. And I even, I even think before I say what I
> say to them because there's always a chance that some-
> one misinterprets, and really deep down I always know
> I want their opinion because I know they are my
> friends, and they are going to say what I want to hear
> and that's not always what I need to hear.
>
> Dr: Well I'm glad. Because I like to think it's helpful.
>
> Pt: It really is. I feel quite good about the whole thing.

The patient here describes being able to say everything "without thinking about it first." He is describing his ability to reveal uncensored primary data that are vital to the diagnostic process; what permitted him to do this was not "wondering what you are going to think about what I am saying to you." This is the aim of medical history taking. Revealing uncensored data was crucial for this patient, who presented with a rash that proved to be sec- ondary syphilis acquired in the course of multiple homosexual contacts. Had the patient filtered out data about his sexual activ- ity, about which he was embarrassed and ambivalent, the diag- nosis would have been made less quickly or, perhaps, not at all. He later died of acquired immunodeficiency syndrome (AIDS), and the need to communicate openly remained vital to his care.

SAGA OF THE FIFTH WHEEL

This section is an aside to address certain concerns of students who are just beginning to learn patient interviewing and physical examination. Often in a hospital setting, where patients are quite ill, the beginning student feels like a spare part, a "fifth wheel," someone who has no responsibility for patients' care. Besides simple inexperience and the anxiety associated with it, this situation leads students to have several other realistic concerns about interacting with patients to whom they are assigned. Three of the major ones are:

1. I don't know enough about pathophysiology to do a good history and physical examination, let alone to "get" the diagnosis.
2. The patients have been worked over 10 times already and are generally tired of it all, and sometimes angry, by the time I come in to examine them.
3. I have no responsibility for the patient, nor the ability to help, so I feel like an interloper—a fifth wheel.

Of course, each of these statements has an element of truth, but none of them need be a major constraint in your interviewing and physical diagnosis experience. Let us deal with each concern.

First, "I don't know enough pathophysiology." It is clear that you are not going to characterize patterns of symptoms as well as or as efficiently as an experienced physician, nor will you be able to pick up subtle physical signs. You might, for example, examine a patient with peptic ulcer before you have studied the gastrointestinal tract in your pathology or introduction to medicine courses. You will complain, "I don't know what symptoms to ask about. I don't know what direction to take." As long as the final *content* of the history (or physical examination) is all that interests you, there is no way to get beyond your lack of knowledge. However, the clinical art (and the point of this book) is to learn the *process* and *method*. Your goal is to learn to talk with patients in a way that maximizes both information gathering and therapeutic communication. The diagnosis (although interesting) is largely irrelevant at this point—you are not expected to make good diagnostic hypotheses without a knowledge of relevant pathophysiology. Your goal is to characterize the symptoms and the person as precisely and objectively as possible and, more importantly, to create an interview situation in which this can occur.

Wolraich and coworkers[108] conducted a study to determine whether improvement in knowledge about medical conditions or disease processes improves the students' interviewing skills. They assigned 10 students to an experimental group that

received some intensive education about diagnosis and management of meningomyelocele; the control group of 10 students did
not receive this information. Each subject in both groups then
interviewed in a simulated clinical situation the mother of a child
with meningomyelocele, and each interaction was rated for
interviewing skills and informational content. They found that
the students' interviewing skills were not affected by an increase
in their knowledge about the medical condition. Other studies
have suggested, in fact, that the interviewing skills of medical
students tend to decline as they progress from their first to their
fourth year of medical education.[109] This is certainly consistent
with our experience as preceptors and attending physicians.
These examples simply point out that, at the very least, the question of whether specific medical knowledge improves the process
of interviewing is an unresolved one.

Second, "The patients have often had numerous other examinations and are sick and tired of it all." The anger your patient
expresses (or just barely conceals) very frequently arises not
from the mere fact of repeated examinations but from the whole
situation—being ill, having a backache that no one pays attention to, uncomfortable diagnostic studies, doctors who are rude
or preoccupied, nurses who seem unsympathetic, and so forth.
The anger is present even before you arrive on the scene.

How do you deal with this? It is crucial to clarify your role, not
just as a student, but as a student learning to do an interview,
someone who will *not* be taking care of the patient on the hospital unit. Then, make sure the patient has really consented to
your interview and examination with a comment or question,
such as "May I talk with you now about the problems that
brought you to the hospital?" If he or she does not wish to talk
with you and says so, let it go at that. For patients who are tired
or in pain, suggest the possibility of your coming in later; if the
patient seems angry, acknowledge the anger. This will give you
a good opportunity to see how effective "interchangeable"
responses can be (see "Levels of Responding" in Chap. 2) in
obtaining information and developing rapport.

Sick people, like anyone else, may have several mutually conflicting feelings at the same time. A given patient may want to be
helpful to a student but be angry about the situation, depressed
about being ill, and simply exhausted simultaneously. You can tip
the balance in your favor: By being honest with the patient and

really listening, you will avoid contributing to the patient's anger and will also tend to defuse it.

Third, "I can't help this patient." The whole issue of responsibility and helpfulness needs another look. The professional role is not something you put on overnight when you get your degree. You grow into it. As a medical student you are demonstrably more a physician now than you were 2 years ago; as a nursing student you are clearly more a nurse now than you were 2 years ago. Although a learner, you are interacting with patients in a professional manner. The information you gather is important. Although the disease data you collect only occasionally contribute to what physicians have already gathered, the personal data you collect will often contribute to the patient's well-being. If the patient has a specific request or complaint, you can discuss it with a unit nurse or with the medical resident. If the patient has a misunderstanding, you can clarify the problem or find somebody else to do so.

Finally, simply listening to patients in an empathic manner can be therapeutic. Listening might not repair the damaged myocardium or lower the blood sugar level, but it will make the patient feel better. That is, after all, what clinical medicine is all about, although the goal of helping another human being to feel better often becomes confused, or at least remote, in a modern hospital. The patient is in a strange environment with a potentially serious or life-threatening illness and is caught in a system, the hospital, that is not always flexible or responsive to his or her needs. If you are willing to take the time to listen, you will be surprised how therapeutic the encounter with you is for your patient, even though you are ostensibly "doing nothing."

CHAPTER 2

Fundamental Skills: Understanding Exactly

> . . . for the moment at least I actually became *them*, whoever they should be, so that when I detached myself from them at the end of a half-hour of intense concentration over some illness which was affecting them, it was as though I were reawakening from a sleep.
>
> William Carlos Williams, *The Autobiography (Reprinted in W. C. Williams, The Doctor Stories, New Directions, New York, 1984)*

Almost everyone agrees that certain attitudes toward patients, such as genuineness and empathy, are praiseworthy. On first hearing this truism, you may think that these basic attitudes reflect the doctor's personality and value structure and are not immediately relevant to taking a medical history. You may not believe that these are skills that can be learned and used. However, these qualities can, in fact, be defined and observed as a certain set of behaviors. These behaviors can be practiced, taught, and learned.

In this chapter, we borrow some concepts from psychologists, particularly Carl Rogers and his followers, who first identified certain observable qualities of the therapist that correlated with good therapeutic outcomes. They called these *therapeutic core qualities*, and the three most important were *respect* (or unconditional positive regard), *genuineness* (or congruence), and *empathy*. They found that the content of psychotherapeutic intervention, such as the specific interventions dictated by a theory, was less important to success than the process of the interactions. Subsequently, other investigators defined specific skills evident in that process. They showed that qualities such as empathy could be broken down into a set of skills in listening to and responding to a patient.[58]

27

These therapeutic core qualities are important links between the art and science of medicine. They improve the interviewer's history-taking ability and the accuracy of the data obtained, and lead to better therapeutic relationships in ordinary practice. In the last chapter, we identified the goal of maximizing objectivity and precision in our communication with patients. In this chapter, we look at some "generic" concepts about how to do this before taking up the actual components of a medical history.

The following two examples serve to introduce these concepts. One is of a practicing physician interviewing a new patient in an office; the other is of a medical intern taking the history of a new patient in the clinic. In the first example, the patient is a 50-year-old woman who complains chiefly of abdominal pain that is worse when she is upset:

Dr: What happens when you get upset? What do you feel like?

Pt: Oh, I just feel *right nervous*, the stomach pains, my arm . . . it pains, it seems like the strength is going out of my arm and hands.

Dr: How often do you get upset?

Pt: Quite frequently.

Dr: What's quite frequent?

Pt: Mostly every day it seems like I'm upset. *I get something on my mind* and that brings on the nauseated feeling.

Dr: So what's the usual sequence? You get upset first and then what happens? You get upset first or does the nausea come on first?

Pt: No. I get upset and then the nausea comes on.

Dr: What are you upset about?

Pt: Well, you know, things you want around the house there . . . it seems like things don't go right around the house. Like I get upset about that.

Dr: Tell me about when you started being upset.

Pt: Oh really, right after my mother passed, really, in April, I've been mostly upset.

Dr: What happened when your mother passed away? I understand it must have been a very upsetting event; was she very close to you?

Pt: Yes, I was really close to my mother, and it seems like

> after she passed, I don't know, something just left out
> of me, I don't know what it was, you know.

In the second example, the patient is a 40-year-old man who came for a checkup. The doctor is inquiring about his family history and found that the patient's father, who had divorced his mother, had died of a ruptured aneurysm in the brain:

Dr: You don't know anything more about that?

Pt: Well my understanding is, the context of this is, that my mother was raised in the Catholic Church, and divorce was a terrible scandal in her mind and she tried to forget about it as quickly as she could. It's such a painful subject that there was never any discussion about who he was and so forth. And as a consequence all I've really heard are niblets, and one of the things I understand is that my father was an alcoholic or at least he had a problem with alcohol, but really caused my mother a lot of problems. So, I don't know if that would be a complicating factor in terms of an aneurysm or not.

Dr: Not that I know of. How about brothers and sisters?

Pt: I have one full natural brother and then four half brothers.

Dr: Medical problems in any of them that you know of?

Pt: No.

Dr: And you work as?

Pt: An editorial writer for the *Journal*.

Dr: And coming through your summer jobs, any unusual exposure to chemicals or mills or anything unusual that you did?

Pt: No, I worked in a bakery.

Dr: Asbestos?

All we have are transcripts of the tape-recorded histories, so we cannot reconstruct the tone or quality of the language, or the nonverbal communication. However, the doctor in the first example (who, by the way, is the medical intern) appears to be connecting with the patient, acknowledging both the facts and the patient's feelings ("I understand it's a very upsetting event"). The doctor in our second example does not appear to be on the same wavelength with the patient; the doctor's agenda has little regard for the other person. The patient has told the doctor that his father died of a cerebral hemorrhage but does not know anything else about it because his parents were divorced. The divorce, the "painful subject," and the history of alcoholism that pours out are ignored by the doctor who abruptly answers the patient's overt question and moves on ("Not that I know of. How about brothers and sisters?"). The second excerpt gives us a feeling that (at least in this interview) the doctor's history-taking skills, in particular, the ability to do it with empathy and respect, are not adequate.

We can define three qualities that enhance communication between doctor and patient:

Respect: The ability to accept the patient as a unique person as he or she is, and to suspend critical judgment;

Genuineness: The ability to be oneself in a relationship and not hide behind a role or facade;

Empathy: The ability to sense the patient's experience and feelings accurately, as well as to communicate that understanding back to the patient.

Respect, genuineness, and empathy are qualities that we demonstrate in relationships with our patients by using certain communication techniques. An important skill in dealing with patients is to maximize your ability to display these qualities through your behavior on any given occasion. When we make patients feel understood and respected, we greatly increase our chances of obtaining accurate primary data. Next we look at each skill and discuss specific ways to communicate to patients that we understand and respect them.

RESPECT

Respect means to value individuals' traits and beliefs despite one's own personal feelings about them and to see patients' habits or feelings as a valid adaptation to their illness or life circumstances. Clearly, this is a crucial issue in medicine. Some patients have habits such as smoking cigarettes, drinking too much, refusing to take medications, and even, at times, being antagonistic to their doctors or to medical students. Other patients have beliefs about their illness that try our patience: the patient with severe emphysema may explain to you that his illness has nothing to do with his 100 pack-year smoking history but was caused by a cold he never got rid of in 1956. Another patient might frustrate you with devastating migratory pains that never go away. Some patients may be unable to keep themselves clean or will be grossly obese. Many will have different value systems from yours or a healthy skepticism about medical technology.

The skill in having respect is to separate your personal feelings about the patient's behavior or attitudes or beliefs from your fundamental concern about helping him or her get well. For example, the patient who believes that his emphysema is unrelated to smoking can still be guided to give a reliable account of his own symptoms. Likewise, while the hostile patient will make you feel uncomfortable, you can still try to respect her reasons for being angry. Moreover, the emphysema patient's denial and the hostile patient's anger may actually be vital to their ability to tolerate being ill; such feelings must be accepted as part of the whole patient, not rejected as threats to the ego of the physician. As Cassell[22] states, "It is useful to remember that when patients argue, object, yell, scream, forget, or anything else from the rich repertoire of behavior that can turn caregivers into combatants, they must have a very good reason for doing it."

Respect involves those skills that demonstrate valuing the patient as a person and as a historian. The following case example, taken from Platt and McMath,[80] demonstrates a lack of respect in several ways:

The interviewer failed to knock at the patient's door. He introduced himself in a hasty mumble so that the patient never had his name clearly in mind. He mispronounced the patient's name once and never used it again. The physician conducted the interview while seated in a chair about 7 feet from the patient. There was no physical contact during the interview. On several occasions, the patient expressed her emotional distress. On each occasion, the interviewer ignored the emotional content of her statements.

> Dr: Exactly where is this pain?
> Pt: It's so hard for me to explain. I'm trying to do as well as I can. (Turning to husband:) Aren't I doing as well as I can?
> Dr: Well, is the pain up high in your belly, or down low?

> Pt: I kept getting weaker and weaker. I didn't want to come to the hospital. I was so frightened (weeping).
>
> Dr: Did the pain come before the weakness or afterward?

The physical examination was brusque; the examiner never warned his patient when painful maneuvers (for example, firmly stroking the sole of the foot) were to be done. At the end of the examination, the physician failed to comment on his findings or his plans. He said in parting, "We'll do some tests and see if we can find out just what's the matter with you," and left the room before the patient had an opportunity to question him.

Notice how the physician seems to have his own agenda, ignoring the patient both as a person, by not acknowledging her emotional distress, and as a historian, by not helping to clarify the nature of the pain and weakness. This vignette illustrates a number of simple things you can do to demonstrate respect for your patient:

1. You can introduce yourself clearly and communicate specifically why you are there. Since you are not the patient's friend, it would demonstrate lack of respect to use his or her first name during an initial interview.
2. You could inquire about and arrange for the patient's comfort before getting started and continue to consider his or her comfort during the course of your history and physical examination.
3. You can conduct the interview while sitting at the patient's level in a position where you can be easily seen and heard.
4. You can warn the patient when you intend to do or say something unexpected or painful, particularly in the physical examination.
5. You can respond to your patient in a way that indicates you have heard what he or she has said.

The previous interview might have gone something like this:

> Dr: Exactly where is the pain?
>
> Pt: It's so hard for me to explain. I'm trying to do as well

as I can. (Turning to husband) Aren't I doing as well as
I can?

Dr: I can see it's hard for you to explain and that you're
trying hard. Perhaps you can show me where you are
feeling it right now.

Pt: It's right about here (pointing) but what really frightened me was that I kept getting weaker and weaker and
I didn't want to come to the hospital (weeping).

Dr: (Handing patient a box of tissues). Here, do you need
one of these? Was it the weakness that frightened you?

Now the physician is focusing not only on the symptoms, but also
on the patient's feelings about the symptoms. In so doing, the
physician is likely to communicate respect for the patient and is
also more likely to acquire accurate data and to do so more
efficiently.

GENUINENESS

Genuineness means not pretending to be somebody or something other than who or what you are; it means being yourself,
both as a person and as a professional. The first time you encounter this concept of genuineness as a problem in medicine may be
in your role as a student. How do you introduce yourself? Should
you introduce yourself as a medical student or as a doctor? As a
nurse practitioner student or as a practitioner? Do you allow a
patient to address you as doctor? How do you respond when
patients ask you medical questions beyond your expertise or
inquire about their own prognosis or care? Or when they say,
"You look too young to be a doctor!" In all these cases, if you
are to be genuine, you must acknowledge what you are: a *student.* You should introduce yourself as a student and, whenever
appropriate, reaffirm to the patient your limited medical knowledge and limited responsibility (but not limited interest!) in the
patient's care. This does not mean you should avoid being helpful, for example, by transmitting the patient's requests to the unit
physicians, obtaining medical information for the patient from
his or her doctor, or encouraging the patient to ask someone else
the question you are unable to answer.

The term "student doctor" may represent a useful concept,
both for you and for the patient. It acknowledges the patient's

need—as well as your own—to perceive you in a professional, helping role, while it also genuinely describes what you are. Student doctor more closely defines your role when you are talking with patients than does the more nondescript term *"medical student."* It also allows you to experience yourself in a more professional light and may facilitate your helping attitude toward the patient.

Interns, residents, and physicians in their practice all experience situations in which patients ask for opinions or require procedures beyond the doctor's capabilities. The doctors are required to call in consultants or refer these patients to specialists. This does not mean abandoning your patients when their problems exceed your area of expertise. Rather, being genuine would mean outlining what you do and do not know, or can and cannot do, and negotiating a plan for future care that involves, for example, consulting a specialist.

Being genuine also means being yourself in another way, that of expressing your feelings while staying within the bounds of a professional relationship. If a patient is in the hospital for a medical or surgical illness but has experienced a recent loss, such as the death of a spouse, it is not only reasonable but even desirable to respond to this fact with a statement such as, "I am sorry to hear that. How has it been going for you?" However, adding that you too have lost a spouse may stress the limits of what you feel comfortable with in a professional relationship. When patients say or describe things that are sad or funny, it is appropriate to respond as a person and not just as a history-taking machine. Demonstrating your interest in the patient as a person is another way of being genuine.

Everyone has bad days, and you may happen to be at a low ebb yourself during your evaluation of the patient. You may have been on call and up all night with a patient in the intensive care unit. You may be having problems in your personal life or eagerly anticipating a weekend of skiing when you leave the hospital. At other times, you may be outraged about the patient's behavior, such as canceling or coming late to appointments. What is the role of genuineness in these situations? Should you hide your feelings, disguise your bad day, or express them to the patient? Genuineness means not pretending, but it does *not* mean that you must share all your feelings with the patient. You must distinguish your genuine *professional self* from the vicissitudes, experiences, or interests of your *personal self.* As you go through medical school and residency, you gradually develop your professional self into a well-integrated instrument of healing. It is this professional self that serves as the standard for your genuineness. For example, the patient who makes you angry by continually canceling or coming late to appointments can be told that you, as a person, are angry about that, but, as a professional, you try to confine your anger to that aspect of the relationship. At the same time, you try to respect the patient by understanding his or her reasons for being late—chaotic lifestyle, three children younger than age 5, single parenting, need to take three buses to get there, and so forth. This does not mean that you are lacking genuineness; rather, you are being your professional, helping self. Understanding is a prerequisite; the more you understand, the more likely that your respect will be genuine.

This discussion leads to two caveats:

1. It is rarely helpful to share your personal anger or disgust with the patient in the name of being honest. You may confront the patient with inconsistencies (to you) in his or her story or point out the patient's erratic behavior, if you believe it will help therapeutically; this is not the same as sharing your own negative feeling.
2. Sometimes physicians are tempted to share their experiences and feelings as illustrations for the patient. This may range from statements like "I have young children too, and I know what you mean," to detailed personal anecdotes. Here again it is crucial to judge your personal revelations in the light of your professional judgment. Ordinarily, comments of rapport and connection are helpful. The type of car you own, the vagaries of parenting, or your opinions about a football team are not really self-revelations. On the other hand, it is rarely part of a genuine doctor-patient interaction to describe intimate experiences or specific political or moral values.

Here is an example of a genuine response by a medical resident who is seeing a woman with asthma, peptic ulcer, and numerous psychosocial problems. She has just related a personal history of child abuse, and continues:

Pt: I can write a book. Well, you know, I'm not any more, but I used to be atheist for a while. God made me. I was

> a little girl, but I think about if you got children, you
> want the best for your children. If we are God's chil-
> dren, why did I go through what I went through? So
> that's why I feel the way I do.
> Dr: I think about that all the time when I see people who
> are sick. They didn't bring it on themselves. It makes
> you wonder. No answer to that one.

EMPATHY AND LEVELS OF RESPONDING

Empathy

Empathy is understanding; it is not an emotional state of feeling sympathy or feeling sorry for someone. In taking a medical
history, being empathic means listening to the total communication—words, feelings, and gestures—and letting the patient
know that you are hearing what he or she is saying. The empathic
physician is also the scientific physician, because understanding
is also the core concept of objectivity. The skill in being
empathic is in learning how to talk to patients to maximize your
ability to gather accurate data.

There are certain ways of responding to what patients say that
will help you demonstrate to them that you understand. The data
about life circumstances and specific symptoms that the patient
gives you will be associated with feelings and beliefs. Remember
the maxim, "You don't speak to patients; you speak to a set of
beliefs about the world."[21] The patient who gives you a detailed
description of his abdominal pain may at the same time feel
frightened because he fears that the pain means stomach cancer
since his father died of stomach cancer. His description will be
filtered through his fears and his belief; unless you attend to the
worry, the patient may not give an accurate account of what he
is actually experiencing. One patient may magnify the symptom
to ensure a complete workup that will not miss cancer; another
may minimize the symptom in the hope of being reassured. If the
interviewer acknowledges the fear, it is easier to find out what is
really going on and get accurate data.

An empathic response can also be important in helping the
patient to clarify what he or she is feeling. At times, the patient
will not be in touch with his or her own feelings. By checking

within yourself—how would you feel, for instance, upon finding blood in your stool?—you can formulate a response. Then, by checking back with the patient—by saying, for example, "That can be pretty frightening."—you as the interviewer can find out whether your assessment of what the patient might have felt is valid in that person's experience of illness.

Levels of Responding

If the patient believes that you are picking up on everything he or she says and are listening attentively with a nonjudgmental attitude, not only will accurate data emerge but feelings and beliefs will also emerge. In formulating a response, it is important to first assess the nature and intensity of any feeling expressed; for example, is the patient upset? And if upset, is he or she slightly upset or furious? Your assessment will include not only what the patient says but how it is said and how the patient looks at the time. Your assessment of the strength of the feeling that the patient is experiencing will influence what you say to the patient.

To talk to patients, you have to learn a professional way of responding, which is different from the way you might respond in social interactions. In social situations, we often ignore or minimize feelings. For example, when people say, "How are you?" or "How do you feel today?" they do not ordinarily expect you to reveal how lousy you are actually feeling. In the clinical setting, however, you really do want to know how the person is feeling; you acknowledge the intensity of any feelings expressed and demonstrate that you understand and accept these feelings.

One way to assess how to respond is to consider four categories or levels of responding: *ignoring; minimizing; interchangeable;* and *additive.*

1. **Ignoring.** You either do not hear what the patient has said or act as though you did not hear. There is no response to either the symptom content or feelings. Examples include:

   Pt: Most days my arthritis is so bad the swelling and pain are just too much.

Dr: And have you ever had any operations?

and

Dr: Do things emotional at work seem to make it worse?
Pt: I think it's . . .
Dr: Do coughing, sneezing, bending, straining at stool, any of those things make it worse?
Pt: I never associated it with those things.

2. **Minimizing.** You respond to the feelings and symptoms at less than the actual level expressed by the patient. Examples include:

Pt: I was in agony with the pain and terribly frightened.
Dr: Well, I'm sure it wasn't that bad.

and

Pt: Most days my arthritis is so bad the swelling and pain are just too much.
Dr: What you need is something to take your mind off it.

3. **Interchangeable.** You recognize the feelings and symptoms expressed by the patient and assess them accurately, and you feed back that awareness at the same level of intensity. Examples include:

Pt: Most days my arthritis is so bad the swelling and pain are just too much. I can't seem to do anything at all any more and nothing seems to help.
Dr: It sounds as though the pain and disability are really getting to you.

and

Pt: I was in agony with the pain and terribly frightened.

Dr: Severe pain can be pretty frightening. Was it the pain that scared you or the thought of what might be causing the pain?

The interchangeable response is the basic goal in medical history taking. This is usually a restatement in your own words of what the patient is trying to describe in order to communicate to the patient that you understand. When you give an interchangeable response, you are likely to find that it has a positive effect on the patient's ability to give an accurate history and talk about what he or she is feeling. This kind of response is essential to being empathic. In the following dialogue, the doctor responds to her patient's concerns even though she does not answer all the patient's questions right away:

Pt: But other than that I'm pretty good but it's my breasts I'm worried about. They started bleeding again, doctor. Why? I want you to take a look today. They're all bleeding in the inside. Is it anything to be concerned about?

Dr: Well maybe I can look and tell you.

Pt: Okay.

Dr: When did that start up again?

Pt: It seems like it will come and it will go, but now they're both all red and I noticed a whole lot of blood just drained out especially this right one, it really hurts down there. This side don't hurt me, but this side hurts me. I don't know.

Dr: So you want me to take a look at your breasts *(interchangeable response).* Is that what's worrying you most today, your breasts? Is there anything else?

Pt: No.

Dr: Okay, come and let me take a look. *(Patient and doctor move to examination table, and she begins checking patient.)* Okay, I can see why you're so concerned; it looks pretty raw here. Okay, this is pretty much like it was before.

Pt: Yeah, but it really does hurt.

Dr: Yeah, I can see that it hurts *(interchangeable response)*. This one is the worst, huh? Remember, how well we were able to clear it up with medication the last time it got this bad?

Pt: Wonder what causes that? That's what worries me.

Dr: Yes most women do worry about things that happen to their breasts *(interchangeable response)*. But this is not serious, although it's very annoying and painful. When bleeding comes from inside the breast, it is serious. But this is from the skin. It's more like a skin allergy. The skin is real sensitive.

Pt: Oh, is that what it is?

Two concise ways of achieving interchangeable responses are through *mirrors* and *paraphrases*. A mirror or reflective response simply feeds back to the patient exactly what is said:

Pt: I feel really terrible.

Dr: You feel really terrible? (mirror)

A paraphrase response conveys the same meaning as the patient's statement but uses different words.

Dr: You're really not feeling well, are you. (paraphrase)

4. **Additive.** You recognize not only what the patient expresses openly but also what he or she may be feeling and is unable to express. One common activity of physicians that involves using additive responses is that of reassurance. This involves making an educated guess regarding what the patient is likely to be worried about and dealing specifically with those worries. Here is an example of an additive response during a follow-up visit by a young man with headaches:

Dr: Well, how are you? Are you having headaches?

Pt: Saturday I had a bad one. I wasn't able to sleep for five nights; my system is so pumped up I can't sleep. The pills did work. I took one a couple of hours before I went to bed and one just when I went to bed.

Dr: You mean the pills I gave you before you went to the hospital? Is it a red and yellow capsule?

Pt: Yeah. I took them two nights and last night was the first night I could sleep without them. I don't like to take a lotta stuff. I was having very strange effects from some of the medication.

Dr: Like what?

Pt: Well, you know everything else about me, I might as well tell you this. Those green pills made me . . . well, I can't describe the feeling it made me feel . . . very strange. They also depressed me, believe it or not, even though you told me that they were antidepressants. I got depressed with them. For 2 days when I was taking them straight and in heavy doses, I found myself breaking into tears in situations . . . I don't even cry when I want to (laughs). It was very, very strange, so I stopped taking them.

Dr: So you're off them now?

Pt: Yeah, off everything now.

Dr: Okay. Can you tell me anything more about this strange feeling you had?

Pt: Ah (patient hesitates) . . .

Dr: *Were you feeling like you were going to lose your mind?* (Additive response)

Pt: Yeah, I felt like I didn't have control over myself. I started to think I would get complications from the illness and how far behind it was making me get in my work because this is a very crucial time in my business. It really opened a lot of stuff for me. I never felt like this before.

The ability to achieve an additive response comes with the experience of seeing patterns of symptoms and of feelings in many patients over time. For a patient with arthritis, an additive response might be:

Pt: Most days my arthritis is so bad the swelling and pain are just too much.

> Dr: It sounds as though the pain is so bad that you think that things won't get much better.

If you have not gotten the sense of the statement quite right the patient may respond:

> Pt: Well, I do feel pretty bad, but I'm still hopeful.

Here is another example of an additive response, this time in an interview with a 50-year-old woman describing her history of depression:

> Pt: You know, sometimes I scare myself.
> Dr: You mean, you think about killing yourself?
> Pt: Yeah, I do.

USING WORDS TO IDENTIFY SYMPTOMS AND FEELINGS

Symptom Words

In order to increase your skill in responding appropriately to your patients, it is necessary to pay attention to words, both your own and those of the patient. Premedical education and medical school can sterilize your vocabulary. You become immersed in the language of medicine, which, although very precise in describing physical attributes, leaves little room for feelings or emotions. It is a language in which adjectives and adverbs carry little weight, and you are usually discouraged from using them in conversation. This socialization into the factual language of medicine can present real problems when you speak with patients. Most vibrant, creative human beings do not happen to be medical students, doctors, or biological scientists. The world of the sick differs from the world of the well, but the difference does not include the sick learning the language of medicine. The most obvious problem you encounter with your medical vocabulary is that patients do not understand the words you use. You may talk about hematemesis rather than vomiting up blood, or paresthesias rather than pins-and-needles sensations in the fingers. Here is an example of a medical faculty member who was trying to ask a patient how much alcohol the patient drank:

> Dr: Okay. Do you use ethanol a lot, little, weekends . . . ?
> Pt: Tylenol?
> Dr: Daily?
> Pt: Ethanol? Alcohol?
> Dr: Drinks?
> Pt: You mean . . . alcoholic beverages? . . . I usually have a drink every night.
> Dr: Okay.

The doctor was thinking "use ethanol" rather than "drink alcohol," and the choice of words created some, in this case, temporary, confusion. Fortunately, the patient acknowledged the misunderstanding. Many times patients do not let on that they have not understood the physician's statement. This is a particular problem with yes/no questions and with explanations and instructions in which no response is sought from the patient.

Feeling Words, Qualifiers, and Quantifiers

Another important result of medical language and thought patterns is our often impoverished ability to describe feelings, qualities, and emotions with any accuracy or precision. Empathy requires both accurate understanding and feeding back this understanding to the patient. This demands that we identify not only facts but also feelings, not only quantities but also qualities, and not only events but also emotions. We must, in a sense, open up our doors and windows to the world; we must relearn and practice using a broad vocabulary of feeling words. Patients use words to quantify many symptoms: how much pain, how much blood, how much suffering, or how much vomiting. Although we are more comfortable with numbers as quantities, the patient who describes the pain as being as severe as the pain he had with his kidney stone is giving us as precise a description as the patient who says that the pain is an 8 on a scale of 1 to 10. Perhaps the description is even more precise, as we may not know what is a "10" for the patient, but we do know that renal colic is one of the most severe pains a person can have.

Table 2–1 presents examples of words that describe various

TABLE 2–1. Descriptive Words for Levels of Feeling

Intensity	Anger	Joy	Anxiety or Fear	Depression
Weak	Annoyed	Pleased	Uneasy	Sad
	Upset	Glad	Uncertain	Down
	Irritated	Happy	Apprehensive	Blue
Medium	Angry	Turned on	Worried	Gloomy
	Testy	Joyful	Troubled	Sorrowful
	Quarrelsome	Delighted	Afraid	Miserable
Strong	Infuriated	Marvelous	Tormented	Distraught
	Spiteful	Jubilant	Frantic	Overwhelmed
	Enraged	Ecstatic	Terrified	Devastated

emotions and their intensity. In giving an interchangeable response to the patient, you must "hit" not only the right feeling, or sensation, but also the right intensity. The patient who says, "I am devastated by this pain" is not likely to believe you have really heard him or her if your response is, "So the pain upsets you a little?" On the other hand, when the patient mentions that "I feel a little crummy today," the doctor is not sticking to his or her observations if the reply is "Sounds like you're feeling utterly hopeless." Once we accept the idea that medicine is about helping people to *feel* better as well as to *function* better, it is easy to understand how feelings reveal important data about the patient, which must be described as accurately and precisely as possible.

NONVERBAL COMMUNICATION

Nonverbal communication is the process of transmitting information without the use of words. It includes *the way a person uses his or her body;* this includes facial expressions, eye contact, hand and arm gestures, posture, and various movements of the legs and feet. Nonverbal communication also includes *paralinguistics* or the *how* of speech; this encompasses voice qualities, the speed at which a person talks, silent pauses, and speech errors. It is probably through the nonverbal aspects of communication that we apprehend another's feelings. We recognize anger not so much by what a person says as by how it is said; speech may slow down and get quiet—controlled anger—or the opposite may occur with shouting and gestures, such as pounding the fist. We can often tell when people lie, unless they are good liars; often they will look away, break eye contact, hesitate, or get "red in the face," that is, an involuntary flush. Common medical examples are the pressure of speech in the anxious or hypomanic person, or the dead voice tone of the very depressed. Patients who are ill often "sound" weak; we may gauge a person's state of health by how he or she sounds ("She's been through a lot of surgery, but she really sounds strong!").

Another component of nonverbal communication involves the *use of personal and social space,* that is, how physically close do we get while talking to our friends, business associates, lovers, and patients. Other factors such as personal grooming, clothing, and odors (for example, perspiration, alcohol, or tobacco) also communicate information about the patient without words and can be helpful to you in your understanding of the patient. For example, if a patient who is normally careful about personal grooming and dress comes in disheveled and unkempt, you are alerted to the possibility of a problem even before the patient begins to speak.

Much of the patient's nonverbal communication, while obvious to you, will be concealed from the patient. This does not mean that the messages sent nonverbally are invalid; in fact, they may be more accurate than the verbal message, because the nonverbal message is often sent unintentionally and uncensored. While it is interesting to note various aspects of nonverbal communication, you may wonder what to do with your observations. The main feature to look for is *consistency;* note nonverbal behaviors and determine whether they are congruent with the patient's verbal message. When there is congruence between verbal and nonverbal messages, the communication is more or less straightforward. However, when there is a discrepancy, an effort must be made to ascertain which is the real message.

Here is an example of a patient who came in for a routine follow-up of abdominal pain and reported first that her husband, from whom she was separated, died recently of some sudden and unknown cause (he was 27 years old). David is the child they had together.

Pt: I want to tell you something before we start.
Dr: OK.
Pt: David's dad died. And now, it's like every week it's something new.
Dr: Oh my. (Note the genuine response.) What happened?
Pt: I don't know. He just went to sleep and never woke up.
Dr: My goodness, when did that happen?
Pt: Last Friday, right before the 9th.
Dr: Oh, I am so sorry to hear that. Ah, how is David doing?

The physician went on to explore how the patient and her son were reacting to this usually sad event, but all the while the patient was discussing things with a bright smile on her face. Although she was separated from her husband, they had remained close and cordial because of David, and her cheeriness seemed inappropriate. What did the smile mean here? What kind of problem did this discrepancy suggest? Indeed, the physician seemed more upset about this news than the patient. It later came out that she was having great difficulty, particularly in communicating to her son appropriate ways to both mourn and remember his father. Although the physician did not confront her early in the interview, he was alerted to a possible problem and later helped guide her toward a more appropriate response.

Often the nonverbal message will be more accurate than the statements made. You may choose in some situations, especially early in the interview, simply to note a discrepancy and use it to help you understand the patient. Or you might use the nonverbal communication to modify your own nonverbal behavior or your conversation or both. For example, if the patient seems tense and anxious, as evidenced by facial flushing or fidgeting, you may modify your voice tone and the way you are sitting in response to the patient's discomfort by speaking in a more soothing way and leaning forward to demonstrate your interest.

At the same time that you are observing the patient's nonverbal behavior, the patient is, perhaps unconsciously, observing your nonverbal behavior as well. As a result, your job is twofold: You should be aware of the patient's nonverbal behaviors as well as your own. For example, if you seem uninterested, as evidenced by never looking at the patient or by looking at your watch, the patient may be unable to provide the details you need. Likewise, if you stand by the door as opposed to sit by the bed, the patient may assume you are in a hurry and, respectful of your time, leave out critical data thought to be unimportant. Attention to your own nonverbal behavior requires a high level of self-awareness as you conduct the interview. It is particularly important to be conscious of how you respond to distractions during the interview, such as an emergency going on across the hall. You need to demonstrate your focus on the patient by maintaining eye contact, an attentive posture, and a seeming lack of awareness that all hell is breaking loose somewhere else.

Gestures

Although many specific gestures have been the subject of study and suggested interpretations, these must always be judged in the context of the entire situation and confirmed with the patient. When the gesture or facial expression appears to imply something different than the words, an effort must be made to ascertain which, the gesture or the words, is delivering the real message. The nonverbal message always adds information. Interpretation is no problem when a gesture "confirms" the patient's statements or the doctor's hypothesis based on them. Consider this example in which a patient is suffering from headaches. The physician learns that the patient has been under much stress recently.

> Dr: So you have a lot of things on your mind.
> Pt: Yes. About them, about some of the members of my family, and, um, mostly it's money worries, mainly money.
> Dr: It's funny, when you say "money worries," you know where you point to?
> Pt: Hah?
> Dr: You point right where it's hurting.
> Pt: Yeah, ah hah . . . That's mostly it, you know.

This type of interpretation, in this example, that financial stress may be causing tension headaches, can be very effective both in demonstrating your empathic understanding and in making more explicit a connection the patient may already experience implicitly.

Here are some examples of possible "interpretations" of various gestures.[85]

- "Steepling" of hands involves joining them with fingers extended and finger tips touching, like a church steeple. Frequently, this indicates confidence or assurance of what is being said.
- Slight raising of the hand or index finger, pulling at an earlobe, or raising the index finger to the lips may indicate a desire to interrupt the speaker.
- Raising a finger to the lips may also indicate an attempt to suppress a comment.
- Crossed arms can be a defensive gesture (indicating disagreement), a sign of insecurity, or simply a comfortable position. Note the manner in which the arms are crossed and muscular tension, especially in the hands.

- Fear or tension leads to the "white knuckle syndrome."
- Crossed legs may suggest a shutting out of, or protection against, what is going on in the interview, or it may be simply a position of comfort.
- Uncrossing of the legs while shifting forward in the chair is likely to indicate that the patient is receptive to what you are saying.

Two particular gestures deserve comment. The first is the helplessness or hopelessness gesture. This is a typically biphasic hand gesture. Both hands are raised briskly to face level, with elbows fixed, palms facing each other rotated slightly outward, fingers spread, and thumb and fingers slightly flexed as though preparing to grasp. This position is held for a second or less, and then the hands fall limply down to the lap. Incomplete variations may be seen. This gesture suggests that the patient feels helpless about the problem or situation. The first part is a reaching out for assistance, while the second part (hypotonia and withdrawal) emphasizes the futility of any help at the moment.[43]

The second gesture is called the respiratory avoidance response. This pattern includes frequent clearing of the throat when no phlegm or mucus is present. A variation of this is the nose rub, which involves a light rub of the nose with the dorsal aspect of the index finger. These indicate rejection or disagreement with statements being made. For example: "How are things at home?" The patient answers "Fine," clears his throat, and lightly rubs his nose. He may actually be saying, "I'm uncomfortable with my response; things aren't really going very well at home."

Paralinguistics

When you hear speech, you don't hear just words; you hear words plus how the words are put together. You hear pauses, tone of voice, and modulation, in addition to specific content. Table 2–2 lists some of what you hear, in addition to the words, when a patient speaks. Likewise, these are the things the patient hears in addition to your words. Paralinguistic cues can contribute significantly to your understanding of the patient and to the patient's perception of you as a helping person.

TABLE 2–2. Components of Paralanguage

Speech rate
  For example: slow, fast, or deliberate
Pause–speech rate ratio
  For example: long or short or inappropriate pauses, mechanical, halting, or flowing
Tone or voice quality
  For example: whiny, flat, nasal, bright, or breathy
Pitch
  For example: high, medium, or low
Volume
  For example: loud, soft, or "wide swings" or "wide variations"
Articulation
  For example: clear, precise, or slurred

Source: Adapted from Cassell.[21]

While we do not have space to comment in detail on paralinguistics, some observations about pausing are in order. The functions of pausing include:

1. Absolute recall time;
2. Language formation time;
3. Censorship of material;
4. Creating an effect (timing); and
5. Preparing to lie.

People rarely need to pause before recalling a place, age, or date fixed in time. For example, a person readily remembers the age at which a parent died but might have to think a moment before remembering a living parent's current age. It is easy to answer a "yes/no" question without pausing, even if giving the incorrect answer: Do you drink alcohol? Yes. No. This has little meaning. How much alcohol do you usually drink in a day? or Tell me about your use of alcohol. These questions demand some thought and integration. Listen carefully to the answer. How much pause is there? How much stumbling or backtracking? In general, it is helpful to listen to the number, quality, and placement of pauses. Frequent long pauses associated with low amplitude and a "dead" tone suggest depression. Frequent pauses over factual answers throughout the history suggest organic brain dysfunction. Pauses over answers in selected areas may indicate sensitive topics, with time required for censorship of material. We return to this aspect of medical interviewing in the sections on truth telling and difficult interviews later on in this book.

CHAPTER 3

The Medical History, Part 1: Getting Started and the Present Illness

> "Never mind," said Holmes, laughing; "it is my business to know things. Perhaps I have trained myself to see what others overlook. If not, why should you come to consult me?"
>
> Sherlock Holmes, *in "A Case of Identity"* from
> *Adventures of Sherlock Holmes*

In the next four chapters we discuss, in turn, the traditional parts of a complete medical history, i.e., the chief complaint, present illness, past medical history, family history, social history, patient profile, and review of systems. In each section we introduce, describe, and illustrate specific skills or techniques useful for that part of the interview—skills particularly appropriate to the interview's content or medical objective (e.g., the review of systems requires a different approach than the history of the present illness). This division of the interview is for simplicity only and does not imply that open-ended questions or interchangeable responses, for example, are useful only in the present illness section. This chapter deals with (1) the setting and how to start, (2) the chief complaint, and (3) the explication of the present illness.

STARTING

The Setting

The setting for many interviews is often a hospital room. It is important to know how to use that environment to enhance communication between you and the patient. The hospital is not the patient's natural habitat; as a result, the patient, who is "dis-eased," may not feel *at* ease. Patients will be similarly uncomfortable, although perhaps less so, in the clinic or doctor's office. When you see a new patient, his blood pressure and pulse will often be elevated, his face flushed, his handshake cool and damp, and his gestures clearly nervous. All these indicate the autonomic response to the stress of illness, seeking help, meeting a new doctor, and the unknown procedures and outcome. If you appear hurried, indifferent, or unsympathetic, the patient may feel even more uncomfortable; this discomfort creates a barrier to effective communication and decreases the accuracy of the data you obtain.

The beginning of the interview sets the atmosphere for the rest of your history and physical examination. This time should be used to establish rapport, demonstrate interest in the patient as a person, and thereby create a base for effective communication. This need not, and should not, take a great deal of time, but it can set the patient at ease. A good history depends as much, or more, on how you ask the questions and the *process* of the interview as on knowing enough pathophysiology to ask the "right" questions.

Establish a sense of *privacy* for the interview. For example, if there is another patient sharing the hospital room, draw the curtain around the bed. While this obviously does not provide a soundproof barrier, it provides the patient with a psychologic sense of privacy. If the patient can walk comfortably, it may be better to interview him or her in a convenient lounge or waiting area, if this will be more private. If the patient has visitors, you might suggest that they wait outside or, if possible, that you will return later to see the patient. Before beginning the history, check to see that the patient is as *comfortable* as possible. Try to seat yourself in a way that will facilitate communication. People have spheres of "personal space" around them: Get close enough for a person-to-person interaction, but do not intrude on the patient's intimate space.

In a small hospital room, it may be difficult to place yourself comfortably so that you strike a balance between being halfway across the room and sitting on top of the patient. If necessary, move the chair around. Try to sit at the same level as the patient; this helps establish good eye contact during the interview. Often it is most comfortable to sit at an angle to the person, rather than facing him or her directly: This allows you to maintain good eye contact but also provides natural opportunities to look away at times. Good eye contact does not mean staring fixedly at the patient, which will only make the individual feel uncomfortable; there are always natural breaks in eye contact. You also can use your body to demonstrate interest: By leaning slightly toward the patient, rather than lounging back in your chair, you convey a sense of involvement with what he or she is saying.

How to Start

As you begin the interview, consider these guidelines:

1. Introduce yourself and explain your role. Although local guidelines differ, if you are a medical student, we suggest you introduce yourself as such or as a student doctor. Besides being genuine and not using the facade of doctor or consultant, you also will be defining your contract with the patient. As Kimball[64] described, the doctor and patient establish a contract in the interview, albeit usually an unspoken one. The patient expects to describe a complaint and then to have the doctor treat it. If you are a student who does not have responsibility to care for the patient, the contract is limited. When, in the course of the interview, the patient asks your opinion about his or her diagnosis or treatment, asks for pain medication, or requests anything beyond your capacity to respond, you can comfortably remind the patient of the boundaries of your contract. You can tell the patient that you will convey the question or concern to the medical resident or nursing staff, or suggest that the patient do so.

2. It is better not to begin by saying to the patient, "I've been asked (or sent) to take a history and do a physical." Such a statement is likely to make the patient feel that you have no real interest in him or her, and it may set the interview off on the wrong track. Although it may be true that you are not interviewing the patient on your own initiative, a better start would be to say, "I'd like to talk to you today in order to get some information about why you're in the hospital and then to examine you. Will

that be all right?'' As part of this introduction, you obtain permission to do the history and examination; by so doing, you demonstrate interest in and respect for the person.

3. Taking notes is essential because you will be writing up the information you obtain. As you begin the interview, inform the patient of your need to take notes and the reason for it; this will also let the patient know what will happen to the information you are obtaining. However, try not to let your note taking control the interview. If you attempt to record what your patient is saying verbatim—with the exception of the chief complaint—the patient is likely to feel that he or she is being interrogated rather than being interviewed. Eye contact is severely limited if you are mainly concerned with recording the data, and you are likely to miss the patient's nonverbal communication, thereby causing difficulty establishing rapport and missing useful data about the person. While you are making notes, look up frequently; this will demonstrate interest in the person and in what he or she is saying. You will find with more experience that only an occasional word or phrase needs to be written down to help you remember, synthesize, and later reconstruct the story in written form.

THE CHIEF COMPLAINT

The *chief complaint* in a standard medical history is the main reason the patient sought medical help. It is usually recorded verbatim in the patient's own words. The chief complaint is often elicited by such questions as:

1. How can I help you today? (If you have responsibility for the patient.)
2. Can you tell me about your trouble?
3. What symptoms made you decide to see a doctor? Come to the emergency room?
4. Can you tell me about your problem?
5. Tell me about the main thing you feel is wrong.
6. What brought you to the hospital? (Although this question may be subject to concrete answers like, "A taxi.")

Consider this example of how one medical resident began an interview with a new patient in an outpatient clinic:

> Dr: I guess the best place to start is to ask you what brings you here today.
> Pt: Well, I haven't had a physical really since 6 years ago, since my daughter was born.
> Dr: I am going to be writing some things down on paper here, okay? Is there any particular reason why you chose now to come in?
> Pt: I figured I kept putting it off and putting it off. I'd make appointments and put them off. There was no particular reason. I just felt as though it was time I suppose.
> Dr: Nothing is bothering you at this point?
> Pt: No, it's just that I am overweight, that's all. I go up and down, up and down.
> Dr: So that was your major concern, the weight problem?
> Pt: Yeah.
> Dr: Can you tell me about that?

The chief complaint here is the weight problem or, stated verbatim, "It's just that I am overweight." It took a little digging to clarify that; we see that the doctor was not satisfied with "There was no particular reason." Sometimes an opening question leads to a clear-cut chief complaint as in the next example:

> Dr: What can I do for you?
> Pt: Um, the reason why I'm here is, in the latter part of July up to now, my bowels wouldn't move and I'd have to, in like 4 and 5 days, I'd have to take either milk of magnesia or a bulk laxative, and I just thought it was maybe something that I was eating, and this still continues until now, and it's the reason why I'm here to see you.

In other cases, the same opening question might lead to a much more complex and rambling answer:

> Dr: Now what can I do for you Mrs. P?
> Pt: Well, first of all, I'm here mainly because I've been experiencing that tired, worn-out feeling most of the time. I can go to bed, say 9:00 in the evening, and get

up at 8:00 or even later and I still feel very tired. And, I don't know . . . I've been still experiencing hot flashes and sometimes now . . . I don't experience them as often as I used to but I still do and especially towards the evening or at night, and it awakens me when I do experience something like that. Maybe that's part of the reason why I felt so tired, I don't know. Anyways, now in the evening when I experience this kind of hot feeling I just get that craving I want to eat, you know, or sometimes it works just the opposite where I feel kind of nervous, I get that nervous feeling, and now last week I had headaches just about every day on arising, I had a little runny nose so maybe, I don't know, maybe I could attribute that to a cold, but I'm just mentioning those things to you. And, sometimes you know my head just feels as though, it feels stuffed . . . when you have a head cold; that's just the way it has felt many times, and I had a hysterectomy, let's see, about 1975 or '76 and since then I just have had no sexual desire or anything, I mean as far as I'm concerned that doesn't mean a whole lot. I know it upsets my husband a bit.

What is the chief complaint? Ostensibly, it is her first statement, "mainly because (of) that tired, worn-out feeling. . . ." but in context, the situation is less clear. What is *really* bothering her most? Why did she come here *today,* as opposed to last month or next week? This particular patient rambles on and on, presenting a type of difficult situation we discuss in Chapter 9. The physician permits this lengthy response, and, in so doing, acquires a wealth of useful information about the patient's symptoms and concerns. The physician will later provide more structure for the patient to clarify her complaints. In contrast, Beckman and Frankel[10] found that in only 23% of office visits did medical residents allow their patient to complete his or her opening statement. Rather, in most cases they interrupted and steered the discussion toward a specific topic, thereby diminishing the chance of getting to the patient's real chief complaint.

It is not just the rambling or discursive patient, however, who presents problems in identifying the real chief complaint; often, the actual reason the person comes to see the doctor lies embedded somewhere else, far from the patient's initial statement.

Here is an example of a patient who presents with chest pain that he has had for some time:

> Dr: I'm glad you came in today. Tell me why you came in.
> Pt: Okay. I been having some problems with my chest; you know it's, it's like pressure and plus I have a knot under my arm, under my armpit.
> Dr: Okay. You have pressure.
> Pt: Yeah, I have pressure, and I don't know if it's because I smoke a lot of cigarettes, or I don't know what it is.
> Dr: Um hum.
> Pt: All I know is it's pressure across my chest. It's not what you call a pain or anything, it hurts; it's pressure all across here.
> Dr: Um hum.
> Pt: And, then, I have this knot under my, under my armpit.
> Dr: Okay.
> Pt: About the size of a half dollar.
> Dr: Okay, let's talk about the chest pain first; when would you say it started?
> Pt: Um, I say about a month ago; maybe it might of been longer but I didn't pay it any attention.
> Dr: Um hum.
> Pt: You know but I can't jog because if I just start jogging, it bothers me in my chest.
> Dr: What made you decide to get it checked?
> Pt: Well, two things actually, I want to get back in shape and I got a note from the Health Department that this test came back positive. See I'm a barber and they test for tuberculosis.

This physician, by asking "What made you decide to get it checked?" not only has the answer to why the patient came in now but an important new piece of data has emerged, namely the positive tuberculin test. We also learn that the patient may believe there is a relationship between his symptoms and the positive test. He really came to the doctor because of the positive tuberculin test, perhaps simply to fulfill a legal requirement for his license and perhaps, in addition, because the positive test made him reinterpret his chest problems as being more serious than they first seemed to be. In any case, if he has no active pulmonary disease, the physician knows that the patient will need reassurance that the cause of his trouble does not lie in the positive tuberculin test.

When you consider why a person might come for medical help at a certain time, it is not enough simply to elicit a certain symptom or symptoms. The symptoms, as in the example above, may have been present for some time. While the answer to these first questions (the chief complaint) frequently contains the core of the patient's problem, sometimes it does not. The *ostensible reason for coming*, as initially stated by the patient in the chief complaint, may not be the same as the *actual reason for coming*.[9] This is most often true with:

1. People who have chronic diseases;
2. People with vague, chronic, and/or recurring symptoms; and
3. People who say they just want a checkup.

Alvan Feinstein[46] used the term *iatrotropic stimulus*, bringing toward the doctor, to indicate why the patient decided to seek care today rather than yesterday, tomorrow, or last year. The iatrotropic stimulus or the actual reason for coming may be of great importance and not immediately evident. If you can answer the question "Why now?" you have probably uncovered the iatrotropic stimulus or the actual reason for coming. Despite the fact that the person has an "acceptable" symptom or disease (heart failure or shortness of breath), it may not satisfactorily explain the whole picture, including why the person sought help today as opposed to last month.

Patients seek care at a certain time for different reasons.

First, the symptoms of the illness may increase to the point that they become unbearable and the person simply realizes he or she needs medical help. We usually assume this reason, and it is often quite true in the hospitalized group of patients with whom you have your first interviewing experiences.

Second, anxiety about the meaning of the symptoms may, for one reason or another, reach the point that the person seeks medical help in spite of the fact that he or she has been sick for a while or may even have a *decrease* in symptoms. Perhaps a television news story about a certain disease or the recent diagnosis of a brain tumor in a friend increases the anxiety about an otherwise trivial symptom.

Third, the symptom in the chief complaint may simply be a "ticket of admission"[4,52] to the doctor's office or hospital; the actual problem may be an entirely different symptom that the patient is at first afraid to mention, or it may be some life stress or crisis.

Finally, if you really listen, the iatrotropic stimulus will come out during the interview. Sometimes it arrives only at the last moment, when you are about to walk out of the room and the patient says, "Oh, by the way, Doc, I'm sure this has nothing to do with it, but. . . ." You can prevent this "door knob phenomenon" by being open ended and empathic in the beginning. The earlier in the interview you ascertain the patient's reason for coming now, the more efficient you are, wasting less time digging for data. Not only will the data be more accurate but so will your diagnosis.

THE PRESENT ILLNESS

The *present illness* is a thorough elaboration of the chief complaint and other current symptoms starting from the time the patient last felt "well" until the present. The best strategy is often, first, to let the patient talk, then to use a variety of nondirective and directive questions to clarify and embellish. Generally you move from open-ended questions to more specific "WH" questions (who, what, when, where, why, and how), laundry list questions (menus), or closed-ended questions, as appropriate.

Questions

Some examples of *open-ended questions* are:

1. Can you tell me more about that?
2. Did you notice anything else?
3. What was the pain like for you?

Another version of these open-ended questions is to restate them as gentle commands, requesting the patient to elaborate:

1. Tell me more about that.
2. Tell me what else you noticed.
3. Tell me what the pain was like.

Nondirective or *open-ended* questions are always a good way to start, allowing the patient freedom to talk and the examiner time to sit back and "size up" the patient. They are especially good for eliciting the less structured data of the present illness and the psychosocial aspects of the patient's problem. These questions allow the patient, who, after all, is the one who "knows," to choose the most important symptoms and to point the way as you develop your interview strategy. The most nondirective of all statements are *minimal facilitators,* queries like:

1. "Yes?"
2. "Uh huh?"
3. "And?" or
4. "And what else?"

Nonverbal cues, such as nodding your head in agreement or smiling, also may serve as minimal encouragers for the patient to continue talking.

Nondirective questioning, however, usually just sketches the picture, without giving precise detail. Patients only rarely spontaneously volunteer all the needed details; a rambling, vague patient may take too much time and still not provide all the information you need, while a shy, reticent patient may say little or nothing. So in a medical interview we move from the general to the more directive, but still open-ended, *WH questions.* These describe the attributes of the patient's symptoms and, as Eric Cassell[21] puts it, create a picture of the "disease process marching through the body." The WH questions are important tools in developing objectivity and precision in the patient's narrative.

Where: Exactly where is it on your body?
or
Show me where it is.

What: What does it feel like?
or
Tell me what it feels like.

When: When does it occur (episodic, inception and duration, fluctuation, and frequency)?

How: How is it altered by season, by time of day, by sleep,

by food, by exertion, and so forth?
or
Describe how your daily activities affect it.

Why: Why does it occur?
What provokes it?
Why do you think you have it?

Who: Who is affected by it (consequences to patient and other people)?

Patient disclosure of relevant clinical information is most strongly correlated with open-ended questions,[88] but other types of questions also must be used to develop fully the patient narrative. *Laundry list questions,* or *menus,* are sometimes useful when a patient cannot find words to express a certain characteristic. For example, "How would you describe this pain—sharp, dull, burning, or tight?" "Would you say it lasted a few seconds, a minute, 10 minutes?" Such questions obviously exclude other descriptive words and are used only when a nondirective approach ("Can you describe the pain?") and WH questions ("What is the pain like?") have both failed.

Directive, or *closed-ended*, questions provide detail; they are good for emergency situations ("What's your name?" "How old are you?" "Are you allergic to any drugs?"), reticent patients, and for structured historic data, such as the past history and the review of systems. They are also useful as *focused questioning* when you have already generated hypotheses in the interview and are trying to build a case for one particular diagnosis (see Chaps. 12 and 13). However, a "high control" interview in which the interviewer asks one directive question after another will produce false or incomplete evidence, not to mention a discontented patient. Some examples of closed-ended questions are:

- Are your parents still living?
- Did you pass out?
- Have you ever been anemic?
- Does this pain occur when you take a deep breath?
- Is there any trouble with your vision?

One does not ask *"yes/no" questions* in situations when information may be sensitive, because a lie will close off all access to

TABLE 3–1. Types of Questions in
Medical-History Taking

Start with	Open-ended questions: General
	Minimal facilitators
	Open-ended questions: Topic
Then proceed to	WH questions
	Laundry lists or menus
	Direct questions
	Yes/No questions
Avoid	Leading questions
	Complex or multiple questions

that information. For example, it is not useful to say, "Do you drink alcohol?" if one suspects alcohol may be a problem; try, "How much alcohol do you usually drink in a day?"

Finally, there are at least two types of questions to avoid. First, avoid *leading questions*, which encourage certain responses from the patient to fit the interviewer's own hypothesis, such as "You're feeling better now, aren't you?" or "That pain wasn't on the left side of your chest, was it?" This type of query suggests to the patient what you want (or don't want) to hear. Likewise, you should avoid *multiple questions*, such as: "Do you have any trouble sleeping and how about coughing?" Sometimes these slip out, because your mind is working too quickly and dragging your tongue along with it. Slow down, wait. Table 3–1 summarizes the various types of queries employed in taking the medical history.

Symptom Description

Throughout the history of the present illness, it is important to describe the patient's symptoms as carefully as possible without jumping to conclusions. For example, "I'm short of breath" is not necessarily dyspnea on exertion or orthopnea; you need more details. It is also important to avoid jumping to conclusions about the meanings of certain words. Many words commonly used to describe symptoms mean different things to different people. Some examples are diarrhea, constipation, tired, dizzy, my side, sick, weak, high blood, low blood, insomnia, gas, and heartburn. The novice has a tendency to establish quantitative ("How many times a day?") aspects of symptoms before establishing the qualitative aspects. The expert interviewer attempts to establish what he or she is dealing with ("Are the stools soft or watery?") before measuring it. One wants to establish the pattern of how things hang together, the *gestalt*; then one fills in the quantitative data. Table 3–2 presents some examples of patient statements, followed by either *quantitative* (prematurely specific) or *qualitative* physician follow-up questions.

It is important not to get caught up in the "New Brunswick syndrome" when taking the patient's history. A friend of ours was living in Canada and his mother from New Jersey was visiting. They were invited to a party and our friend noted that his mother was carrying on a long, animated discussion with a woman with whom he thought she had nothing in common. Afterward, he asked his mother what they were talking about. She said, "Well, we were sharing a lot of memories of our childhoods in New Brunswick." They had carried on a long, gratifying conversation despite the fact that one was talking about New Brunswick, New Jersey, and the other was referring to the Canadian province of New Brunswick. The same words mean different things to different people. This does not present too much of a problem at a cocktail party, but it can be deadly in the medical history. This is what we mean by *precision* in obtaining data: we must describe exactly what occurred and not suffer from the New Brunswick syndrome of medical words.

The symptom called "dizziness" presents a prime example. A patient comes in and says, "My main problem is dizziness. It just

TABLE 3–2. Patient Complaints and Possible Quantitative or Qualitative Physician Questions

Complaint	Quantitative Questions	Qualitative Questions
I've been having chest pain.	How long have you had it? How often does it come?	What does it feel like? Where exactly is it located?
My side hurts.	How long have you had it?	Show me where.
I have diarrhea.	How many times a day?	What do you mean by diarrhea?
I vomited blood.	How much?	What did it look like?
I can't walk as far as I used to without getting tired.	How far can you walk?	What do you mean by "tired?"

came on me about a month ago, and it's been getting worse now. I'm so dizzy I can hardly stand up sometimes. What's wrong with me, Doc?" The first thing that is wrong is the word "dizziness." According to Reilly,[86] there are at least four common syndromes or symptoms vaguely labeled with this word. These include:

1. Vertigo, a definite rotational sensation or sense of environmental motion;
2. Presyncope, the sensation that loss of consciousness is about to happen;
3. Disequilibrium, the sensation that balance, especially during walking, is impaired; and
4. Lightheadedness, a vague head sensation that is not vertigo and not presyncope.

There are also other symptoms as well, such as weakness, fatigue, or anxiety, that some persons idiosyncratically label as dizziness.

The following exchange, adapted from Reilly,[86] shows an example of a doctor trying to find out precisely what a patient means by dizziness:

Dr: Can you describe what you mean with words other than dizzy?
Pt: I feel out of balance. I feel like I might fall down even. I haven't yet, but I get awful woozy when I walk.
Dr: Is it mainly when you walk that you have trouble, or do you get this feeling sometimes when you are sitting or resting?
Pt: I guess it is mainly when I am up and around.
Dr: Can you tell me, then, how you feel bad when you walk? Try not to say dizzy.
Pt: Well, I feel I'm unsure of myself. I can't trust my walking.
Dr: Does everything around you spin or move, or do you feel like you're spinning?
Pt: No, not exactly.
Dr: Do you feel like you are going to faint?
Pt: I feel like I will fall, not faint.

Notice the mixture of open-ended and directive questions that the physician uses to characterize as precisely as possible what the patient is actually experiencing. There is much more to find out about this symptom, but from the exchange so far the patient appears to be describing disequilibrium, rather than vertigo, pre-syncope, or lightheadedness.

Another example of the New Brunswick syndrome arose in the following interchange with a patient who came to the doctor because of her cough. Note how the clinician begins with an open-ended question, specifying only that the doctor wishes to hear about the cough, then follows up with WH questions until the symptom is known precisely.

Dr: Tell me about the *cough* that you've been having.
Pt: It's just worse at night, I can't get no sleep.
Dr: What happens?
Pt: I'm up on three pillows. I'm just miserable that's all.
Dr: You go up on three pillows to try to prevent the cough?
Pt: Yes.
Dr: How is it miserable?
Pt: Well, if I lay flat I can't breathe, and then I start gasping and gasping for breath, and the only way I can stop is when I sit up and watch TV or something.

The patient in this example actually suffered from congestive heart failure with orthopnea: She became short of breath when she lay flat in bed. She experienced a tightness in her chest and a sense of "gasping" for breath that she chose to call "cough." Later in the conversation, the doctor learned that she had anginal chest pain and dyspnea on exertion as well as these nocturnal symptoms.

In this next, longer example, the physician wants to pin down the exact timing of the onset, duration, periodicity, and pattern of chest pain. The doctor is concerned that the symptom in this 62-year-old smoker may be caused by coronary artery disease and knows that only precise symptom description will guide the diagnostic process. Each time the patient gives a somewhat vague statement, the physician follows up with an attempt at clarification (these are preceded by an asterisk).

Pt: . . . and little bit too fast, it might just be my imagination though, I don't know.
Dr: Uh huh. When did this all start?

Pt: Well, just since the weather has been hot, like it is, you know.

°Dr: Several weeks it's been going on, would you say?

Pt: Uh huh, just—now the chest pain is not continuous, like, during the day, I don't have to be doing anything, I can just be sitting.

Dr: And where do you feel it?

Pt: It's in here. And like full, just too full, it's fullness in here.

Dr: And then how long does it last when it comes?

Pt: Not too long.

°Dr: Minutes, hours?

Pt: Not hours, just maybe a half hour, or something—you know, it doesn't last.

°Dr: Do you do anything that seems to relieve it?

Pt: No, I don't take anything, just sit and be quiet, or either I'll rest. Like, the neighbors, like I told you, were throwing out those old chairs—that recliner, I could use it, so he helped me with it, he put it over the fence and helped me with it into the house and that helps a whole lot. I go in and stretch out on that.

Dr: Uh huh.

Pt: And rest seems to help, when it starts acting up, whenever I could or would be doing around the house, I let it go and just rest.

°Dr: Does it sometimes come on while you are doing something?

Pt: Yea, mostly, if I'm doing something like trying to sweep or clean in the house or something like that.

°Dr: How about with walking?

Pt: With walking sometimes, and like mostly. I'll go up to the mall every day and that way I am inside walking and they have benches, I'll sit . . . when it starts acting up.

°Dr: And then how long does it take to go away once you sit?

Pt: Once I sit, oh, I'll say, half an hour to an hour.

°Dr: And it will take a half hour or an hour to go away?

Pt: Uh huh.

°Dr: Or do you sit for that long even though it's gone before that?

Pt: Uh huh. I just sit for that long until it eases.

°Dr: And it takes a half hour to an hour for it to ease up?
Pt: Uh huh.
Dr: Do you have any other symptoms along with it when you have the pain?
Pt: No.

Notice how the clinician in this example tries to establish a pattern of chest pain brought on by exertion and relieved by rest. Perhaps the most critical detail to establish if one suspects coronary artery disease, is the length of time it takes for the "pain" (in this patient, a "fullness" in the chest) to ease once the patient rests. In typical angina, the pain ceases after several minutes or less. This patient is not typical. It is likely that had the response been "Less than 5 minutes" to the question "And then how long does it take to go away once you sit?" the clinician would have let it go at that.

Summarization, Confrontation, and Clarification

A summary is a technique by which the clinician feeds back to the patient the high points of what has been said thus far. Frequent summaries ensure that the interviewer has the story straight, help terminate one area of the history and launch another, and help the interviewer remain organized. A summary may be as simple as repeating a particularly important statement to see if you have it right, such as: "Okay, as I understand it, the pains you had in 1985 were exactly like the ones you're having now. . . ." In other cases, a brief summary helps one get back on track if the patient is wandering and switching topics, such as: "Okay, we'll get to the cough in a minute, but I need to understand your chest pain better. You said it was like a heavy pressure right in the center of your chest, and it lasted about 5 minutes. . . ."

Summaries are also very useful as transitions from one part of the interview to another. This allows both you and the patient to keep track of where you have been and where you are going. Here is an example of a summary that leads into a transition from the history of the present illness to the past medical history:

Pt: So that's about how it happened.
Dr: Okay, let me see if I have it straight. You felt perfectly

> well until 2 days ago when you began to notice an
> uncomfortable feeling right in the middle here around
> your belly button, and this has gradually gotten worse,
> and you are now also having diarrhea. (Patient nods.)
> OK, I think I understand pretty well what's been going
> on the last 2 days. How about in the past, have you had
> any problems with your health in the past?

Sometimes as you try to summarize, you note discrepancies in the patient's story; and because you want to know exactly what happened, it is often necessary to point out those discrepancies. When you do this, you are *confronting* the patient. This rather dramatic word arose from interviewing techniques in psychotherapy. It has connotations of pointing out falsehoods, rationalizations, or neurotic conflicts, and in its everyday usage often implies opposing sides. In the medical interview, however, *confrontation* is often simply an attempt to compare statements that are not consistent; you heard one thing and now it appears the patient is describing the experience differently or contradicting an earlier statement. Which version is right? An example is:

> Dr: Now let me see if I can understand this. You said before
> that you were coughing up some bloody stuff with that
> heavy cough last year. But just now you said, when this
> cough developed yesterday, it was the first time you
> ever saw blood come up. Did I misunderstand you?

A *clarification* falls somewhere between a summary and a confrontation. You say what you heard, but ask for more detail, perhaps to resolve some ambiguities in the story, as in the example of our patient with chest pain.

EXAMPLES

We conclude this chapter with three examples of beginnings of interviews. In each case, we have labeled the physician's statements or questions with the term that describes the technique being used. Note the importance, in this part of the interview, of social greetings, nondirective questions, clarification, minimal facilitators, and summaries.

Example 1

Dr: Okay, hello again. I'm Dr. Block. Tell me what I can do for you today. (social greeting and nondirective question)

Pt: Well, I have a terrible vaginal itch, and I don't know whether it's the vaginitis or whether it's the urine, urinary tract infection. My regular doctor treated me for vaginitis.

Dr: That was Dr. Hill? (clarification and facilitation)

Pt: Uh huh. Then I got, um, a urinary tract infection and then the vaginitis came back. But during the whole ordeal, I've never got any relief.

Dr: During the treatment for the vaginitis, during the treatment for the urinary tract infection, you still had this terrible itch? (summary and clarification)

Example 2

Dr: Good morning. (social greeting)

Pt: (Patient is seated on end of exam table) Good morning.

Dr: Why don't you have a seat back over here, and we can talk a little bit first. Tell me why you came today. (seeing to the patient's comfort and nondirective question)

Pt: Um, to get my blood pressure checked.

Dr: To get your blood pressure checked? What do you know about your blood pressure? (reflective response and nondirective question with topic specified)

Pt: Well, I have heard various things over the past couple of years, really, that it has been high, and um . . .

Dr: For several years? (clarification and facilitation)

Pt: (Nods) And I went about, oh, it was quite a while ago, maybe 5 or 6 months ago to the health center, um, and the doctor told me it was high and also, but he could not treat me until I lost approximately 38 pounds, so I haven't been able to take the weight off and I was kind of, well, he did not give me any special diet to follow or you know, what I should cut out of my diet, and I was very discouraged by it, so when I went to the emergency room because I cut my finger, um, the nurse told me that my blood pressure was very high and I should have it checked, and since I don't have a family doctor, she suggested I come here.

Example 3

Dr: It's nice to see you again. What brings you here today? (social greeting and open-ended question)

Pt: Doctor, I'm not well.

Dr: I take it you have not been feeling really well for a while. (summary based on previous knowledge of this patient)

Pt: No, well, I haven't been feeling very good for about the last, oh, I'd say about a week, about a week now.

Dr: Uh huh. (facilitation)

Pt: About a week now, I haven't been feeling good.

Dr: What have you noticed? (nondirective question)

Pt: Oh, some soreness in here right through here, and some pain in my arm and a, a, a strangulating feeling right in here and a burning in the, in the middle, right here and a burning in my throat, a little bit, and dizzy—I felt real dizzy when I was on the scale out there, you know, and I called you and the nurse, and she helped me and I wasn't real bad and you know, I told her to open a window and she said first "do you want me to open a window" and I said "yeah and I want to get near the air."

Dr: Does that help? (clarification)

Pt: Oh yeah.

SUMMARY OF FACILITATIVE TECHNIQUES

We now summarize some techniques presented in the first three chapters that help any interviewer obtain accurate and precise data during the initial part of the medical history.

1. Maintain an attentive body position and minimize distractions, achieving a sense of privacy for both you and the patient.
2. Take notes, but maintain enough eye contact so as not to "lose" the patient.
3. Use language the patient can understand. This means translating certain terms as they may appear in an outline of a history or present themselves in your head into words that are familiar to the patient.

4. Structure questions to go from general to specific subjects, using open-ended questions to introduce the history or each part of the history and then proceeding to more specific questioning.
5. Use minimal encouragers or facilitators, such as silence with or without a head nod, but almost always looking at the patient; repeating a key word or the last word before the patient pauses; or saying "Uh huh," "And?""And what else?" or "For example?"
6. Proceed to WH questions to characterize symptoms.
7. Employ menus or direct questions when necessary for specification or efficiency.
8. Strive for *interchangeable responses* to encourage more information and show that you are listening; this means restating what the patient has said using a combination of your own words and those of the patient to show you "understand exactly" (see Chap. 2).
9. Avoid leading questions that reveal the answer you expect or desire, or multiple questions that confuse the patient.
10. Give the patient time to answer in his or her own words. This means waiting a little and not being afraid to endure silence as you wait.
11. Clarify and maintain direction for both yourself and the patient by using summaries, clarification, and, when needed, confrontation.
12. Feed back positives (e.g., the patient's strengths as you can see them) to help develop the relationship, support the patient, and elicit more information. For example, say, "It sounds as though you've been coping really well, despite a lot of pain for some time now. Now let's talk about what happened just yesterday to make things worse. . . ."
13. Keep a simple "roadmap" in your head (or on a note card) of where you intend to go in the interview and to remind you of where you are.

In the next chapter, we consider the more structured aspects of taking the medical history.

CHAPTER 4

The Medical History, Part 2: Past History, Family History, and Review of Systems

> To hold a true belief about an event in one's past experience is not sufficient for remembering it. There is still a distinctive factor lacking . . . Now it sometimes happens that a belief . . . transforms itself into a memory.
>
> Alfred Jules Ayer, *The Problem of Knowledge*

Once you have elicited the chief complaint, iatrotropic stimulus, and the complete description of your patient's present illness, other parts of the history, while tedious at first, are, in a sense, easier because they deal with structured data and are specific questions about predetermined topics. The skill lies in being precise about important details, while avoiding overinterpretation and overdescription of unimportant data; later, you will be able to relate pertinent information from the past medical history or the review of systems (ROS) to your patient's current illness. The trick is to emphasize the relevant features of past health and medical care experiences without getting too overwhelmed with a mass of detail. Feinstein[46] has spoken of the "Scylla of overdirection" and the "Charybdis of digression." By this he means the ability to keep your inquiry open ended enough to avoid missing the important events without getting bogged down in endless details about unimportant events.

This chapter and the one following cover parts of the medical interview that fill in the total picture of your patient's health and illness experience. These aspects of the interview provide important details that enhance your evaluation of and response to the person's current illness. In this chapter, we discuss obtaining past

75

medical history, family history, and ROS. These components help complete the picture by providing you with information about the context or setting in which the illness occurs, including the previous state of the patient's health as well as the presence of risk factors that have implications for both the current diagnosis and the prevention of future ills. We cover the patient's personal profile or social history in Chapter 5.

THE PAST MEDICAL HISTORY

You can begin your inquiry with a quite general question, such as,

- "How has your health been in the past?"

Another possibility is:

- "Tell me about any serious illnesses you have had in the past, starting from when you were a child."

A third possibility is:

- "Now I'd like to ask you about any illnesses or medical problems you've had in the past. How has your health been?"

Or one can provide a transition from the present illness, such as,

- "Okay, I think I understand what's been happening in the past few weeks, how about your health in the past?"

Patients may answer in quite general terms, such as, "I've always been sickly," or "Well, I used to have stomach problems," or they may begin to discuss particular symptoms. You must try to focus the inquiry on (1) discrete episodes that (2) caused substantial disability or a difference in the usual health pattern, and attempt to determine (3) the name that they have given, or their doctors have given, to these illnesses. You should never simply accept a diagnosis that a patient relates to you as being, in fact, the correct medical diagnosis. This is true even when a patient says she was hospitalized and was told her problem was a "heart attack" or "pneumonia." Many patients will tell you they have had "four or five heart attacks" in the past when, in fact, they have never suffered a documented acute myocardial infarction; this problem arises because their use of the term *heart attack* is not the same as your use of that term. A good question to ask is, "What exactly were your symptoms that made the doctor think that?"

There is no point, however, in obsessively trying to confirm every item of the past history by grilling the patient on obscure details. Your time and energy and those of the patient are limited. Consider how asking about "ancient history" is apt to make the patient feel:

> It's bad enough that I don't know all my family's medical diseases or of what my grandparents, whom I never knew, died, but I begin to feel positively stupid when at the mature age of forty-four I do not know whether as an infant I had measles or chicken pox. I may do a little better with more recent conditions but the feeling sinks again when it comes to medications I've taken that have given me trouble. "Those little red pills" seems an insufficient answer, and the recording physician's dubious look does not help much . . . By this point in the interview when I am asked questions about the specific timing and location of my varying symptoms, I begin to answer with a specificity born more of desperation than accuracy."[41]

Many adult patients have one or more chronic illnesses, and often each of these can have several exacerbations or require hospitalization at different times. It is necessary to consider the relevance of these illnesses to the current one. Consider the patient who has rapidly progressive congestive heart failure symptoms, has no clear evidence of ischemic heart disease, is not hypertensive, and who was referred to a medical faculty member. The referring doctor thought the patient might have a congestive cardiomyopathy because of a dilated heart, predominance of severe right-sided heart failure, and symptoms that appeared to begin rather suddenly 1 year before. However, the past medical history revealed quite frequent episodes of "acute bronchitis" and "pneumonia," and the ROS also yielded the information that the patient had a chronic "cigarette cough," usually producing a fair amount of sputum each morning. The patient was found to have chronic obstructive pulmonary disease with heart failure on the basis of cor pulmonale. She had not (nor had her physician!) related her recurrent lung problems and cigarette smoking to the illness at hand. When the doctor made this connection, it became clear that the present illness really extended much further into the past than was initially thought to have been the case.

After you acquire general information about the person's past health, you should fill in important categories of past medical history (as shown in Table 4–1). Old records can and should be obtained when, on the basis of your complete evaluation, you believe the information will be relevant to caring for the person's present illness or for his or her future general medical care.

The exact date or even year, if it is remote, is generally not important. Inquiry that is too precise will lead both to frustration and to answers that are likely to be falsely precise (that "specificity born of desperation"). A "hysterectomy in the early 1960s" is usually adequate; it does not matter whether it was 1962 or 1963. You should try to clarify what your patient means by the term *allergy*. A person may tell you he is allergic to flu shots because, after having one, he went on to have several colds that winter, or a person may tell you that she is allergic to aspirin because it gives her stomach discomfort. The first case is a personal attribution of a poor outcome, while the second case illustrates a side effect rather than a true allergy to aspirin. Be sure to ask specifically about allergies to medications. You should inquire what medications the patient is currently taking (or supposed to take), but also broaden your inquiry to include any regularly used drugs, such as oral contraceptives (which the patient may not consider a medication), cold preparations, pain relievers, or laxatives obtained without a prescription. Remember also to ask about vitamins or mineral (for example, iron) tablets, because many people consider these "natural" products and not

TABLE 4–1. Past Medical History

Serious illnesses, from childhood through the most recent one
Hospitalizations for these problems
Surgical procedures
Accidents or injuries
Pregnancies, deliveries, and complications (women)
Immunizations
Allergies
Medications currently used (including over-the-counter drugs and vitamins)

medication; they may not mention them unless specifically asked.

When you do your write-up, keep two things in mind:

1. Transfer data relevant to the current problem into the history of the present illness.
2. Make liberal use of quotation marks to indicate what the patient says but what you have not actually confirmed such as "hysterectomy," "allergy," or "slipped disc" (see Chap. 7 on recording the history).

Here is an example of a past medical history obtained from a 39-year-old woman at her first office visit for evaluation of headaches. She was found to have elevated blood pressure. Note the ease with which the clinician prepares the patient for the introduction of each new topic:

Dr: Okay, let's talk about your past health. Did you have any unusual childhood illnesses, rheumatic fever, scarlet fever, diphtheria?

Pt: Bronchitis.

Dr: Bronchitis. What do you mean by bronchitis?

Pt: Well, I'm not sure. That's what my mother told me. I guess I used to get sick a lot when I was a kid.

Dr: Were you ever hospitalized? Any serious illnesses or operations?

Pt: Uh huh.

Dr: What have you been hospitalized for?

Pt: When I've had D & Cs done, and I had my appendix out with part of my ovary.

Dr: Part of your ovary came out and . . .?

Pt: Well, I have a history of cysts growing on my ovaries.

Dr: Were you followed by a gynecologist?

Pt: Yes, Dr. Smith here in town.

Dr: Now, you mentioned you have two children. Any problems with your pregnancies or with childbirth?

Pt: With my little girl, yes. I had a lot of water, plus I had a bladder infection.

Dr: Did you have high blood pressure with that?

Pt: No, but I was sick a lot, nauseated a lot. It was like morning sickness but I had it for 8 months with her.

Dr: Doctor put you to bed at all?

Pt: No.

Dr: Any other hospitalizations, any other medical problems in the past that you had that you can remember?

Pt: No, just the D & Cs and the children and that one operation I had.

Dr: Do you have any known allergies?

Pt: I am allergic to goldenrod.

Dr: To what?

Pt: Goldenrod. Wool. I have hay fever. Anything like flowers—I get around them, I constantly sneeze my head off or get stuffed up. Roses, stuff like that. Right now, I'm having a time because we went up to the lake and we have a lot of goldenrod growing wild.

Dr: Do you take anything for it?

This is an example of a fairly typical and complete past history relevant to the present problems. Notice how the physician asks exactly what the patient means by *bronchitis*. Although the patient is not sure, she later reports symptoms of allergy; symptoms of allergy plus a childhood history of bronchitis suggest atopy, with the bronchitis perhaps representing episodes of childhood asthma. The patient has now "outgrown" her asthma but still has an atopic disposition as evidenced by the hay-fever symptoms. The physician also uncovers the history of fluid retention during pregnancy. This could have been a sign of toxemia, possibly of relevance to her hypertension now. Notice how the doctor asks specifically if the patient had high blood pressure. He also tries to determine if the previous physician treated the patient for hypertension without informing her of this by asking, "Doctor put you to bed at all?" Another way to ask this (especially if you have no idea what the therapy might have been) would be, "How was that treated?" The question regarding whether the patient takes anything for her hay fever is relevant for at least three reasons:

1. The physician can avoid the embarrassment of recommending something the patient has already tried.
2. Knowledge of what the patient has tried and the success

of the treatment indicates something of the severity of the symptoms.

3. Some decongestants raise the blood pressure when they are used by susceptible individuals or to excess.

Our final example is that of a patient who was being seen for back pain and reported a past history of phlebitis. What follows is the physician's search for the evidence (in how the patient was diagnosed and treated) that he did, indeed, have phlebitis:

Pt: But I have more trouble in my left leg than I do in the right leg, normally with this phlebitis that I had.

Dr: Were you ever admitted to the hospital for phlebitis and given intravenous medicines?

Pt: It's so long ago I don't remember.

Dr: Did you ever take a blood thinner?

Pt: Yes, Coumadin.

Dr: You were on Coumadin at one time. Did they ever do any x-ray studies of your legs with a dye. Did they ever put a . . .

Pt: I had the fibrinogen test. I had a series of tests.

Dr: Fibrinogen scans . . .

Pt: Yes, I had a series of tests done.

Dr: Did they ever do a venogram?

Pt: I don't know what that is.

Dr: You would remember it. A venogram is where they put a needle into a vein in your foot, and they inject a dye.

Pt: No, they didn't do that.

Dr: So you haven't had a venogram done.

Pt: I was taking iodine and had to take the iodine every day and come to the hospital every day for a month. I think that was the fibrinogen test.

Dr: The fibrinogen scan. Did you ever have, I imagine you would have had, something called a Doppler study.

Pt: I don't remember.

Dr: Or IPG, that's where they use sound waves to look for clots in the legs.

Pt: Is it a machine?

Dr: Yes.

Pt: I was on a machine in the emergency room one night.

Dr: On a machine for . . .

Pt: . . . for phlebitis.
Dr: Checking your legs, or do you mean one of the IV machines?
Pt: No, it wasn't IV.
Dr: Is it a machine where they ran a little microphone like thing?
Pt: No, they put little things on like they're going to take your blood pressure. They put them on my legs.
Dr: So they were studying blood clots. So, you have been on . . . were you only on the Coumadin one time?
Pt: Twice.
Dr: Twice. And you were hospitalized both times?
Pt: No, I wasn't hospitalized.
Dr: You weren't. You were never hospitalized before you were put on Coumadin.
Pt: No. I was in the emergency room and then I went to the doctor's office.
Dr: And they put you on Coumadin. You never had any heparin.
Pt: No I didn't have heparin. I had Coumadin. The little white pills.
Dr: Right. That's interesting.

The Family History

The family history is the systematic exploration of the presence or absence of any illness in the patient's family that may have an impact on the diagnosis of the present illness or on other concurrent illnesses, or that influences the patient's health or risk of future disease. This simple statement obscures two important questions: (1) what "illnesses" are relevant? and (2) what do we mean by "family"?

First, what illnesses and conditions are relevant? Relevant illnesses include:

1. Frankly hereditary diseases, such as sickle cell anemia or dyslipoproteinemias;
2. "Familial" illnesses, such as coronary artery disease, adult-onset diabetes mellitus, or carcinoma of the breast, in which the genetic transmission is not clear cut but in which familial clustering may become manifest in the presence of appropriate environmental stimuli;

3. Family "traits," such as short stature;
4. Illnesses such as manic-depressive disorder or alcoholism, which may not only be familial but also profoundly affect the patient's past and present environments; and
5. Current illnesses that suggest a common infectious or toxic exposure among family members.

Second, for familial hereditary disease by family we generally mean (of first importance) the patient's parents, siblings, and children and of somewhat lesser importance the patient's grandparents, cousins, aunts, and uncles. The spouse is a vital member of the patient's family but is of no importance to familial disease. Sometimes we must distinguish family from household, such as when one is considering environmental (toxic exposure) or contagious illness, perhaps even broadening the definition to include the patient's place of work.

The family history always enriches our understanding of the patient, whether in "getting" the diagnosis or in managing the illness; but because time and energy are limited, the potentially enormous amount of information must be tailored to the specific situation. How much we want to know depends on the patient, the type of problem, and the ability of the patient to give the information. For example, a family history of breast cancer is obviously of less relevance to a 10-year-old boy with tonsillitis than to a 45-year-old woman with a breast mass. A seriously ill patient may have a very relevant family history but be too sick to give any but the most critical data about the recent progression of symptoms. This might be the situation, say, in a patient with an acute myocardial infarction who has a strong family history of coronary artery disease; if there is no ambiguity about the diagnosis, the family history can wait until the patient feels well enough to remember and discuss the details. These details will be vital as the patient recovers, because how the patient feels about his or her future will be colored by recollections and beliefs about family members who had or have the same diagnosis.

A good way to start the routine family history is:

- "Are there any illnesses that seem to run in your family?"

or

- "Has anyone in your family been seriously ill?"

- "How about your parents? Children?"

It is almost always helpful to ask,

- "Has anyone in your family ever had anything like the symptoms you are having now?"

or, if you know the diagnosis, then you can ask,

- "Has anyone in your family had heart attacks?"

    In the case of an acute, possibly contagious illness, helpful questions to begin with are:

- "Has anyone else at home or work been sick lately?"

or

- "Have you come into contact with anyone who has similar symptoms?"

Here is an excerpt of a routine family history that will give you some sense of the flow of this part of the medical interview. Notice how the physician first introduces the new subject area (a transition) and then goes on with a specific question:

Dr: Okay. I think I understand the symptoms. Now I'd like to find out a little about your family. How about your parents, are they still living?

Pt: They're deceased.

Dr: Do you recall what they passed away from?

Pt: My mother had a heart attack 2 months ago.

Dr: How old was she at that time?

Pt: 63, I think.

Dr: How about your father?

Pt: About 7 years ago.

Dr: What did he pass away from?

Pt: Lung cancer.

Dr: How old was he?

Pt: Oh, I'd say 57.

Dr: Brothers or sisters?

Pt: Yes, I have nine brothers—I mean I have five brothers and three sisters.

Dr: Do they have medical problems that you are aware of?

Pt: No.

Dr: Is there any history of high blood pressure in the family?

Pt: My mother.
Dr: Your mother, okay. How about diabetes?
Pt: No.

The physician begins with a general question asking first about problems or illnesses, then follows up with some very specific yes/no questions about illnesses that one tends to see in families, such as hypertension and diabetes, or illnesses of particular relevance to this patient, who has hypertension.

But we observe something else here. There is no way to avoid the fact that some of the information we obtain is at once medical and social. Because the family is a social unit, the information we obtain in this part of the history invariably has some social aspects to it. The fact of the matter is that the information we seek in the family history is almost never neutral information: Everyone has feelings about his or her close relatives, especially parents and children. There is no way to avoid this; we can, however, acknowledge it, be prepared for it, and deal with it in a compassionate way during the interview.

In the previous example, notice that the patient's mother is very recently deceased. This is certainly not emotionally neutral information. The physician here faces a choice about how to proceed, whether or not to explore the patient's feelings, simply to make an empathic statement, or to continue getting information. In this instance, the physician continues to get more information and this appears to be useful. Had the patient's mother died at a late age after increasing illness or disability, the physician would expect the patient to have different feelings than if she died suddenly at a relatively young age. A potential problem here is that the physician takes his or her patient's word for "heart attack" and learns little more. There are many possibilities: Was it sudden? After many previous attacks? Was she sickly for years, perhaps with rheumatic heart disease and a final "attack"? And what of the resulting effects on a patient with a sickly mother? The physician will, later in the interview, return to her loss and deal with it more effectively and empathically.

What the patient "knows" about his or her family shapes the patient's beliefs and worries about health, health risks, and current symptoms. A patient with chest pain may believe that she has a bad heart like her mother, even though she is young and suffering from a totally different type of problem. A patient approaching the same age at which a parent died may have special concerns about his or her own health. Consider this family history in a 41-year-old woman who came because "it's been a while since I had a good checkup":

> Dr: Your parents still living?
> Pt: My father is living. My mother died when she was 42.
> Dr: How is your father? Is he in good health?
> Pt: Uh huh.
> Dr: How old is he?
> Pt: He was born in 1919.
> Dr: So he's 71.
> Pt: Yes.
> Dr: Any brothers or sisters?
> Pt: Two sisters. Both are in good health as far as I know. I don't keep very good contact with them, because I live here and they live out of state.
> Dr: Any medical problems? You said there are some medical problems that run in your family. What are they again?
> Pt: My mother had a bad heart. Most of it is in my mother's family. Like my grandmother died, she had cancer. She had diabetes too. When my mother died, she had had a plastic valve put in, then slowly deteriorated. She had sclerosis of the liver and a bad heart. She lived about a year after she had the plastic valve put in.

Again, this information is two sided; a woman who dies at the age of 42 after having an artificial valve, probably had rheumatic, or possibly congenital, heart disease. While there is some chance that the daughter may suffer from a similar problem, of more relevance is whether the daughter believes herself to be at risk. Note that she is 41 years old and her mother died at age 42. If she is found to have no signs of heart disease, it will be important to reassure her that her symptoms are totally unrelated to what went on with her mother.

Even the most straightforward questions tend to produce double-edged information:

> Dr: You said you've been pregnant five times?
> Pt: Yes.

Dr: Do your children live at home with you?
Pt: Yes.
Dr: Five of them?
Pt: Yes.
Dr: How old are they?
Pt: 20, 15, 13, 10.
Dr: That's four children.
Pt: Oh, I lost one.
Dr: Did he die of disease?
Pt: No, he died—he had a little growth on his eye and he died in surgery.

The physician dedicated to using a mechanical set of family history questions could have simply ignored the fact she gave only four ages. While the death of her child seems to have no strictly "medical" bearing whatever, a parent who has lost a child will certainly have feelings attached to the memory of the event and also may have negative feelings about the medical system, which, in a sense, caused her child's death.

Yet another problem in doing the family history is that while you wish to raise awareness or simply obtain neutral information, you may increase anxiety. In asking about family diseases, whether or not they are frankly hereditary, there is an implication that the history matters to the patient's current medical problem. It is helpful to be reassuring about this and to emphasize the "routine" nature of the inquiry. If you do not know whether there is a connection between the patient's family history and his or her present illness, say that you do not know but explore how the patient would feel if there were a connection. Do not raise anxiety unnecessarily. Here is an example of a physician who stumbles on anxiety-provoking information in asking a routine family history question:

Dr: Yeah, Okay. Very good. Now your mother and father what did they . . . Are they still alive?
Pt: Um, my mother is alive, my . . .
Dr: Age?

Notice how the physician hesitates over the initial question, realizing that the first thing he needs to know is if the parents are living; then barely listening to the response, the doctor asks another question. The dialogue continues:

> Pt: She is 64.
> Dr: She have any illnesses you know of?
> Pt: Uh . . .
> Dr: Heart disease, lung disease, anything?
> Pt: No, nothing of that sort; she's had a well-known skin cancer and uh, and she seems to have a recurring, it's a problem with her back, but actually it's a nerve that has to be blocked every once in a while.
> Dr: Okay. Your father?
> Pt: I never really knew that much about my father, but as I understand it he died of a cerebral hemorrhage.
> Dr: How old was he?
> Pt: Oh, he must have been in his late 40s.
> Dr: Was an autopsy done or anything to find out . . .
> Pt: There was so little . . . there was a bad occurrence, bad divorce between our mother and father when I was real young and I never saw him after age 9 months really. So I'm very hazy on the particulars of this.

The physician here stumbles on two kinds of loaded information; one, that the father died of a cerebral hemorrhage at an age that happens to be about the same age as that of the patient; two, that the patient does not know much because of "a bad occurrence." The physician ignores the latter and goes after the theory that the hemorrhage was caused by a congenital berry aneurysm, of relevance to this patient because such a condition can be hereditary.

> Dr: But nobody knew whether it was traumatic; did he get hit or anything?
> Pt: I don't know the details, to tell you the truth. He had, well, I just don't really know enough to talk about it.
> Dr: Cerebral hemorrhage at a young age would be an unusual thing. No other causes being known.
> Pt: I could find out more, my mother may know more about it.
> Dr: If she knew, it would be important to you . . . if she would know, for instance, if he had an aneurysm in his

> brain that burst, which is one of the ways you can have a cerebral hemorrhage at a young age. I think that would be very important, for instance, for your general health information so perhaps you can find out. Okay? Do you know anything more in terms of other problems?

Note the physician's graphic description of "an aneurysm in his brain that burst" and the implication that this "would be very important" while quickly moving on to "other problems." The patient now goes on to talk about "the painful subject" while the physician completely ignores the affective content of the interview.

> Pt: Well, my understanding is, the context of this, that my mother was raised in the Catholic church and divorce was a terrible scandal in her mind, and she tried to forget about it as quickly as she could. It's such a painful subject that there was never any discussion about who he was and so forth. And as a consequence, all I've really heard are niblets, and one of the things I understand is that he was an alcoholic, or at least had a problem with alcohol, but really caused my mother a lot of problems. So, I don't know if that would be a complicating factor in terms of aneurysm or not.
> Dr: Not that I know of. How about brothers and sisters?
> Pt: I have one full natural brother and then four half brothers.
> Dr: Any medical problems in any of them that you know of?
> Pt: No.

This example, part of which was presented in Chapter 2, demonstrates a doctor's insensitivity to the patient's feelings and self-disclosure. It also shows that by pursuing an item of family history the doctor can increase the patient's anxiety and raise new questions in the patient's mind about his own health. A person who tells you that his sister had breast cancer, that his father who smoked two packs of cigarettes per day for all of his adult life developed lung cancer, or that his uncle who was an asbestos worker died from mesothelioma, may feel that he is at high risk for developing cancer. The more you press for details about such illnesses in relatives, the more your patient may feel there is a connection with the illness he or she suffers at present. If your patient does not smoke and has no asbestos exposure, he or she may need reassurance that the family history does not presage a personal risk of lung cancer or mesothelioma.

You can avoid creating anxiety by being clear about why you need the information, sensitive to the patient's responses, and informative in your explanations.

1. You make it clear that family history is a routine part of your complete medical interview.
2. You listen carefully for any emotional overlay or any connections made by the patient between family illnesses and his or her own.
3. You demand no more detail than is required for your care of the patient. There is no point in close questioning about diseases of grandparents or in trying to determine whether a "heart attack" in an uncle was really a myocardial infarction.
4. If the patient does become anxious, you direct your attention to the anxiety. This usually means allowing the patient to express his or her concerns directly, for example, that the patient's mother died at age 42 from heart disease and now the patient herself is 41 years old and not feeling so well. Such an age coincidence is not at all uncommon, and often the patient will not have consciously made that connection. In such a case, anxiety may be "free floating," and you may need carefully to point out the coincidence of ages while also explaining the total difference in circumstances.

Another source of anxiety rises from the psychological bias called "availability" (see Chap. 14). An unusual illness that happens to occur in a family member is highly visible and "available" to the patient. Therefore, it has a greater impact on his or her fears than we might feel is justified. We look at the disease statistically and understand that it is not familial and that the chance of its occurring twice in a small number of people is extremely remote. However, as a medical clerk, resident, or practicing physician, you will find that availability plagues you all the time, just as it plagues your patients. After you diagnose your first case of glioblastoma multiforme, you will likely over-react to your next group of patients who complain of headaches. For the same reasons, you must be especially sensitive to the anxieties of the dizzy patient whose sister has multiple sclerosis or of the mother of a child with vomiting and recent varicella infection whose nephew had Reye's syndrome.

THE SEARCH FOR OTHER ACTIVE PROBLEMS AND THE REVIEW OF SYSTEMS

The review of systems demonstrates your responsibility for the total patient, and the review may uncover significant problems or symptoms not otherwise elicited. It is neither a refuge nor a burden. Some physicians who feel uncertain about how to conduct an interview, or about their ability to integrate data, take refuge in a long, detailed ROS that uses up an inordinate amount of time and energy. They seem to be asking about every possible symptom individually and in great detail, behaving as though it is possible to get "all" the information simply by asking "all" the questions. Such a marathon is exhausting for both patients and doctors. Other physicians look upon the ROS as a *pro forma* detail, something of little value that must be done; in other words, a burden.

It is easier to understand the ROS by first concentrating on the function it serves rather than on its content or the method by which you perform it. The function is simply to uncover any additional active medical problems and symptoms that may or may not influence or be related to the ones for which the patient came to see the doctor. The doctor may ask questions that serve this function at any time during the interview. The ROS proper may be "emptied" when the relevant information is obtained elsewhere. This search for *other active problems* (OAP) may be accomplished by asking nondirective questions at the end of the "present illness" segment of the interview. For example,

- "Can you think of any other symptoms that you've had lately?"

or

- "Do you have any other illnessness that have been acting up lately or are under treatment?"

In this way other problems that relate to the present illness are uncovered early in the interview, thereby avoiding last-minute surprises during the eleventh hour of the ROS. For example, a patient may be admitted to the hospital with pneumonia but may also suffer from chronic renal failure, diabetes, or hypertension. These chronic illnesses are also current problems and clearly affect the situation at hand. Another good screening question is:

- "What medications do you take?"

Whatever the patient responds to this, it is often good to ask,

- "Are there any other medications? How about over-the-counter or nonprescription medicines? Aspirin? Vitamins?"

The past medical history sometimes also presents opportunities to explore OAP and the ROS. If the patient reports any chronic illnesses or ill-defined symptoms in the past, it is a good idea to ask if these or similar symptoms are occurring now.

Platt and McMath[80] observed more than 300 clinical interviews conducted by medical residents and delineated five syndromes of "clinical hypocompetence." One of these syndromes is called *flawed database* and is illustrated by the following case:

> The clinical interview took 44 minutes to complete. Time allocation was as follows: introduction—1 minute; definition of chief complaint (cardinal symptom) and development of present illness—15 minutes; major past medical events, health hazards (smoking, alcohol, medications), and family illnesses—8 minutes; and review of systems—20 minutes.

In this case, the interview was structured in such a way that its efficiency in generating data was very poor. A large portion of it was devoted to a review of systems; this is generally unnecessary when one uses earlier parts of the interview to develop an understanding of the patient's life, habits, interests, and other active medical problems, as well as a skillful exploration of the current illness. The authors point out that a more functional allocation of time might be:

- introduction (1 minute);
- understanding the patient's life, habits, and interests (5 minutes);

- definition of chief complaint and present illness (15 minutes);
- definition of other active medical problems (5 minutes);
- major past medical and family history (8 minutes);

and

- ROS (3 minutes)

At first glance, a 3-minute ROS seems surprising if not downright impossible, but as you gain skill in asking open-ended questions early in the interview, the ROS will get shorter and shorter.

As you gain experience, much of the ROS may be conducted while you perform the physical examination. As you examine the patient's ears with your otoscope, you might ask if he or she has had any problems with hearing, ear infections, and so forth; as you examine the eyes, you might ask if he or she wears glasses. This method of doing an ROS, however, requires a high level of competence in performing the physical and the ROS so that you do not miss anything. An additional problem is that the patient may believe that you are asking your question (e.g., "Are you having any headaches?") because of something that you see during the physical examination. This may create anxiety, which could change what would otherwise be neutral and accurate information. It is important to preface your examination, or at least your questions, with a comment that you will be asking routine questions for the sake of completeness rather than questions specifically related to the patient's illness or physical findings.

Some practicing physicians approach the ROS with a standardized questionnaire that the patient fills out prior to seeing the doctor (see Chap. 12). The use of such an instrument, however, does not replace a ROS section of the interview but merely changes its character. Instead of asking about symptoms, the physician must review the questionnaire and ask for more detail about all those items for which the patient has indicated a "yes" answer. The clinician also must determine that the patient has, indeed, understood the written words well enough to answer the questions accurately. This is a perfectly acceptable format, but it is useful for the beginning physician to learn to ascertain a complete ROS without the benefit of such instruments. Then, after you have developed a comfortable style, you might create a personalized questionnaire for future use. You must still check out *pertinent negatives*, the symptoms a patient *does not* have that would, if he or she had them, support one of your diagnostic hypotheses. If a patient presents with cough, e.g., a pertinent negative might be a lack of shortness of breath.

Several guidelines are useful in learning about and conducting a good ROS.

First, it is not necessary to ask detailed questions about every symptom related to every organ system. You can expand the net of your inquiry by first emphasizing symptoms related to the patient's principal complaint and by starting with general as opposed to yes/no questions. For example, you can ask, "Are you having any trouble with your vision?" rather than "Is your vision decreasing?" or "Do you see double?" In other words, ask the patient about general difficulties with each system, then focus in on details of existing symptoms, and finally check out pertinent negatives.

Second, the ROS obviously should be abbreviated or eliminated in emergency situations; it also can be completed at a later date if the patient is too tired or too sick to respond to a tedious inquiry at present.

Third, anyone, even someone in perfect health, is likely to have some positive responses on a complete ROS. In the case of each positive response, you should obtain enough detail to indicate whether positive symptoms are significant or trivial. As a general rule, significance relates to severity and duration: the more severe and the more chronic the symptom, the more likely it is to be important.

Fourth, the use of ambiguous terms such as *indigestion, bowel trouble,* or *fatigue* is adequate for initial screening. For example, "Do you have any stomach or bowel trouble?" If there are any positive responses, the symptoms must then be defined more precisely.

Finally, the separate ROS section of the history should be at the end of the interview so that you have had time to "size up" the patient and ascertain how much direction the patient will need to volunteer important symptoms, whether there is denial on the one hand or obsession with the trivial on the other.

The following transcript, taken from a real patient history, provides an example of a ROS. It is neither completely comprehensive nor ideal but simply a reasonable example conducted by a medical intern. As you read through this interview, think about how you might have phrased these questions, whether you feel important information is missing, and whether you feel any questions are excessively detailed:

Dr: I'm going to ask you a bunch of questions I ask everybody. They are very general questions and some of them have short answers. Do you find that you get fevers often?

Pt: No.

Dr: How about chills? Have you had any chills recently?

Pt: Yes, but I just took that as being, you know my hormones for my hysterectomy. That's what I took it as being.

Dr: Okay. Do you get night sweats?

Pt: Yes.

Dr: Do you soak through all your bed clothing?

Pt: No.

Dr: How much do you weigh now?

Pt: 202.

Dr: How much did you weigh a year ago?

Pt: About 180–190.

Dr: What is the most you have ever weighed?

Pt: This.

Dr: You certainly aren't losing weight right now. Is that right?

Pt: Right.

Dr: Do you get headaches?

Pt: Sometimes. Maybe I'd say once a month. Maybe once every other month.

Dr: Do you have problems with your vision?

Pt: No.

Dr: Do you ever have double vision?

Pt: No.

Dr: Ever see spots in front of your eyes?

Pt: No.

Dr: How about blurry vision?

Pt: No.

Dr: Have you ever passed out?
Pt: No.
Dr: Blacked out?
Pt: No.
Dr: Do you often feel lightheaded?
Pt: No.
Dr: Do you hear ringing in your ears?
Pt: No.
Dr: Do you get a pain in your throat?
Pt: No.
Dr: Sore throats often?
Pt: No.
Dr: Does your neck hurt?
Pt: No.
Dr: Have you noticed any lumps or bumps anywhere in your body?
Pt: No.
Dr: Do your joints ache?
Pt: Yes.
Dr: Which ones?
Pt: Here.
Dr: Okay, you are pointing to your left knee and your back. How about other joints in your body?
Pt: No.
Dr: Do your muscles ache?
Pt: I just thought that it was my muscles in my leg.
Dr: Okay, fine. Do you get short of breath when you exercise?
Pt: I haven't exercised.
Dr: How about just walking around town?
Pt: No.
Dr: Can you climb stairs without becoming short of breath?
Pt: Yes.
Dr: Do you get pain in your chest?
Pt: No.
Dr: Have you ever gotten pain in your chest while you were exercising?
Pt: No.
Dr: Have you ever felt your heart fluttering or racing very quickly?
Pt: I don't think so.

Dr: Do your ankles swell on you?

Pt: No.

Dr: Are you able to lie flat in bed without becoming short of breath?

Pt: Yes.

Dr: Do you ever wake up in the middle of the night short of breath?

Pt: No.

Dr: Do you have to cough often?

Pt: No.

Dr: Ever cough up blood?

Pt: No.

Dr: Have you noticed any change in bowel habits, your bowel functions?

Pt: Yes.

Dr: How have they changed?

Pt: I don't pass my bowels as often as I did before I had surgery.

Dr: How often do you pass your bowels now?

Pt: Maybe twice a week.

Dr: Is the stool shaped as it was before or is it different? Is it thicker or thinner?

Pt: Thicker. Yeah because a lot of times I have to chew some Feenamints to make it go myself.

Dr: Do you have diarrhea intermixed with this at all?

Pt: No.

Dr: Have you noticed any tarry black stools?

Pt: No.

Dr: How about blood in your stools or on your stools?

Pt: No.

Dr: Have you had any belly pain?

Pt: Yeah.

Dr: Where does your belly hurt you?

Pt: Right where I had my incision. Sometimes like only when I laugh.

Dr: It hurts you along the incision?

Pt: Uh-huh.

Dr: How about somewhere else in your belly?

Pt: Right here.

Dr: Okay, you are pointing to your right groin area.

Pt: It's just like—mostly like when I see something real

> funny and just like when I laugh. There is not any pain, it's just there. I just get a pain when I start laughing.
>
> Dr: Have you noticed if you are very thirsty often? Do you find yourself drinking a lot of fluids?
>
> Pt: Sometimes.
>
> Dr: Do you think that you get cold more easily than some of your friends? Do you find that you put on heavy clothing when other people are not wearing jackets and things?
>
> Pt: No.
>
> Dr: Does the heat bother you more than you think it bothers other people?
>
> Pt: No.
>
> Dr: What is your energy level like?
>
> Pt: So-so. It's moderate.
>
> Dr: Do you become fatigued easily?
>
> Pt: Sometimes.
>
> Dr: How's your appetite?
>
> Pt: Great.

What are the good and not-so-good features of this ROS? Among its good features are its completeness (almost every organ system is covered) and the way in which this section of the interview (which is likely to differ from the more open-ended style of the earlier phases) is introduced. Also, the physician asks one question at a time and gives the patient time to respond. However, there are some problems. For example, the physician introduces a little medical jargon with the use of the terms *night sweats* and *change in bowel habits*, although many patients will understand these terms. The more striking problem (and one common to ROS) is the combination of lack of detail for some problems and the presence of overly elaborate detail for others. For example, the patient's complaints of headache, joint pains, and thirst are not further characterized; the clinician seems to have dismissed these symptoms as unimportant without additional information. On the other hand, there seem to be too many questions on cough and various types of shortness of breath where one question, such as, "Do you have any trouble breathing?" would do.

The trick is to achieve a balance between overly general questions that yield meaningless information and excessively detailed negative responses. The purpose of the ROS is to uncover problems that the patient has not brought up, either because the data have been forgotten or are considered unimportant. Because the physician is asking questions presumably unrelated to the main problem, the ROS is serving as a screening device. These questions are not hypothesis driven, and the probability that a positive response indicates significant pathology is low. Another way of putting this is that the *positive predictability* (how often a certain symptom or symptom complex actually signifies a certain disease) of ROS responses is less than the positive predictability of spontaneous statements that arise in the course of the patient's elaboration of the present illness. We discuss these issues more in Chapter 12. In our interview example, the clinician seems to assume that the symptoms of headache, joint pain, and thirst are unlikely to indicate important disease.

CHAPTER 5

The Patient Profile

Dialogue . . . can exhibit the object from each point of view, and
show it to us in the round, as a sculptor shows us things, gaining
in this manner all the richness and reality of effect that comes from
those side issues that are suddenly suggested by the central idea
in progress, and really illumine the idea more completely, or from
those felicitous after-thoughts that give a fuller completeness to
the central scheme, and yet convey something of the delicate
charm of chance.

Oscar Wilde, *The Critic as Artist. Part II*

The patient profile, also called the social history, is that part of
the medical interview in which we attempt to learn something
about who the patient is as a person and how the patient's lifestyle influences his or her health. Illness is not simply disordered
pathophysiology; illness happens to a person and involves
changes in the person's feelings and abilities. Moreover, getting
sick, seeking care, getting well, and staying well, all have social
determinants. "Patienthood is a psychosocial, not a biologic
state. A person becomes a patient by consulting a physician, or a
surrogate for one, in the officially legitimated health care system."[40] Knowledge of the patient as a person enriches the overall
experience of seeing patients as well as one's understanding of
the individual patient; it is essential to the biopsychosocial
approach to the patient. Therapeutic decisions involve not only
medical judgments but emotional, philosophic, social, ethical,
and interpersonal considerations as well.

The importance of the social history may not be readily apparent in the acute hospital setting where the diagnostic and therapeutic objectives are set on an hour-to-hour (if not minute-to-
minute) basis. In this artificial setting, knowing who the person
is or what the illness is like for the person seems much less important than knowing about the disease process. This artificial set-

101

ting is irrelevant when it is time to discharge the patient, and the home situation becomes critical.

- How many stairs will he or she have to walk up?
- Is the patient able to prepare or have access to the low-salt food required by patients with congestive heart failure?
- How will he or she juggle the complicated medication schedule?
- How much will the patient's employment allow changes in lifestyle necessitated by the illness?

In practice, your objective is not only to get the patient out of the hospital but also to help him or her be well enough to stay out of the hospital. To do this, you need to understand the impact of the disease on the person and on that person's style of living.

- For stress-related illnesses, what is the impact of the patient returning to the same stressful situation that may have occasioned the hospital admission in the first place?
- What about diseases that are clearly occupational, such as back injuries in a young mother or carpal tunnel syndrome in a heavy equipment operator?

Moreover, while early in medical training, physicians tend to be preoccupied only with physical factors; the person's decision to become a patient is very much a social decision. A person may well be ill, but a person does not become a patient until he or she consults a physician or other health care practitioner. This decision is influenced by patients' access to care, by what others in their group say about the symptoms, by their experiences with others who had the same symptoms (relatives or friends), and so on. Numerous investigators have documented the importance of these factors in the patient's timing of request for help. Consider, for example, the "social" nature of rashes: people seek help for rashes on exposed skin earlier than for rashes obscured by clothing. School nurses send home children with "pinkeye," and this usually mild and self-limited illness shows up promptly in the clinician's office. Some individuals become patients when their symptoms become acceptable as new diseases or become fashionable because of news stories; a recent example is premenstrual syndrome. The publicity about AIDS causes many people at risk for HIV infection to seek care for mild symptoms that they would have ignored otherwise. Some patients do not seek care of their own "free will" but are forced to come by spouses or parents; interactions with such patients are often difficult until they become willing participants. Adolescents and the elderly are often considered less than autonomous by parents or relatives, but they must be approached as adults in the physician-patient relationship. In such instances, the physician must work to establish the "contract" with the patient—assuming he or she is competent—as opposed to the usually well-meaning family member.

We segregate the social history into its own small section of the written case history as if the social history were something distinct or even optional, but this is an arbitrary separation for the sake of organization only. You are continually acquiring social information throughout the history from "small talk," the patient's manner of dress and speech, payment method, or insurance information that may appear on the chart. In the hospital, there is less access to this kind of information—there is a sameness to how people look lying in bed in hospital gowns. But what ward the patient is on, whether he or she has a private physician, and whether the patient normally uses clinics or emergency rooms as opposed to private practitioners, all yield clues. Another important aspect of what might be called social history is knowing enough about the patient to assess educational level and intelligence, both of which are critical to your ability to communicate successfully. Much of this is done automatically in the course of conversation. You want to converse at your patient's level of comprehension and not to speak in a manner inappropriate to his or her life experience.

Just as it is a mistake to believe that there is such a thing as a "complete" review of systems (ROS) (there are always more questions you could ask), it is also a mistake to believe that there is a "complete" social history (there will always be more about the person that you do not know). You have time constraints. How do you limit the inquiry so as to avoid a lengthy assessment? What is relevant and what should be obtained in the limited amount of time that you have? What information must be obtained when the patient is admitted or on the first office visit,

and what can wait to be developed over the course of a hospitalization or long-term relationship with the patient? You need to
know enough, at least, to answer these three questions:

1. How does the patient's lifestyle support or mitigate this
   illness?
2. How does the lifestyle contribute to or limit the severity
   of illness?
3. How will the lifestyle interfere or help with getting well?

The connection of certain illnesses with a patient's lifestyle or
personality is obvious, such as the development of recurrent viral
infections among child care workers. At times, the social history
is critical to making the diagnosis (AIDS and personality disorders are excellent examples); at other times, keeping the patient
well depends on his or her ability to, for example, follow a special
diet or complex regimen of medications.

WHAT GOES INTO THE PATIENT PROFILE

You can begin the patient profile with questions such as:

- "Can you tell me a little about yourself? Your family?
  Your work?"

or

- "How have things been going for you otherwise? At
  home? At work? In your marriage?"

Try to develop a picture of the patient as a person.

- What is this person like?
- Who is he or she?
- What is a typical day like?

Often one of the most useful parts of an entire history is a
detailed description of what the patient usually does on an ordinary day and exactly how this is modified by the illness. For
example, in the case of a person who may be suffering from
dementia, the description of a typical day may be more revealing

than mental status testing, particularly when the dementia is mild. The description may be more important as well, since what really counts is how the patient functions in his or her environment, not on a mental status test.

The degree of completeness that you need depends on the situation. Some of it may emerge in the course of the interview without specific questioning. Much of it is acquired not on the first day of hospitalization or during the first office visit but over time as you get to know the patient and understand what is relevant to his or her care. Keep in mind that the idea is to find out the patient's strengths and weaknesses and the nature of his or her support system, if any. How has this person coped with illness or other stress in the past? How does he or she keep distress within manageable limits? Remember that more intimate data are more easily and reliably obtained when you know the patient better, whether later in your initial history, later in the interview, later in the hospitalization, or years later in your relationship with the patient. Tailor what you need to know to the situation at hand.

A complete patient profile could be structured as summarized in Table 5–1. This is not an outline of questions to ask but a framework in which to organize information. The areas included are the basics, such as demographic information; risk factors, such as diet; relationships with significant others; and health

TABLE 5–1. Elements of the Patient Profile

Basics
    Demographic data: age, sex, race, ethnic group, religion, marital status,
        education, and area of residence
    Occupational history
Risk factors
    Cigarette, alcohol, and drug use
    Diet
    Daily activities and exercise
    Recreational interests
Relationships
    Marital and other significant relationships
    Family and household composition
    Support system
Cultural and health benefits
    See Chapter 14

beliefs. Any category, whether or not it is labeled as a risk factor, may contain a "factor" that puts that person "at risk." For example, a 20-year-old inner-city black man is at risk for violent death. Age, race, and area of residence are risk factors every bit as predictive of morbidity or mortality as smoking habits. We consider these categories below in some detail.

The Basics

DEMOGRAPHICS

The patient's age, education, race or ethnic background, religion, and residence are among the most fundamental data you need. These characteristics affect risk of various diseases, beliefs about the causes of illness, and the ability to participate in recommended therapy. Often this information is provided for you on the "front sheet" filled in by office or hospital personnel when the patient registers or is admitted.

OCCUPATION

Data about employment, school, or retirement are vital to understanding the patient and to building an understanding of the patient's support system. For married women, it is better to ask "Do you work outside your home?" than "Do you work?" Are there financial problems related to the patient's job or lack of a job? Is the retired person actively involved in hobbies or volunteer work? How does the patient cope with being a working wife and mother? How does the patient unwind from the rigors of daily living?

There are three essential points to a basic yet quick occupational survey that should be included in any complete medical history.

1. The physician should inquire about the patient's occupation and construct a short list of jobs he or she has held, particularly those held for a long time.
2. The ROS should include one key screening question about exposure: "Do you now (or did you sometime in the past) have exposure to fumes, chemicals, dusts, loud noise, or radiation?"

3. Some attention should be devoted to exploring any temporal relationship of the current medical problem to activities at work or at home, including job-related stress.

The key details are what the person actually does on the job. For example, a patient who "works for the phone company" may be a manager, install telephones, or do maintenance on poles out-of-doors. Similarly, a "steelworker" may operate heavy equipment, drive a truck, or work in a blast furnace. Each job is different and exposes the patient to different risks, ranging from chronic stress to serious accidents. By not considering occupational exposures, clinicians miss the opportunity to diagnose certain acute and chronic illnesses. Table 5–2, adapted from Goldman and Peters,[51] presents various examples of environmental causes of medical problems.

TABLE 5–2. Examples of Environmental Causes of Medical Problems

Effects	Agent	Potential Exposures
Immediate or Short-Term		
Dermatoses (allergic or irritant)	Metals (chromium or nickel), fibrous glass epoxy resins, cutting oils, solvents, caustic alkali, or soaps	Electroplating, metal cleaning, plastic, machining, leather tanning, or housekeeping
Acute psychoses	Lead (especially organic), mercury, carbon disulfide	Handling gasoline, seed handling, fungicide, wood preserving, or viscose rayon industry
Asthma or dry cough	Formaldehyde, toluene diisocyanate, or animal dander	Textiles, plastics, polyurethane kits, lacquer use, or animal handlers
Pulmonary edema or pneumonia	Nitrogen oxides, phosgene, halogen gases, or cadmium	Welding, farming ("silo filler's disease"), chemical operations, or smelting
Cardiac arrhythmias	Solvents or fluorocarbons	Metal cleaning, solvent use, or refrigerator maintenance
Angina	Carbon monoxide	Car repair, traffic exhaust, foundry, or wood finishing

TABLE 5–2. Examples of Environmental Causes of Medical Problems

Effects	Agent	Potential Exposures
Immediate or Short-Term		
Abdominal pain	Lead	Battery making, enameling, smelting, painting, welding, ceramics, or plumbing
Hepatitis (may become a long-term effect)	Halogenated hydrocarbons (e.g., carbon tetrachloride) or virus	Solvent use, lacquer use, or hospital workers
Latent or Long-Term		
Pulmonary fibrosis	Asbestos, silica, beryllium, coal, or aluminum	Mining, insulation, pipefitting, sandblasting, quarrying, metal alloy work, or aircraft or electrical parts
Chronic bronchitis or emphysema	Cotton dust, cadmium, coal dust, organic solvents	Textile industry, battery production, soldering, mining, or solvent use
Lung cancer	Asbestos, arsenic, nickel, uranium, or coke-oven emissions	Insulation, pipefitting, smelting, coke ovens, shipyard workers, nickel refining, uranium mining
Bladder cancer	β-Naphthylamine benzidine dyes	Dye industry, leather, rubber-working, or chemists
Peripheral neuropathy	Lead, arsenic, n-hexane, methyl butyl ketone, or acrylamide	Battery production, plumbing, smelting, painting, shoemaking, solvent use, or insecticides
Extrapyramidal syndrome	Carbon disulfide or manganese	Viscose rayon industry, steel production, battery production, or foundry
Aplastic anemia or leukemia	Benzene or ionizing radiation	Chemists, furniture refinishing, cleaning, degreasing, or radiation workers

Source: Adapted from Goldman and Peters.[51]

Risk Factors

Cigarette, Alcohol, and Illicit Drug Use

These habits are often listed as part of the social history. While these data may be obtained in that part of the interview, smoking and casual use of alcohol more properly belong in the medications or ROS part of the interview. Illicit drug use and alcohol abuse are illnesses in their own right and are also "social" problems for the patient, the family, and society at large. One should ascertain the amount, frequency, situations of use, and reasons for use. We consider the drug and alcohol history in detail in Chapter 9.

Diet

You may not learn much detailed, practical knowledge about nutrition during your medical education. Your patients, on the other hand, may have strong beliefs about the role of diet in their illnesses. Many will have tried specific weight reduction plans and will ask your advice about them. You also will be recommending changes, such as salt restriction or reduction in saturated fats, for treatment of your patients with chronic diseases such as hypertension and certain health risk factors such as elevated total cholesterol. If you have no idea about the person's basic eating habits, you will be unable to give specific advice. The nutrition part of your patient profile is important, and sometimes, in health maintenance and prevention, it yields your most effective interventions for the patient.

You should find out how many meals per day the person usually eats and roughly at what time. You also should learn what sort of snacks your patient eats on a daily basis. You will encounter obese patients who tell you, truthfully, they eat only one meal per day. They attempt to cut down and lose weight but are continually frustrated in their efforts. "I hardly eat anything, yet everything I eat turns to fat. . . . I just can't lose a pound." This problem may arise from their one-meal-per-day habit, which promotes frequent (sometimes continual) snacking during other times of the day. This snacking may be an almost unconscious background phenomenon that the person fails to consider and "count" as a meal. Another factor contributing to this failure to lose weight is that very obese people tend to be sedentary. They need relatively few calories and so will find it difficult to "cut down" to a level of intake below the calories they are burning up daily. Finally, while these behaviors contribute to the difficulty in losing weight, many obese patients do, in fact, have relatively low caloric requirements on a genetic basis.

Another aspect of dietary history is a picture of dietary composition, particularly with regard to fats, salt, food groups, foods never or rarely eaten, and foods eaten in excess. You should find out roughly:

1. The proportion of red meat in the diet, as compared to poultry or fish;
2. Other saturated fats in the diet (butter or margarine, dairy products, and cooking oils);
3. Some indication of indigestible fiber intake (grains and leafy vegetables); and
4. Preferences for salt cooked in food and/or added to food ("Do you add salt when you cook or at the table?").

Specific food intolerances, food allergies, the condition of the patient's teeth, ability to shop and prepare food, and income all affect dietary habits. Ethnic and cultural influences may be very resistant to change. Perhaps the most accurate and efficient way to assess the patient's dietary habits is to ask, "Tell me what you've eaten over the last 24 hours beginning with just before you came to the office (for outpatients) and working back." And then, "Is this a typical day for you?" or "How is it different?" The question "Tell me about your diet" may be misinterpreted if the patient is not on a (weight reduction) "diet." Details are important. If the patient has "toast" for breakfast and a "sandwich" for lunch, find out what goes on the toast and between the slices of bread.

Some consideration also should be given to caffeine in the diet. It is not uncommon to find patients who drink several cups of coffee per day routinely, in addition to frequent cola beverages, and who increase this intake during periods of stress. Caffeine usage may be a crucial factor for patients who come in with upper gastrointestinal symptoms, headaches, irritability, palpitations, fatigue, and lightheadedness.

Daily Activities and Exercise

Knowledge of the patient's demographic characteristics and occupation will give you some clues to the patient's lifestyle. How he or she spends a typical day reveals even more about factors that may contribute to illness or facilitate getting well. For example, the sedentary retired salesman will need an explicit and graded exercise program with frequent monitoring of his progress as he recuperates from a heart attack. People who are constantly on the go, eating on the run, and rarely preparing their own food may need to undertake major and difficult changes in lifestyle in order to treat their obesity and hyperlipidemia.

Exercise history is an important feature of the patient profile. Vague answers, such as, "I like to play tennis" or "I have a rowing machine at home," are not necessarily indicators of regular aerobic exercise. Perhaps the patient has not had time for tennis since the summer of 1986 or the rowing machine sits unused in the basement. To monitor health effects, you must inquire specifically about regularity and duration, as well as type, of exercise. As you do this, you also are assessing the potential for various types of trauma that result from sports and exercise programs, from stress fractures in joggers to major knee injuries in skiers.

Relationships

Marital and/or Significant Relationships

As you begin to understand the patient's lifestyle, you also will be developing a sense of the patient's relationship with his or her spouse or significant other. You may not need to ask direct questions about this. Because patients may regard this sort of information as intimate and possibly unrelated to their illness, it is best to ask questions in a somewhat indirect and open-ended manner, which permits the patient to answer in their own terms, revealing as much or as little as they wish. Start with questions that relate the patient's illness to the current state of the relationship, such as,

- "How has your doing home dialysis affected your husband?"

Then proceed to more intimate questions, such as,

- "How have 20 years of married life been?"

Such questions allow the patient to say anything from "Okay" to "Well, we've had our rough spots but things are pretty good right now" to "To tell you the truth, I keep wanting to leave him, but I can't." Still more specific questions, such as

- "What are some of the good and bad things about your present relationship?"

or

- "What would you change?"

are useful once the patient has indicated an interest in discussing the relationship. Sexual behavior and illness influence each other in many ways and may affect significant relationships. We consider the sexual history in detail in Chapter 9. In addition to the impact of illness on relationships and of relationships on illness, certain diagnoses and clues to diagnoses reside in the patient's relationships history. For example, a personality disorder is a historical diagnosis;[94] the criteria for making this diagnosis lie in the patient's history of difficult relationships with family, friends, and employers.

Support System

It is helpful to find out the family composition and who lives at home (e.g., parents, grandparents, siblings, spouse, or children) and their ages. Persons who are widowed face special problems in coping with stress and, indeed, have higher rates of illness and death, particularly in the first year of widowhood. As you get to know the patient better, you can begin to discuss the stresses and satisfactions related to his or her family's functioning. With the answers to these questions, you have begun to develop an idea of the patient's support system.

- Are there family members nearby who are willing and able to help in time of crisis?
- What kind of help does the young mother have with her new baby?

- Who will care for the elderly, demented patient when her husband (who normally cares for her) has his hernia surgery?

Most chronic illnesses, any illness that results in disability, as well as psychiatric disorders, require the physician to know who is available to help the patient get well and stay well. When there is no family or the family has limited financial or emotional resources, it is necessary to involve social agencies to provide services ranging from transportation to doctor's appointments to meals in the home.

Beliefs

CULTURAL AND HEALTH BELIEFS

Illness may affect the patient in many ways—both trivial and profound. There are the day-to-day problems, such as getting up and down steps for a patient whose surgery or illness limits her ability to do so in a house with its only bathroom on the second floor, or the widower who eats out and must limit his sodium intake. Illness produces hardships of a different sort when it takes away the patient's ability to earn a living or renders the aging spouse unable to care for his or her mate. Illnesses also have an emotional impact; a woman with a localized breast cancer and a man with an uncomplicated acute myocardial infarction may well have the same good prognosis, but in our society, a diagnosis of cancer is usually more devastating than a diagnosis of heart disease. For some, illness has positive consequences, such as for the person who believes physical suffering leads to spiritual enlightenment. For others, illness may represent a concrete sign of their failure to pray correctly or to have sufficient faith in God to be "healed." We consider sociocultural aspects of illness and the impact of the patient's health beliefs in Chapter 14 on negotiation and the healing connection.

SOCIAL HISTORY EXAMPLES

Next we consider some examples that demonstrate the importance of the social history or patient profile in the diagnosis and management of medical problems. In this first example, a 61-

year-old black woman with known diabetes and hypertension urgently scheduled a visit to her family physician, complaining of chest pain, headache, and increasing concern about her blood pressure. The physician, confused about which problem was really the chief complaint because the symptoms were chronic and the blood pressure was well controlled, asked the patient to clarify her concerns:

> Dr: Uh, what, what would you say is the thing that's worrying you the most right now?
> Pt: Well, mostly, is how, getting those bills paid. See, I'm on, I'm on assistance.
> Dr: Oh, I see. Tell me more about this worry. Did something new happen?
> Pt: Mostly it's a gas bill and then, um, see I own a house. I have the taxes, keeping up with them, and, ah, just finances generally.
> Dr: Did you recently get your gas bill?
> Pt: Yes I did.
> Dr: When did that come?
> Pt: Yes, ah, it came the other day.

In this instance, the "social" problem was *the* problem. Notice how the physician went after positive or confirmatory evidence that there were, indeed, data to support the notion that it was her inability to pay the gas bill that was really bothering the patient. This does not mean that the patient did not have "real" chest pain, headaches, and high blood pressure; but it was very helpful in answering the "why now" questions, that is, *why* the patient sought care *now* for symptoms that had not changed.

Next, consider this example in which another kind of social determinant of the decision to seek care becomes apparent.

> Pt: See, um, I used to, okay, I used to do hair, I'm a barber, I'd do a lotta hair, so I had to go to, uh, um, I had to go to the clinic. Okay, now barbers every time they get their license renewed, they have to go to the health department.
> Dr: Right.
> Pt: Right. Okay and they gave, uh, they gave me some pills

> to take because they gave me a test, um, humm, and it came back positive . . .
> Dr: Um humm.
> Pt: You know they gave me some pills to take, they say I have to take them for a year.
> Dr: Um humm.
> Pt: But before the end of the year, after I run out, I'm supposed to come back and get some more . . .
> Dr: Right, I see . . .
> Pt: And I didn't.

Here, this patient who has chest pain is probably concerned that his failure to follow-up on recommended treatment for what was a positive tuberculin test may be the etiology of his current symptoms. The only reason he had the tuberculin test in the first place was to satisfy the state licensing requirements to be a barber.

Here is another example, in which the patient describes a bout of gastrointestinal symptoms:

> Dr: Do you think that a week ago when you had this vomiting that you had some kind of virus or flu bug?
> Pt: I could of had a little bit of a slight—I ate some food that wasn't real fresh and it could of been that, plus maybe—I don't know what it was. It could of been the food I ate.
> Dr: How was it that you ate some food that wasn't so fresh?
> Pt: Well, my refrigerator is bad and it's been so hot. I don't have the money to fix it.

The physician is rightly concerned about how it was that the patient came in contact with possibly offensive food; a bad refrigerator is a "social" problem that can lead to disease. Let us close with an example of a patient who has numerous influences on his lifestyle that are contributing to his illnesses, which include obesity, headaches, and secondary syphilis:

> Pt: The thing that is interesting to me is I am busy and I am constantly on my feet and I must put in at least 4 miles

each day, but it doesn't affect my weight because of the types of things I eat. I don't eat heavily, it's just the things I eat.

Dr: How do you mean?

Pt: When I have not eaten for a whole day, I go to some deli and grab a creampuff and go to bed. That gives me sugar and sugar helps me. Sugar really helps me keep elevated. I have a terrible—well, I have to drink orange drink. I don't eat breakfast, as a matter of fact, I only eat one meal a day, but it's a junk meal. And I'm very hooked on, I have to have a sugar-type drink in the morning to get elevated. Could use one now!

Dr: Now that you know all these things, is there any way you can change something? Like when you go to New York, you can find some time for yourself, even if it's sitting down for 10 minutes instead of 10 seconds?

Pt: I lived there for 2 years, and when I started the business, I didn't realize at the time that the business was going to grow as quickly as it did, and I found out I was going to New York more and staying in hotels. Hotel living is disgusting. All I want to do is—my day starts at usually 6:30–7:00 o'clock in the morning and sometimes ends at 10:00 or 11:00 at night. And all I want to do is go back to the hotel, shove some sugar in my face, and go to sleep. This is the part where it gets into the personal part of it. My lifestyle changed quite a bit; a lot of things changed for me. I have always felt that I had very strong religious convictions and things like that. When I moved to New York, my lifestyle totally changed. I had to be very social; I wasn't a very social person. I wasn't a party person, I wasn't a drug person. But I went to parties where everybody was having sex with everybody else and you really didn't even get to know the person. You may never see them again and that type of thing. Well, all these things happened to me in this period. And I have to be honest with you, they frightened me, but I enjoyed them. I knew they were wrong, but there was a part of me that enjoyed them. So I was getting very confused. I felt that it was time for me to come back.

Dr: You felt that this was a way of coming back home?

Pt: Exactly. What happened to me recently was that because of me going back to the way I wanted to be and things not working out the way I thought they should, so I figured why should I make sacrifices and be this person. You know, and not getting the results I want from it. I'll go back to being the other person. And I went back to being the other person and I got (laughing loudly) a social disease! Now you know my life story. That's it in a nutshell.

Note how the physician, even in this more structured part of the interview, skillfully uses open-ended questions ("How do you mean?") and interchangeable responses ("You felt this was a way of coming back home?")

This patient (whom we met briefly in Chap. 1) had numerous social influences contributing to his diseases. He probably acquired syphilis at a party at which he had multiple sexual partners. He was finding his obesity difficult to control and was experiencing constant fatigue and stress-related tension (muscle contraction) headaches. His syphilis, which had advanced to the secondary stage with the development of a rash before it was diagnosed, required hospitalization and became very public evidence of what the patient saw as religious transgressions. He became dreadfully afraid that he had been exposed to the AIDS virus during his contacts with homosexuals who had numerous sexual partners. His anxiety, and his guilt, about possibly contracting a lethal disease made it very difficult for him to work as hard as he felt he needed to in order to keep his business going. He did, indeed, develop AIDS, and he died about 2 years later.

CHAPTER 6

The Transition to the Physical Examination and Closure

"Your escape plans have melted!
You haven't a chance,
for the next thing you know,
both your socks and your pants
and your drawers and your shoes
have been lost for the day."
The Oglers have blossomed
like roses in May!
And silently, grimly, they ogle away.

Dr. Seuss, *You're Only Old Once: A Book for Obsolete Children*

Medical interviewing, unlike other forms of the helper-client interaction, usually also involves a physical examination. The history and physical examination are different parts of the same process; a process that also includes negotiation, education, and clarification of plans. If we focus on data gathering, it is difficult to pinpoint exactly where the history ends and the physical examination begins, or vice versa. For example, from the first moment the patient walks into your office or you walk into the hospital room, you begin to make observations about the physical condition of the patient: You observe skin color, affect, behavior, and mental status. The entire "mental status examination," although part of the interview in that it involves no touching, is really more properly considered as part of the systematic "physical examination." On the other side of the coin, as you are doing the physical examination you continue to interact with your patient, hoping to obtain not only physical but also personal and symptom information.

TRANSITION TO THE PHYSICAL
EXAMINATION

It is difficult, at first, to go from talking to touching. Early in your medical experience, it is especially difficult to unglue yourself from your chair and approach the patient. You can handle this transition with a statement such as "I'd like to examine you now—if you're not too tired." In the hospital, paying attention to the patient's comfort, such as offering some water or changing the window blinds, may be appropriate.

Ordinarily when in the clinic or in your office, you will be interviewing a patient who is fully clothed. Although having a patient disrobe and putting on an examination gown prior to the medical history is often conducive to good office functioning, it is rarely conducive to patient comfort. It undermines respect for the person. Thus, the patient should be fully clothed, and you will be faced with telling him or her to get undressed when you are ready to start the examination. You should be quite direct and clear about what is going to happen and why.

> *First,* give the patient an opportunity for the last word. For example, "I think that's about it for now. Is there anything else we haven't covered or that you'd like to tell me before I examine you?"

> *Second,* tell the patient clearly what the game plan is. For example, "Next I'm going to do your physical examination, and then after that, we can sit down and talk about your problems and what tests you might need."

> *Third,* be very specific about what clothing the patient should remove, where he or she should sit or lie, and in what position. For example, "I'm going to step out of the room for a moment now. Please get undressed down to your underpants and put on this gown. Put it on with the opening toward the back. And then sit on the end of the table up here."

Here is how one physician begins an examination of a patient that the physician is seeing for the first time. Note the explicit directions as well as the review of systems (ROS)-type question the physician asks at the beginning of the examination:

> Dr: Do you have any questions before we do your exam?
> Pt: No.
> Dr: Okay. Why don't you climb up here, and just sit there, just step around, and come around there. Okay. I am going to cover you and you can just sit there first. I am going to check your thyroid and your lungs and your heart, and examine your breasts. Have you had any thyroid trouble?
> Pt: No.

It is best for you to leave the room, or to pull a curtain across the room if one is available, while your patient gets undressed. In the hospital, of course, this is usually not a problem, but, even there, patients may want to use the bathroom and/or to remove a dressing gown or robe. In office practice, when you are doing only part of a physical examination, it may be appropriate for the patient to remove only his or her shirt or unbutton several buttons. For specific parts of the examination, ask the patient to disrobe that area or, alternatively, say, "I'm going to untie (or unbutton or remove) . . . ." If a female patient has large breasts, ask her for assistance in moving the breast in order for you to listen to the heart. This helps the patient to feel more like a participant and less like a victim.

CONVERSATION DURING THE PHYSICAL EXAMINATION

While maintaining a conversation during the physical examination allows you to continue to gather data, it may serve other essential functions as well. You can use your communication skills to put the patient at ease, encourage the patient to feel like an active participant in his or her own care, and diminish the perception of a difference in power between the physician and patient, which becomes more marked during the physical examination. Here is how one patient described it:

Whether it be horizontal, or in some awkward placement on one's back or stomach, with legs splayed or cramped, or even in front of a desk, the patient is placed in a series of passive, dependent, and often humiliating positions. These are positions where embarrassment and anger are at war with the desire to take in what the doctor is saying. In this battle learning is clearly the loser.[41]

You also can use conversation to show the patient that you remember the complaint about abdominal pain while you are doing the abdominal examination, or you may use "small talk" to distract the patient so the patient's muscles will relax, making the abdominal or pelvic examination easier for the patient and more accurate as well.

Keep talking during the examination to gather further information, reassure the patient, and explain what you are doing. It may not be possible as a beginner to make comments while you also are concentrating on the sequence of things to do and the techniques for doing them. It is not difficult, however, to make such observations as:

- "I'm going to look into your ears now."
- "I'm feeling for your thyroid gland. Can you swallow now? I know it's difficult to swallow like that when someone asks you. Good."
- "I'm going to do a rectal exam now to check your prostate gland. It will make you feel like you are going to have a bowel movement, but don't worry, you won't."

It is also easy for you, and is reassuring for the patient, to indicate that parts of your examination are normal. It is usually not particularly helpful to comment on every little thing you do, but if you know the patient is concerned about a particular system, it would be helpful to note your findings about that system right away. For the patient who comes in with chest pain, a comment that the heart and lungs sound normal can be quite reassuring for the patient (who need not be bothered at this point with the academic information that the heart may sound normal even when there is heart disease). Here is an example of how a physician spoke to a patient during the parts of the physical examination that involved listening to the lungs and heart, and palpating the breasts and abdomen. Notice the insertion of a few ROS-type questions as the physician examines a part, education about self–breast examination, and attention to the patient's comfort ("Tell me if I hit any sore places."):

Dr: Okay, I am just going to loosen this (unties gown in back). How long have you been smoking?
Pt: About 3 years . . .

Dr: And you want to quit.

Pt: Well, yeah, I been thinking about it.

Dr: Take a deep breath, Okay, out, good, and again . . . Good. Now I am going to ask you to slip your arms all the way out and I am going to listen to your heart . . . Okay. Sounds good. Now I'm going to check your breasts. I want you to put your hands up like this (doctor demonstrates) and I'm just going to look at them first to see if there are any bumps . . .

Pt: Uh mm.

Dr: Okay, have you ever tried it?

Pt: No, not really.

Dr: We recommend that everyone do it once a month; the best time is right after your period has stopped. Do your breasts get sore before your period?

Pt: Yes.

Dr: Okay, well some women do and that is why it is best to wait until after your period starts when usually the lumpiness goes away and they're not tender to touch . . . I am going to ask you to just hold this up . . . and I want you to put your arms up over your head. What you do when you are checking is to do exactly what I'm doing . . . Go all around the outside of your breasts like this . . . up here is breast tissue and also up here . . . so you are going to go in kind of a circle like this . . . then spiral in until you get every part including under the nipple. Okay? Now I'd like you to lie down and we'll check your breasts again . . . we always check them in two positions . . . And I am going to check your heart . . . Do you have any indigestion or trouble with your bowels? Now tell me if I hit any sore places.

The pelvic examination is a particularly personal and anxiety-producing experience. You should explain clearly what you are about to do and what the patient is likely to feel. Ask the patient if she has had a pelvic examination before. Whether she has or not, it is very reassuring to say something like "I'm going to pretend that this is your first pelvic and explain everything that I'm doing." The less experience the patient has had either with pelvic examinations or with you, the more reassurance she will need. You should first touch the patient's inner thigh and then firmly but gently conduct the examination. You should describe the anatomy to the patient as you are doing the examination. As you become more experienced, you will be able to help her relax her muscles through your calm tone of voice, your gentle palpation, and your instructions about deep, slow breathing.

Here is how one physician introduced a patient (who requested a diaphragm for birth control) to her first pelvic examination; everything is described with a relaxing, almost hypnotic, tone of voice, the physician's gestures are slow and deliberate (no sudden moves), and the physician continuously looks at the patient's face to gauge her reactions:

Dr: The next thing I am going to do is a pelvic exam. These are all the things I am going to use, but I am not going to use all of them on you. Okay. These are the slides on which the Pap test is done, and these are the swabs that I use to do the Pap test. They're just like long Q-tips, okay, and this also, which I will roll around the cervix just like that (demonstrating), see it is not sharp . . . We usually do a culture for infection at the same time . . .

Pt: A culture?

Dr: Yes, and that is to check for infection. This instrument is cold, and that is really the worst thing about it. It is called a speculum and this is inserted very gently into the vagina and then opened very gently like that (demonstrating) so that I can see your cervix and see that it is normal. Okay? (Patient nods.)

Dr: What I will ask you to do is to put your feet into these things which are called stirrups, these metal things, that is good, and now I want you to pull yourself all the way down to the end of the table like that, and practically feel yourself like your bottom is coming off the end of the table. Okay? That's fine. I am going to put this pillow under your head right there, okay, and I am going to shine a light on you so that I can see what I am doing and as I do things I will tell you what I am doing. Okay? Are you more or less comfortable?

Pt: I guess so.

Dr: All right, it is not very comfortable, that is true. Okay. Now what I am going to do is to look at the outside of you first. If you can just kind of relax, that's good. Now what I am doing is checking the labia, or lips. Good. Now you are going to feel my finger at the edge of the vagina, feeling where your cervix is. Do you know what your cervix is?

Pt: No.

Dr: Okay, that is the opening to your womb or uterus. Okay, I am just kind of locating it first, and that is just my finger again. Okay, now you're going to feel the cold metal which I tried to warm up a little bit, but usually it's still cold. Is that okay?

Pt: Mm hmm.

Dr: Now I insert it just until I can see your cervix so that I can do the Pap test. Okay, now I can see your cervix very clearly now . . .

Pt: Is that where I put the diaphragm?

Dr: Exactly, that is exactly where to put the diaphragm. Okay, now I am just using one of those long Q-tips to do the Pap test, okay?

Pt: Mm hmm.

Dr: And now I'm going to use one of those scrapes and sometimes you feel that scraping feeling, but usually what you feel is the pressure of the speculum being in place there . . . Now I am just spraying those glass slides that I just took and that preserves them so they can be checked later. And now I am taking the speculum out. Are you still with me?

Pt: Yeah.

Dr: Okay, the next thing I am going to do is check your rectum and that will make you feel as though you have to have a bowel movement, right, that is just my finger in your rectum. That's kind of an uncomfortable feeling with some people. It feels completely normal. Now I am going to just check back inside your vagina, okay, and where my fingers are is where you put the diaphragm. Now I am going to ask you that when you go home you practice feeling where your cervix is. I am touching it right now. On you, it is a little bit off to your left side, okay, and it feels like the tip of your nose when you touch it. Okay. When I put one hand over here and between the two hands I can feel where your uterus is . . . And I am touching it right now and it feels

> normal. Now I am checking on each side for your ova-
> ries . . .
> Pt: Can you feel all that?
> Dr: You can feel all that, especially in someone like you,
> because you are very relaxed and I can feel everything.

Notice how the physician keeps talking, but frequently checks back with the patient, and is educating the patient all the while about her body and about the normality of the findings. Indeed, the proof that the technique is effective is in the patient's pleasure and wonderment ("Can you feel all that?") at the ability of a pelvic examination to tell a physician so much and at her ability to completely relax her muscles.

Your continued "interview" with the patient during the physical examination provides clarification and reassurance. The new information aspect will gradually develop as you become more comfortable with the procedures of physical examination, so that concentration on the actual techniques can sink into the background and you are able to concentrate more thoroughly on your immediate observations. Until you are experienced, do not try to do the complete ROS during the physical examination. However, if you are looking at the eyes, for example, and this reminds you of an eye question you forgot to ask, go ahead and ask it. The physical examination is also a good time to find out more about the person's life and lifestyle. Such "small talk" yields pertinent information as well as makes the patient more relaxed by distracting him or her from what your hands are doing.

USES OF THE PHYSICAL EXAMINATION

What are the purposes of the physical examination? What diagnostic or therapeutic value does it serve?

First, of course, more data that complements and supplements the history is obtained during the physical examination. The examination yields a different kind of data, *signs* rather than *symptoms*. The signs serve to confirm or disconfirm the hypotheses that we are beginning to develop from the history, or perhaps the results of the examination will suggest entirely different hypotheses. The physical examination, in this sense, should be as flexible and targeted as the history. In the physical examination, we should not obsessively attempt to make all possible observations but only those that are relevant to the problems at hand.

Table 6–1 lists frequently observed errors in performing physical examinations; the observations are based on a study of medical house officers.[107] Some are errors in technique, simply not performing the procedure correctly; some are procedures omitted inappropriately; some are errors in classification or detection, missing a sign that is really present or asserting that a sign is present when it really is not; and some are problems in interpretation, recognizing the sign but failing to recognize its value or meaning. These will be useful to review. It is comforting to know that other students and young clinicians have the same problems with physical examination as you do. Physical examination courses have, in the past, emphasized students "doing it" on their own, usually examining hospitalized patients, and then reporting findings to their preceptors. The preceptor had little opportunity to observe the student and to teach correct techniques in this process. Skillful physical diagnosis requires not just experience (it is easy to perform the same egregious errors habitually!) but also guided instruction. Request that your preceptor observe your examinations periodically, even if you do not think you need it.

Second, the physical examination also serves as a screening device through which we can obtain information about asymptomatic disease or about problems not mentioned by the patient during the interview. In this sense, it is somewhat like a physical version of the ROS. A few parts of the physical examination serve an especially important screening function; that is, they permit the detection of completely asymptomatic disease. In adults, these are:

1. Taking the blood pressure;
2. Breast examination in women;
3. Examination of the skin for suspicious lesions;
4. Pap smear for cervical cytology in women; and
5. Rectal examination with a test for occult blood in the stool.

Third, the physical examination, as we have indicated earlier, also provides an opportunity to continue the interview under new circumstances. It allows us to ask specifically about things

TABLE 6-1. Errors Most Frequently Made in a Physical Examination

Type of Error	Head and Neck Examination	Chest Examination	Abdominal, Genital, and Extremity Examination	Neurologic Examination
Technique	Bimanual palpation of head and neck Determination of tracheal position Measurement of jugular venous pressure Hepatojugular reflux venous pulse waves	Palpation of expansion Percussion of diaphragm movements Auscultation for low sounds and murmurs	Palpation of spleen Deep abdominal structures Popliteal pulses Testes Percussion of liver and spleen and auscultation for bruits	Visual fields Calorics Corneal reflexes Tendon reflexes and Babinski testing
Omission	Auscultation of neck vessels Inspection of retina, cornea, lens, and iris Inspection of nasal cavity	Auscultation of lateral chest and apices Cardiac auscultation in various positions Use of Valsalva and respiratory maneuvers Following radiation of murmurs	Palpation of spleen in right lateral decubitus Palpation of prostate, ovaries, and kidneys Measurement of liver size by percussion Pelvic and rectal examination	Testing olfaction Hearing Corneal reflex Sensation Calorics
Detection	Thyroid nodules Tracheal deviation Bruits Oral ulcers Scleral icterus Breath odors	Decreased expansion of chest Palpation of crepitus from rib fracture Decreased breath sounds Bronchial breathing Cardiac dullness Mitral diastolic murmurs, grade 1 aortic diastolic murmurs, S_3, S_4, grade 1 systolic numbers Fine rales	Minimal splenomegaly Palpation of enlarged kidney, gallbladder, and accurate identification Small hernias and prostatic nodules Aortic aneurysms 3- to 5-cm masses	Organic mental syndromes Aphasias Mild paresis Conjugate and disconjugate occular defects
Interpretation	Tracheal deviation Jugular pressure Skin turgor Venous pulses	Bronchial breathing Systolic murmurs Use of ancillary signs such as fremitus or whispered voice	Abdominal tenderness Transmitted pulsation versus aneurysm in the epigastrium Masses, intraabdominal wall versus abdominal wall Venous flow patterns Liver size	Eye signs Patterns of sensory loss or weakness Reflex differences between sides

we observe and, thus, generate new information. Our examination of a certain part of the body, for example, the ears, may stimulate the patient to remember an ear pain or ear infection he or she had not discussed when asked about past illness. Likewise, we have an opportunity to ask about old surgical or traumatic scars. We can inquire further about specific limitations caused by pain or weakness during the musculoskeletal examination of persons who have joint or muscle complaints.

Finally, the physical examination itself has a therapeutic role. Simply touching the patient—the "laying on of hands"—may cause him or her to feel better and be reassured. Tactile communication opens up a channel of interpersonal response that can be very important in healing. In particular, specific attention to the painful areas of the body demonstrates that you have listened, understood, and are concerned about the patient's suffering.

Your systematic touching of the patient, however, does present certain risks. Such contact is a violation of taboos in our society outside the realm of intimacy. You have a privileged role that is charged with meaning for the patient. The patient is ill and vulnerable; you are powerful. In a sense, the patient sees you as holding the keys to health or illness. You may be viewed as the messenger who carries bad news or good news, the seer who understands secrets of the body, or the conduit of power over illness. This charged relationship leads to several risks in doing the physical examination:

1. Inadequate preparation without appropriate attention to the patient's comfort and modesty may result in feelings of exposure or violation for the patient.
2. Appearing to neglect the patient's major concern while exploring physical findings in another area (such as examining the ear of a patient who comes in with a stomach complaint) may lead to feelings of being ignored or misunderstood.
3. Instilling fear or anxiety when a certain area of the physical examination is emphasized (such as prolonged listening to the heart) may lead the patient to believe something may be drastically wrong.

All of these dangers can be minimized by adequate preparation and explanation to the patient.

TOUCHING

We referred earlier to the fact that performing a physical examination actually has therapeutic value in itself. Patients very commonly will not be quite satisfied until you have examined them—perhaps only taking their blood pressure and listening to their heart—even when they return to your office for a follow-up visit during which no examination is medically necessary. There are two components to the therapeutic value of examination, one arising from cultural expectations about what a doctor in our society does, and the other arising from the more elemental fact of touching itself.

You often have patients who say, "My stomach has felt terrible for weeks, but this morning, just as I was coming in to see the doctor, it's not hurting anymore. . ." This phenomenon of the tooth feeling better on the expectation of seeing a dentist or the pain disappearing just prior to a visit with the doctor is part of the symbolic healing dimension that permeates all patient care situations. Another aspect of this dimension is the therapeutic value of diagnostic tests. Some patients will find that their back pain improves after being assured that their lumbosacral spine x-ray results are normal. Other patients sometimes overtly confuse diagnostic studies with therapeutic procedures, for example, "I've felt good ever since I had that x-ray."

Everyone knows that doctors do physical examinations and can "read" the clues that they find. The physical examination is part of the *therapeutic context* of medicine in our culture. Therefore, it can have a strong symbolic effect that may contribute to healing but that also may cause iatrogenic, i.e., from the doctor, suffering. For example, the doctor who lingers a long while over a cardiac auscultation, announces gravely that the patient has a heart murmur, and then tells the patient that he or she had better see a cardiologist has caused some unnecessary anxiety. This may in some cases be inevitable, but it can always be minimized by a full, empathic explanation to the patient.

The laying on of hands aspect has always been an important component of healing. Healing by touch was once thought to be a divine attribute of kings. Most traditional forms of medicine involve some component of touch in their armamentarium. The contemporary holistic health movement has spawned many forms of therapy that rely on touch, methods ranging from reflexology to the school of therapeutic touch. Some observers believe that a major factor in chiropractic's appeal and success has to do with the physical contact involved in the chiropractic examination and spinal adjustment.[26]

We cannot speculate here on the full meaning of touch, but it clearly has great psychologic benefit if used appropriately. Whether, or by what means, this translates into physiologic benefit is unknown. Certainly, we cannot equate all touch: A cursory auscultation of the heart is far different from a detailed, careful musculoskeletal examination. Touch that arises because you and the patient are "connecting" and you feel you need to reach out (as when you put your hand over the hand of a crying patient) may well have far different therapeutic value than the touch involved in routine diagnostic procedures.

Our goal here is to emphasize the potential value of touch and to point out that, in general, you should not shy away from physical contact with your patient. You should see it for its symbolic value, even when you believe it will have no diagnostic value. The physician who pays special attention to touching each patient as he or she makes hospital rounds will likely find that this brief physical contact will help establish better understanding and more empathic communication. This kind of touching may be as simple as putting a hand on the patient's shoulder as you speak with him or her, listening to a heartbeat even though the monitor is on and there is almost no "practical" reason for doing so, or stopping for a moment and placing your hand on the patient's hand as you make a routine inquiry. Doctors who do this find that their patients perceive that their physician spends considerably more time with them and explains things much better. This occurs even though these physicians spend exactly the same amount of *clock time* and explain things in exactly the same way as other physicians who never make an effort to touch their patients unless it is necessary for a diagnostic procedure.

ENDING THE INTERVIEW

This section could be subtitled "How to get out of the room without leaving a lot of loose ends and with a good feeling on your part and that of the patient." You have completed the physical examination, and now, in a sense, you "reconvene" the interview in order to terminate it. The goal of a good closure is no different from the goal of your entire interview and will be easier to attain if the patient understands from the outset the purpose of the interaction and who you are. The purpose of the interaction will vary, depending on whether you are a student in a physical diagnosis course with a one-time "shot" at the patient, a clinical clerk with major responsibility for communicating with the patient, or the resident or attending physician with a long-term role in the patient's management. Overall, the patient (and you) should expect nothing more than to feel understood and not be abused in any way. In history taking, this means that you have gotten the story straight and that the patient has not been forced to expose himself or herself either personally or physically without your appropriate concern for his or her comfort, privacy, and modesty. The techniques of being accurate, empathic, respectful, and genuine apply to this part of the encounter as they do to all the other parts.

It is always a good idea to give the patient the opportunity to have the last word:

- "Anything else?"
- "Do you feel there is anything about what you have told me that I have not understood?"
- "Is there anything else you'd like to tell me or ask me?"

As in all other aspects of clinical examination, what you do to close the encounter depends on:

1. Who you are—your status, how much responsibility you have in the care of the patient, as well as your own style;
2. Who the patient is—his or her expectations and needs (emotional and physical); and
3. What the illness is—simple versus complicated, mild versus severe, benign versus malignant, acute versus chronic, and curable versus terminal.

In your role as a student learning about medical interviewing or taking a physical diagnosis course, when you close any encounter with a patient you should:

1. Provide a summary of what the patient has told you.

2. Be sure to let the patient have the last word or ask any additional questions.
3. Give a pleasant thank you and goodbye.

This is fine with most patients, especially if you have been careful all along to clarify your role. If a patient asks a question you cannot answer about the disease or about his or her medical care, you should say something like "I am not able to answer that, but it is a good question to ask your doctor." This is a truthful answer whether the reason that you are unable to answer is that you do not know or you do know, but the question is more properly answered by the patient's physician.

Once you have responsibility for a patient's care, the more typical closure implies a contract between you and the patient. It acknowledges responsibility for solving problems and providing care. In this general context, ending a patient encounter, whether it be a complete history and physical or a short office visit, should include these actions on the part of the physician:

1. **Share findings:** By this we usually mean the physical findings and your diagnosis, differential diagnosis, or hypotheses. As a student, you are unable to share much, as you are often unsure about your findings or diagnosis. When you become a physician, the question is always *what* to share. What you share depends on the one hand on the patient—how sick he or she is, how knowledgeable, and whether or not he or she has other sources of information. What you share also depends on the illness; some findings are pertinent to the illness, while others are incidental or may be trivial. Avoid discussing what is interesting to you but may be irrelevant to the patient.

2. **Devise a problem list with priorities:** This is painstaking and difficult at first but becomes easier with experience. How you do it is not the subject of this book, but it is important to realize that the doctor's priorities often differ from those of the patient. Patients may be interested first in feeling better, second in their overall prognosis, and third in the specific diagnosis. Clinicians do share these same concerns but often (especially while in medical school or in training) are more interested in making

the diagnosis than in treating the symptoms. Treating the symptom is often not the same as treating the disease. Many trivial illnesses (e.g., simple upper respiratory tract infections) do not in themselves need specific medications but have symptoms that patients want treated. On the other hand, many significant illnesses (e.g., hypertension) have no symptoms but demand, from the doctor's point of view, specific therapy.

3. **Agree on a plan of action and clarify responsibilities:** Determine what will happen next and who will do what. The physician may agree to order and interpret tests, talk with consultants, write prescriptions, or do procedures or an additional history and physical. The patient may agree to take the medication, modify diet, keep the following appointment, or report further symptoms. Responsibilities are often blurred, especially in the patient who says, "I'm in your hands, Doc." Ideally, medical care is a partnership in which you negotiate an agreement or contract with the patient, but the character of that contract depends on the patient's illness (emergency care versus chronic antihypertensive therapy) and on the patient's acceptance of responsibility (see the discussion about negotiation, Chap. 14).

4. **Educate the patient:** The physician should tell the patient as much as the physician knows about the problem, within the limits of what the patient wants to know and can accept and understand. This is easier to say than to do and is not a one-shot thing. Rather it is a process over time as the physician learns about the patient and his or her problems. It is different for each physician, each patient, and each illness.

To conclude this chapter, here is an example of the closing minutes of an office visit (the patient suffers from back pain):

Dr: I don't find anything on my exam. I don't find anything that makes me think you have a pinched nerve. I think periodically you may be getting some nerve irritation and that's accounting for the pain that's shooting down your legs. What I think we should do, I want to check your x-rays that you had. I want to review those. I think we should prescribe bed rest for a while and just get you off of your feet. At least for a short time. Maybe 3, 4, or 5 days. Is that, are you able to do that?

Pt: Yeah.

Dr: You don't live by yourself?

Pt: No. I live with my daughter.

Dr: Okay, fine. I'm going to give you a couple of different medicines. I'll refill the Darvocets, but I only want you to use that as needed. I'm going to give you another medicine called Motrin. Are you able to take aspirin?

Pt: Yes.

Dr: So, I'm going to give you Motrin, which is an anti-inflammatory medicine. I don't want you to expect any overnight relief from the Motrin, because it takes several days, sometimes up to a week. So I'm going to give you the Motrin, Darvocet, and I'll give you a prescription for something called Pericolace, which is a very mild laxative and stool softener to make sure while you're . . . while you're down in bed rest that you don't get constipated. Do you have a heating pad at home?

Pt: Yeah, I have a moist heating pad.

Dr: Wonderful. You can use that every hour if you like, but I don't want you using it for more than 20 minutes at a time. But you can use it up to 20 minutes out of every hour. All right? So, I want you to stay in bed. Well I actually would like you to stay in bed for a week. I want to see you next week, preferably on Friday.

Pt: What about my physical therapy?

Dr: I want to lay off that. I think physical therapy is very, very important in the treatment of backache, but I think you never had a good trial of bed rest.

Pt: No, because I was going to physical therapy.

Dr: The only time I want you up is to go to the bathroom, and I really don't want you sitting up in bed. Do you have a firm mattress?

Pt: Well, I haven't been able to get in bed since October.

Dr: Well, that's where I want you.

Pt: I have like a loveseat pullout bed and it's low to the floor so I, my legs . . .

Dr: Well, then you need to get a board or something and put it under that sleeper.

Pt: It's like a board.

Dr: Okay, if it's very hard and firm that's good.

Pt: Okay, it's like that.

Dr: It doesn't sag anywhere . . .?

Pt: No, it's straight, and it's real low to the floor.

Dr: Fine. That's where I want you then, other than going to the bathroom and eating your meals, flat on your back. Okay?

Pt: Now will you explain to me again what the Motrin is?

Dr: Motrin is an anti-inflammatory drug. It's an arthritic drug.

Pt: In other words, it's supposed to help the pain in the back?

Dr: A lot of the pain in back injuries is due to irritation of the tissues and this will quiet down that irritation of the tissues, that in conjunction with, first of all, the rest. I didn't feel too much muscle spasm in your back now.

Pt: Well, that has quieted down some. I had quite a bit in October. It sort of quit, but I still have the pain.

Dr: There's your prescriptions, here's the Darvocets, only take that as needed for extra pain. The Motrin I want you to take one, four times per day; breakfast, lunch, dinner, bedtime, and you should take that continuously . . . I want to see you next week, preferably on Friday, that will give us a full week. Okay? And we will see in a week, see how you are doing and, as I said, in the meantime, I'll review the x-rays. Okay? Anything else?

Pt: I wanted to mention to you. I had gone for a Pap smear and they said the Pap smear was normal, I mean I don't have cancer . . .

Notice how the physician shares the findings and clarifies the plan of action, including what the physician will do and expects the patient to do. Note, too, how the patient at the last minute brings up her concern about cancer possibly being the cause of her pain. The physician can now offer her appropriate reassurance that the etiology of her pain is not cancer; moreover, the physician will know that the patient's fear of cancer may reappear if the pain does not improve. It is not at all unusual for critical information like this to surface at the close of the interview when the patient feels comfortable and can see that he or she is being listened to. It is vital, therefore, that you demonstrate your open-ended attitude even as you close the encounter, as this physician did with the remark "Okay? Anything else?"

CHAPTER 7

Recording the Medical History: Creating a Text

> The point of all this is that medical histories are created, not found. Furthermore, whatever we physicians compose and record as history is not "reality" in any global sense, but one version of reality, one that we choose to construct.
>
> William J. Donnelly, *Righting the medical record. Transforming chronicle into story, JAMA* 1988;260:823–825

After you have interviewed and examined your patient, you walk away, perhaps carrying pages of cryptic and chaotic notes. You have the story firmly, or perhaps, not so firmly, in your head, as well as a few inklings of a differential diagnosis. The most important part of your patient's work up is actually complete at this point, but before progressing further, you must put together the story on paper. Your next job is the "write-up." From the morass of your patient's symptoms and experiences, how do you do this? What do you write down? What do you choose to include in the permanent medical record?

Since this text is limited to the skills of patient interviewing and does not deal with physical diagnosis or diagnostic workup, in this chapter we consider how to record the patient's medical history. We present, in some detail, how to conceptualize, format, and write that history. However, the medical record is, in fact, a literary genre with its own objectives and standards of practice. In this genre, a patient history does not normally stand alone. Its proper format also includes physical and laboratory data, an assessment or formulation (e.g., what the doctor's hypotheses are), and a plan for diagnosis and/or therapy, not to mention subsequent entries like flow sheets and progress notes. Consequently, to give a more complete picture of the medical record, we also present some guidelines for the other, nonhistory elements of your write-up.

This chapter consists of four major sections. In the first, we consider a few basic concepts about medical recording. What is the purpose of a medical record? Whose story is it, the doctor's or the patient's? The second section presents a basic outline for constructing the written history and physical examination. We consider next the problem-oriented method of medical record keeping, commenting on some of its advantages and disadvantages. The final section is in two parts. The first part is a complete transcription (with annotation) of a medical interview as you might hear it, were you sitting in with the doctor and patient. This is followed by a sample write-up based on the transcribed interview and a subsequent physical examination.

WHAT GOES INTO THE WRITTEN HISTORY

Just the Facts?

Recording the history is not a question of "just the facts, ma'am." It is the end product, if you will, of a long process of selection, interpretation, and editing. What you write on paper is a result of at least four levels of selection and interpretation.

- The *first* level is the patient's experience, that is, the "facts" as they actually happened and what it was really like to experience the headache or dizziness.
- The *second* level is the patient's conceptualization of the experience, that is, how the patient put together the facts to make a story that provides some coherence and meaning to the experience. The patient started to construct this story before your interview, but your questions and selective attention helped create the current version.
- A *third* level is the "clinical tale," the story you generate by means of the medical interview. Because you speak a medical language and live in a medical culture, you are able to reconstruct the patient's story so that it has some new characters (e.g., groupings of symptoms) and a somewhat different plot development.

- *Finally,* you select some of this story to record in the chart. To do this, you must apply certain canons of literary form. There are rules and guidelines appropriate to the patient write-up just as there are rules and guidelines appropriate to other types of writing, such as the short story or the nonfiction essay.

When we call the final product the medical history, it is easy to forget the interpretive and selective process that goes into producing it. The doctor is not simply a passive secretary or scribe. It is both inefficient and virtually impossible to repeat everything the patient says. Nor is the doctor simply a reader presented with a clear-cut, unambiguous text. However, it is useful to use the metaphor "interpreting a text" to describe diagnosis and problem solving in the doctor-patient interaction. In recent years, several medical thinkers have emphasized this interpretive or hermeneutic function of medical practice. This serves to highlight important features of medical practice that are obscured when we think of medicine as "hard" science (another metaphor!) and diagnosis as an exercise in logic or decision analysis. Gogel and Terry,[50] for example, suggest that, among the metaphors we commonly use in clinical medicine (like **medicine is war** or **the body is a machine**), we should also include **the doctor is a literary critic** and **the patient is a complicated text.**

What does this mean? What seems at first glance to be "just the facts" is actually an interpretation of the facts. You are interpreting the patient's story much as a literary critic interprets a text. The quality of your interpretation depends on your skill and experience as well as the text's underlying "readability." The context in which you see a patient or read a sentence can be a major determinant in your interpretation. No single interpretation of a book or of a patient's illness is final; there should be continuous re-evaluation. In medicine as in literary criticism, a "true" interpretation is validated through open discourse among peers and consultants.

Another helpful metaphor is **the doctor is an editor.** The doctor uses conventions and rules to create a case history out of the sprawling "first draft" presented by the patient. Form follows function. These rules ensure that the functions of the medical record are accomplished efficiently and effectively. But what are the functions? What is the purpose of a permanent medical record?

FUNCTIONS OF THE MEDICAL RECORD

1. **Memory aid.** Originally the medical record served only as a stimulus to jog a clinician's memory. Doctors kept brief notes on little cards. The complete information, though, was not on the card but in the physician's mind. That is where clinical understanding and integration took place. Even though today we have complete and well-organized (and sometimes computerized) written records, the doctor's mind, not the medical chart, is still where the patient's "complete" database is kept. We remember many details about our patients' lives and experiences that we do not write down; and we think many thoughts that we dare not write down.

2. **Communication.** The medical record, while a memory aid, also serves to communicate with other health professionals. In the modern hospital or clinic setting, health care is a team activity. Perhaps 20 or 30 people have legitimate access to an inpatient chart. Most of them will want to communicate their findings and their treatments to other members of the team. This communicative function leads to certain conventions regarding which observations are important to record and the form in which they ought to be recorded. The need to communicate also raises important questions about confidentiality. There is, after all, information about your patient that might be helpful to you as the physician but which need not or should not be communicated to others, even if they are also on the patient's health care team.

3. **Evaluation and research.** Thirdly, medical write-ups are used in evaluation. An attending physician evaluates his or her students and residents, at least in part, on the basis of their patient records, and hospital quality assurance and utilization review committees monitor the performance of physicians by reviewing their charts. The medical record also serves as a data source for clinical research. Retrospective chart reviews still serve as the

backbone of clinical epidemiology, even though variations in available data, recording styles, and legibility present great methodologic problems.

4. **Legal and administrative document.** Finally, the record serves a legal and administrative function. It is a written document that can be used as evidence in court. Various quality control and cost-containment strategies require that charts be reviewed and decisions be made partly on the basis of recorded data. Third-party insurers also use the chart to verify diagnosis and to establish that certain services were provided.

FORMAT OF THE WRITTEN HISTORY

Table 7–1 presents elements usually contained in a medical write-up. Although there is broad consensus on these major features, detailed conventions about the way they are put together vary from hospital to hospital. Some hospitals have specific forms to use, at least for the more "objective" parts of the write-up, such as problem lists and physical examination. The following discussion is a relatively generic one into which most hospital-specific formats should fit.

Identifying Data and Chief Complaint

The write-up begins with a succinct statement that identifies the patient and tells why he or she is seeking medical help. Often

TABLE 7–1. Elements of the Medical Case Description

Identifying data and chief complaint
Present illness
Other continuing (or active) medical problems
Past medical history
Family history
Social history and patient profile
Review of systems
Physical examination
Laboratory data
Assessment (impressions and differential diagnosis)
Plan

the patient's chief complaint, stated in the patient's own words, is the most effective descriptive statement to use. For example:

> Mr. Steven Maringo is a 47-year-old construction worker who came in because "I've had a sore throat for a month and it won't go away."

> Ms. Alice York is a 41-year-old chemist at Alcoa, with a history of "ulcers," who came in now because "I've had a burning pain under my ribs all week."

> Beth Salisbury is a 10-year-old fourth grader who came in because "my ear hurts" since yesterday.

> Mr. Fred Jones is a 32-year-old computer programmer referred by Dr. A. Zinger for evaluation of a persistent "washed out" feeling and lower extremity weakness.

When a patient has been referred, as in the last example, it is important to record that fact. The patient may not have a chief complaint as such; the patient may be coming for a routine checkup or for a driver's license examination. Whatever the reason, it should be recorded in the patient's own words.

Other particularly relevant data also may be included in the introductory statement. For example, "Mr. Fred Jones is a 32-year-old, black, unmarried, computer programmer who works at Ibex Industries . . ." However, one should not try to pack this sentence with too many identifying features. Is the fact that Jones is unmarried or black relevant to his persistent "washed out" feeling? Perhaps so. But a thousand other features might be relevant as well. While it is best to strive for simplicity here, many hospitals have their own conventions about how to begin the write-up. Some, for example, might insist that all patients be identified by race and occupation, in addition to age and sex, no matter what their medical problems are.

Present Illness

This section should reflect your interpretation and organization of the patient's story. While the diagnoses may be in doubt, you should have a good grasp of the patient's problem(s), and organize the present illness description accordingly. The description should be succinct, with emphasis on:

1. Time course;
2. Symptom characteristics (see Chap. 2); and
3. Functional deficits.

Use the patient's own words and "voice" when possible, but remember that you are the author here. If the patient rambles or has 13 different complaints, that is no reason for you to ramble or to produce an over-long Present Illness section. Your organization and choice of material here should reflect your thinking about how the symptoms fit together, not the patient's.

For example, consider the transcription of an opening statement presented in Chapter 3. The written Present Illness section might begin thus:

> Mrs. P has been feeling "tired" and "worn out" even when she gets as much as 11 hours' sleep. Sleep is interrupted by "hot flashes," although these are less frequent than previously.

The writer may choose to put the patient's concerns about nervousness and loss of libido under the other Active Problems section (see below) or may include them in the Present Illness section if they are believed to be part of the same problem (a depressive disorder, for example).

You will frequently encounter patients who have had multiple hospital admissions, and who have records that are quite complete—perhaps someone with ischemic cardiomyopathy and obstructive pulmonary disease who is well known to your hospital's emergency room or a patient with metastatic breast cancer, admitted frequently for courses of chemotherapy. It is tempting to construct the "present history" of such a patient from old chart data, with little input from the patient herself. For example:

> Mrs. Ely was first found to have carcinoma of the breast in May 1985, after which she underwent a left simple mastectomy, followed by a course of local irradiation. In June 1986 she was noted to have bone mets in T4 and L1 . . . (a series of medical interven-

tions) . . . and today (in November 1989) is admitted to be evaluated for chemotherapy.

This is not a history of an illness; it is a chronicle of medical events. Does the patient currently have symptoms? Why is chemotherapy being considered at this point in time, rather than last year or next month? The patient's voice is absent. Medical records can provide supplemental information that sheds light on the current problem, but it is never appropriate to construct a narrative based on data from old records and call it "present illness." If the patient cannot speak coherently and if there is no other informant, then the writer does not complete the Present Illness section. In all other situations, this section is primarily the patient's story, not gleanings from an old medical chart.

Other Continuing (or Active) Medical Problems

It is useful to consider this a separate section, although sometimes it may form an integrated text with the Present Illness section. Patients often have complex and chronic medical problems. A given episode of illness may well be an exacerbation of a chronic problem or interact with another ongoing disease. Because of this, it is important to select continuing problems from the Past Medical History and to provide details about their current status. In the example above, if Mrs. Ely was admitted for symptoms of pneumonia, her history of chemotherapy would certainly be relevant, and it should be recorded thoroughly in this part of the text.

Past Medical History

This section begins the more standardized or routine part of the write-up. By definition, it includes only those problems not directly (or obviously) relevant to the illness at hand. The format, as described in Chapter 4, should be as follows:

- Serious illnesses, from childhood to the present, including hospitalizations;
- Surgical procedures;

- Accidents and injuries;
- Pregnancies, deliveries, and complications;
- Allergies, including type and known allergens;
- Current medications, including over-the-counter drugs, giving specific dosages and schedule (these may also be listed under Other Continuing or Active Medical Problems); and
- Health maintenance data, including immunizations and screening tests.

Family History

The family history is best presented in a genogram that shows relationships in a diagrammatic form (Fig. 7–1). Squares represent males, circles females. A diagonal line or "X" indicates that the person has died. Diseases may be indicated above or below the symbols. Alternatively, the family history can be presented in tabular form. This method is more efficient if the patient does not have much medical information about his or her family. Relationships can be indicated by abbreviations, for example, MGM for maternal grandmother, PGF for paternal grandfather, and so forth. Such a family history can look like:

MGM (d. age 60s), unknown cause

MGF (d. age 70), heart attack

PGF (92), arthritis, forgetful

Social History and Patient Profile

The object of the "social history" is to give a picture of the patient as a functioning person and to record medically related, and health-related, behavior. The harried physician should avoid leaving the person out entirely and recording only whether the patient smokes tobacco or drinks alcohol. On the other hand, the writer should avoid becoming too discursive and/or personal. Some considerations about how much personal data to include are presented in the next section. Approach writing the Patient Profile with a standard outline in mind, similar to the outline

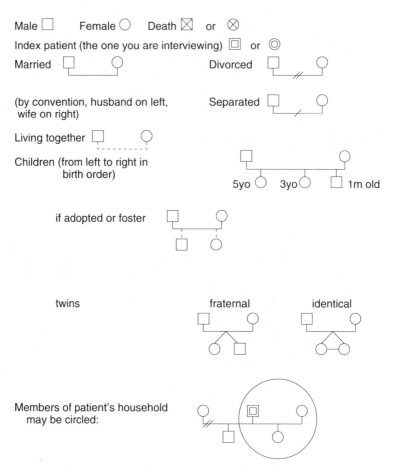

FIGURE 7–1. The genogram. If you are required to draw a genogram—essentially, a diagram of the patient's family tree—here are the basics. Such a diagram may work for you as a convenient shorthand to lay out the essentials of the family history. The symbols used are indicated above.

used during your interview, even though, in a given case, you need not necessarily write something for each item.

- Brief biography (e.g., place of birth, education, military service, and years in this locality);
- Current marital, family, and home situation;
- Occupation and occupational history, including toxic exposures and stresses;
- Lifestyle (e.g., religious affiliation, personal interests, hobbies, travel, and exercise);

- Diet and nutrition;
- Personal habits (e.g., use of tobacco, alcohol, and addictive "recreational" drugs);
- A typical day's activities (which may be placed under Present Illness when a change in functional status is an important descriptor of the illness); and
- Relevant feelings and beliefs (e.g., work satisfaction, perceived stresses, beliefs about the illness, and attitudes toward health care)

Review of Systems

Data obtained in the Review of Systems (ROS) section of the interview may be:

1. Incorporated into the written Present Illness if it is relevant to the current problem(s);
2. Placed in a structured system-by-system ROS section; or
3. Simply left unwritten.

Beginners should write a fairly comprehensive ROS to develop the discipline of thinking about each system in turn (see the case write-up at the end of this chapter). More experienced clinicians will usually write a few positive findings and pertinent negative findings. They will then indicate that the rest of the ROS was "unremarkable" or "negative."

Physical Examination

The "write-up" in Chapter 7 uses a fairly standard format for organizing the data. You begin with a statement about the patient's general appearance and continue with vital signs (respirations, blood pressure, pulse, and temperature) and the results of the examination of skin, head, eyes, ears, nose, throat, neck, lymphatic system, chest, back, breasts, heart, abdomen, rectum, genitourinary system, extremities, musculoskeletal system, nervous system, and, finally, mental status. While mental status data are generally collected by talking as opposed to touching, they should be recorded as a separate system toward the end of the physical examination.

Laboratory Work

Results of diagnostic studies may be included as part of the initial write-up if they are "routine" or are available shortly after your interview and physical examination. In such cases, the results are part of the database on which your assessment and plan are based. There is no standard method of recording laboratory or x-ray findings. Perhaps the most efficient and efficacious way is to use the appropriate flow sheets and not place this data in the midst of written text. Nevertheless, it can be useful to have a "snapshot" of basic studies (complete blood count and differential, urinalysis, serum chemistries, chest x-ray, or electrocardiogram) in the database to help buttress your initial assessment. Each institution has its own recommended set of routine laboratory work for new patients or for patients admitted to the hospital. However, in recent years the emphasis has been on rationally choosing diagnostic studies to test hypotheses rather than on using an "optimal" routine set of studies.

Assessment and Plan

The best way of organizing your assessment and plan is to use principles derived from the problem-oriented medical record system described below.

RECORDING PERSONAL INFORMATION

Some medical writers believe that, because of its many functions, the medical record has become distorted, a source of misinformation rather than information.[20] They point out that errors (e.g., mistakes in clinical judgment and laboratory errors) tend to be perpetuated when so much emphasis is placed on the written word. A wrong diagnosis, once written, is difficult to eradicate. Other writers urge that we attempt to transform the medical record from a "chronicle" full of organ and biochemical data to a true "clinical tale" or story by injecting the personal dimension.[36] Of course, because the record is accessible to many people in clinics or hospitals, we are at risk of compromising confidentiality by recording personal data.

What personal data should or should not be recorded? Here

are some guidelines that attempt to steer between the Scylla of biochemistry and the Charybdis of disrespect and sentimentality.

1. Important data about the patient's attitude, style, expectations, and/or health belief system should in some way be indicated in the record. While it is always useful to have this sort of knowledge about the patient, it is not always important to write it down. Unless a patient's histrionic or dependent style is out of the ordinary range, privacy and efficiency dictate silence. But if you need to communicate a patient's style to others, because it plays a significant role in how you interpret the story or in your approach to therapy, then it should be written. The same is true about the person's idiosyncratic beliefs.

2. There are certain personal data that should rarely be placed in a permanent medical record, even though they may be important to the patient's care. These include, for example, explicit description of sexual habits, embarrassing personal idiosyncrasies, or a criminal record. One also should be cautious about recording suicide attempts and hospitalizations for mental illness. These will be discussed further in the section on confidentiality (see Chap. 15).

3. The person can enter the record through the use of his or her voice. Include the patient's own words whenever possible, not just in the chief complaint. It is often particularly useful to include similes or metaphors that the patient uses to describe his or her experience. For example, recording that the patient describes the headache as "a deep pain like someone is twisting a screwdriver inside my brain," tells a lot about the patient and is less judgmental than writing "patient describes the headache in a bizarre fashion."

4. Distortion can be minimized by avoiding language that "pathologizes." As Donnelly[35] points out, in medicine we preferentially use words that turn people, experiences, or feelings into "pathologies." The plain language of human experience does not seem "medical" enough for us. We like to use "depressed" rather than "sad," and rarely do we describe patients as "discouraged" or "courageous." To make the record more personally

descriptive, avoid words like: apathy, anxiety, denial, depression, and manipulative. Try instead to use words like: determined, discouraged, hopeful, optimistic, brave, fearful, sad, or hopeless.

5. Much personal information can be packed into behavioral or functional descriptions. By simply describing how the patient spends his or her day, what his or her hobbies are, or what he or she does on weekends, you can sketch important features of the person without getting too "personal." These statements fit well into the medical record. The operative principle is to be descriptive, not judgmental.

PROBLEM-ORIENTED RECORDS

In 1970, Lawrence Weed[106] introduced the problem-oriented medical record (POMR), and this approach found widespread acceptance during the next decade. The main elements of the POMR system are:

- A *database* that includes the written history, physical examination, and laboratory data.
- A *problem list* that displays the names of identified "problems," not simply medical diagnoses. This list includes both current and inactive problems, and is updated regularly.
- A *standard format* for writing about each problem in one's own formulation or in daily progress notes. The format requires that a note be divided into four sections:

   A. Subjective, recounting symptom or personal data.
   B. Objective, dealing with physical signs or laboratory data.
   C. Assessment, expressing the clinician's analysis of the problem.
   D. Plan, stating the measures to be taken. Hence, the acronym *SOAP* notes or **SOAP** format.

- *Devices* such as flow sheets to simplify, organize, and display data.

One main thrust of the problem-oriented system was to humanize medical care by focusing attention on medical problems rather than solely on medical diagnoses. For example, symptoms like "abdominal pain" or "swollen elbow" are perfectly appropriate to list as problems in an initial evaluation. Subsequently, the patient might be found to suffer from splenic flexure syndrome, which would then explain the abdominal pain and replace the annotation "abdominal pain" on the problem list. Alternatively, the patient might be found to have inflammatory bowel disease with an associated arthritis. This diagnosis could explain two problems, abdominal discomfort and swelling of the elbow. Frequently, however, the doctor might find no ready diagnostic explanation. No diagnosis is made. Yet abdominal pain is still a problem.

In Weed's formulation, problems also could be personal, social, financial, or functional difficulties, not just somatic symptoms or medical disorders. Poor vision, unemployment, marital discord, and cigarette smoking are all separate problems, some of which may be amenable to the traditional method of differential diagnosis and some of which may not be. Since a separate SOAP note had to be written for each problem, the Weed system forced the physician to address each problem on a regular basis and not let some of them fall by the wayside. Moreover, the overall organization minimized the possibility that information would slip through the cracks and get lost. Separating "subjective" from "objective" data also was intended to humanize clinical practice by forcing physicians to take subjective data seriously. Subjective data had to be considered, written in the note, and presumably used in making one's assessment.

Twenty years later, it appears that Weed's contribution is more in his philosophy of medical recording and in the broad outline of his approach rather than in POMR's specific details. Some of these concepts are widely used, but the full POMR is rarely found. Unfortunately, even when POMR concepts are used, clinicians tend to distort them, so they no longer serve to humanize care (even if they do help in organization and jogging the memory).

The difficulties with POMR are both structural and cultural. The structural concern is that the system is cumbersome. Modern hospital patients often have six or eight active problems. It is difficult and time and space consuming to write a daily SOAP note on each one. Medical outpatients may have an equal number of problems, and there is even less time for charting in the clinic setting. The cultural problem is that, given our disease-oriented medical culture, we tend to restrict problems to medical diagnoses, thus losing the system's main advantage. Students and interns may write elaborate SOAP notes on "diabetes," but they rarely indicate that "marital discord" is an active problem, and they almost certainly never SOAP it. Moreover, the subjective category, rather than emphasizing the critical importance of patient reports as it was intended to do, plays second fiddle to the objective category. We seem to treat subjective data as less scientific—and, therefore, less worthy—than objective data. Often problems are discussed in SOAP notes with no entry under "subjective" at all.

We subscribe to the Weed philosophy and believe that medical write-ups and records should include at least these features:

- The clinician should develop a well-rounded database on each patient. The database should include a patient narrative that reflects the patient's personality. It may be written over a period of time, however, and need not (should not) be a one-shot database.
- The clinician should think in broad human terms when identifying problems and include the types of situations and disabilities that Weed originally intended. This means that a symptom or a situation that constitutes a problem for the patient should be listed, even if we cannot comfortably fit it into a diagnosis.
- The clinician should keep a complete, frequently revised problem list on each patient.
- The clinician should respect subjective data and use them regularly in writing progress notes. The term "person-oriented" data is perhaps more appropriate than "subjective" because so much of our objective data today is heavily encrusted with interpretation and is, therefore, also in a sense subjective (cf. "Interpretation versus Observation" in Chap. 1).
- The clinician should use flow sheets and other devices in the record to jog his or her memory and to enhance patient care.

CASE EXAMPLE

The following example presents a transcription of an actual diagnostic medical interview, and a write-up of the same patient as recorded in the medical chart. The patient came to the clinic for a general checkup and was seen by a medical intern. The typescript is slightly altered to protect the patient's privacy. This particular interview is not presented as an ideal or exhaustive medical history but simply as a good example of a careful and empathic doctor-patient encounter. We have provided at various points in the text some comments that identify specific skills the doctor used at that juncture. In the write-up, we have suggested (in brackets) additional data that perhaps should have been obtained but were not. As you read through the interview and write-up, think about both content and process (skills). What are the good features? Not-so-good features? How is the interview incomplete? How could you have done it better?

The Interview

Typescript	Comments
Dr: I guess the best place to start is to ask you what brings you here today.	Opening.
Pt: Well, I haven't had a physical really since 5 years ago, since my son was born.	
Dr: I am going to be writing some things down on paper here, okay? Is there any particular reason why you chose now to come in?	Acknowledges note taking. Open-ended question. Probe for iatrotropic stimulus.
Pt: I figured I kept putting it off and putting it off. I'd make appointments and put them off. There was no particular reason. I just felt as though it was time, I suppose.	
Dr: Nothing is bothering you at this point?	
Pt: No, it's just that I am overweight, that's all. I go up and down, up and down.	
Dr: So that was your major concern, the weight problem?	Summary statement. Interchangeable response.
Pt: Yeah.	
Dr: Can you tell me about that?	Open-ended question.
Pt: Well, I've always been big. All the women in my family are big. It's never slowed me down or anything, but I would like to just like firm up, maybe my thighs and my stomach. From after having children I don't know, they say everything takes time, you don't put it on right away, but I guess I'm impatient.	
Dr: How much do you weigh right now?	The doctor inquires in detail about the symptom—what,

Typescript	Comments
	how much, when, or why?— developing accuracy and precision.
Pt: I don't basically know. Last time I weighed myself I weighed 200 pounds and that was like about 2 months ago.	
Dr: Say a year ago, what did you weigh?	
Pt: A year ago I weighed about 230 pounds.	
Dr: 230 pounds? So you have actually lost 30 pounds between then and now?	The doctor checks back with patient, confirming data.
Pt: Yes.	
Dr: Have you been on a diet?	
Pt: No.	
Dr: How have you lost the weight?	
Pt: I don't know. In the last, I'd say the last 6 months or so to a year, I've been getting to the point I'd go all day without eating. I'm real active. I'm very active.	
Dr: Can you tell me about the activity?	Open-ended question with topic specified.
Pt: Well, I do a lot of tennis. I have dance class. It seems like I don't want to stop to fix nothing when I'm working in the house. I won't stop to fix nothing to eat. I'll just keep on going.	
Dr: Is that a conscious effort on your part, to try to lose weight?	
Pt: I don't know if it's subconscious or conscious. I really never sat down and thought about it.	
Dr: Was that something you're attempting to do? That's one of your goals?	
Pt: Yeah, something like that.	
Dr: How many children did you say you had?	A series of closed questions.
Pt: Four.	
Dr: Before you had your first child, how much did you weigh?	
Pt: I weighed about 140 pounds.	
Dr: And how old were you then?	
Pt: I was 18.	
Dr: How many years ago was that?	
Pt: Thirteen years ago.	
Dr: When would you say that you had gained the majority of weight between then and now?	
Pt: When I had my second child.	
Dr: How much did you weigh at that time, before the second child?	
Pt: Before? Before my second child, I weighed around 150 to 160.	

	Typescript	*Comments*

Dr: What do you think it was between then and now that's made you gain the weight?

Pt: Nerves made me do a lot of eating. Then a lot of marital problems.

Dr: Do you want to discuss that a little bit more?

Open-ended question, leading to further exploration of possible emotional etiologies for weight change.

Pt: Oh, it was just a thing, me and my husband were—just like any other marriage I guess—good times, bad times—but more bad times than good. I had gotten to the point that I felt as though, I got all these children, what am I worth? You know, that kind of depressed me a little bit and I started gaining all that weight. After I had my last child I don't know, something just hit me, and I came up out of that.

Dr: When was that?

Pt: Five years ago.

Dr: So, how would you describe your general mood now?

Open-ended question, topic specified.

Pt: Fine.

Dr: You don't feel anything is wrong?

Pt: No. I very seldom—last time I got depressed was one day about 3 months ago 'cause there wasn't no jobs and that's about it. But depression, I can't remember at all when I last felt depression. I feel good about myself, good about my surroundings, 'cause you know you are only doing the best you can.

Dr: What do you think has brought about that change?

Pt: I don't know what it was really. I really don't. Well, after me and my husband had separated, I started feeling good about myself because for one, I got to the point, well, the children have to depend on me now, because I was doing a lot of depending on him.

Dr: When exactly was that?

Pt: That was about 3 years ago.

Dr: So since then you have generally felt better about yourself.

A summarization of the patient's statement.

Pt: Yeah.

Dr: Can you describe your eating habits over the past several years?

Pt: Okay, well, I eat breakfast. I eat sometimes a large breakfast and during the midday I'll

Typescript	*Comments*
drink tea, eat some fruit, drink milk. I drink a lot of milk. I might sit down and eat dinner about—lunch, I don't even worry about lunch 'cause I never see it. I eat dinner about 6 or 7 o'clock in the evening. In the last couple months I stopped snacking on a lot of sweets. Before I used to crave them at a certain period of the time, mostly when it was my menstrual period. I'd crave a lot of sweets. Lately I just don't even care for sweets too much. But I still drink a lot of milk, as long as it's cold. I'll drink a lot of milk.	
Dr: So you eat basically two meals a day.	Checking back about important data.
Pt: Yeah, sometimes one.	
Dr: And you don't do much snacking between meals.	
Pt: No.	
Dr: Now besides this weight problem, which seems to be improving, do you have any other complaints?	The doctor asks about other current problems—perhaps an iatrotropic stimulus as yet unmentioned.
Pt: None whatsoever.	
Dr: None whatsoever?	With a mild confrontation the doctor elicits a new concern—edema.
Pt: Yeah—now, weird as it might sound, now my ankles—on my right leg, my ankle will not swell up, but my left leg swells up. And I was taking water pills there for awhile from a doctor.	
Dr: How long has this been going on?	Beginning of questions defining and categorizing causes of edema.
Pt: I'd say for 3 months.	
Dr: When is the ankle swelling worse? Is it during the morning when you wake up?	
Pt: No, during the evening.	
Dr: As the day wears on?	
Pt: Yeah, as the day wears on.	
Dr: When you wake up in the morning, are they decreased?	
Pt: Yes.	
Dr: How many pillows do you sleep on?	
Pt: One.	
Dr: Do you ever wake up in the middle of the night gasping for air?	
Pt: No.	
Dr: How many times do you go to the bathroom at night?	

Typescript	Comments
Pt: About once.	
Dr: And that's your only other major complaint at this time?	
Pt: Yes.	
Dr: Have you had any change in bowel habits?	Beginning of some ROS-type questions, probing specifically for symptoms of thyroid disease.
Pt: No.	
Dr: Constipation? Diarrhea?	
Pt: No.	
Dr: Change in your voice?	
Pt: Yeah, my voice has gotten heavier.	
Dr: How long has that gone on?	
Pt: I'd say in the about the last year and a half.	
Dr: Any change in your skin or your hair?	An open-ended question with topic specified.
Pt: My hair has gotten longer.	
Dr: Besides longer, the quality of your skin or your hair?	
Pt: My skin is getting—I don't know—a couple of years ago I just looked like I was older and maybe I just started taking better care of myself.	
Dr: Okay, but you wouldn't say that there was any thinning or thickening of your skin or anything like that?	
Pt: No.	
Dr: Do you ever feel hot in a room where everyone else is cold or cold whenever everyone else is hot?	
Pt: I can't stand heat. I cannot stand heat at all. Summertime I stay in the house until the evenings. I've always been like that. Cold weather I love.	
Dr: Do you have any allergies?	Beginning of past medical history.
Pt: I have bronchitis.	
Dr: But any drug allergies that you are aware of?	
Pt: No.	
Dr: Any medications that you are taking?	
Pt: No. I'm allergic to penicillin.	
Dr: Okay, you are allergic to penicillin.	
Pt: Yeah.	
Dr: What does penicillin do to you?	Note the clarification—what does "allergy" mean?
Pt: I broke out in hives.	
Dr: Do you know of any medical problems that you have had in the past? Any high blood pressure?	

Typescript	Comments
Pt: No. I have low blood. I'm anemic.	
Dr: You're anemic?	
Pt: Yes.	
Dr: How long have you had the anemia?	
Pt: Since I've had my first child.	
Dr: Have you taken anything for it?	
Pt: I used to take iron pills there for awhile. That was about 10 years ago, then I just stopped because they made me feel tired.	
Dr: How's your pep and energy been?	
Pt: Fine.	
Dr: Any shortness of breath?	
Pt: No.	
Dr: Any problems with your heart?	
Pt: No.	
Dr: Heart attacks?	
Pt: No.	
Dr: Heart murmurs?	
Pt: No.	
Dr: Rheumatic heart disease?	
Pt: No.	
Dr: Have you ever had any strokes?	
Pt: No.	
Dr: Problems with your lungs?	
Pt: No.	
Dr: Asthma? Tuberculosis? Bronchitis?	
Pt: Bronchitis.	
Dr: How does that show itself?	The doctor asks for primary observations; the doctor does not accept interpretation.
Pt: Last time I had—it showed itself bad—it was like 10 years ago and I was in the hospital for that.	
Dr: Do you have any cough now?	
Pt: Yeah, 'cause I smoke.	
Dr: Do you cough up any sputum?	
Pt: Yeah.	
Dr: How much sputum?	
Pt: Not very much.	
Dr: What would you think? More than a shot glass?	
Pt: No.	
Dr: And what does it look like, the sputum?	
Pt: It's white.	
Dr: Any other problems? Stomach ulcers?	
Pt: No.	
Dr: Seizures?	
Pt: No.	
Dr: Problems with your kidneys or liver?	
Pt: No.	

Typescript	Comments
Dr: Any operations in the past?	
Pt: I had my tubes tied 5 years ago.	
Dr: Was that with your last child?	
Pt: Yes.	
Dr: Did you make that decision?	
Pt: Yes.	
Dr: How do you feel about that decision?	The doctor elicits the patient's feelings about a potentially sensitive issue (which might bear upon her weight problem).
Pt: At that time I felt good. Then a couple years ago I met this friend and I felt bad about it because I wanted to have another child. And I snapped out of that real quick.	
Dr: But you've gotten over that?	
Pt: Yes.	
Dr: Any other operations that you remember?	
Pt: No.	
Dr: Tonsils?	
Pt: No.	
Dr: Appendix? Gallbladder?	
Pt: No.	
Dr: So you have five children now?	Beginning of the "social history," but notice how much you already know about this person from the manner in which the present illness inquiry is conducted.
Pt: Four.	
Dr: Four children.	
Pt: Yes.	
Dr: And are they all living at home with you?	
Pt: Yes.	
Dr: What are their ages?	
Pt: 13, 11, 8, 5.	
Dr: Are they all in good health?	
Pt: Yes.	
Dr: Are you fortunate enough to have a job right now?	Notice how well this question is put *(respect)*.
Pt: No, not right now.	
Dr: What type of work did you do in the past?	
Pt: I've done various things. I drove a bus, did maintenance work, cashier in a store.	
Dr: How long have you been unemployed?	
Pt: For about 2 months now.	
Dr: Any prospects?	
Pt: No, just a lot of applications in. That's about it.	

Typescript	Comments
Dr: How does that feel? You must be upset.	Attempt at interchangeable response.
Pt: Not really. Something will come up. Something's bound to come up.	
Dr: So you are optimistic?	Successful interchangeable response.
Pt: Yeah.	
Dr: You said you smoked cigarettes. How much do you smoke?	Transition to new topic.
Pt: I smoke—a pack will last me about 2 days.	
Dr: How long have you smoked?	
Pt: I've been smoking since I was 16.	
Dr: Right now, you're 31?	
Pt: Right, I'll be 32 in July.	
Dr: Drink any alcohol?	
Pt: No.	
Dr: Have you ever?	
Pt: Yes, I stopped drinking when I was 18.	
Dr: Why was that?	
Pt: I was pregnant with my first child.	
Dr: Do you use any other type of drugs?	
Pt: No.	
Dr: Are your parents living?	Beginning of family health history.
Pt: My mother is.	
Dr: How old is she?	
Pt: 60.	
Dr: And your father?	
Pt: He's deceased.	
Dr: How old was he when he passed away?	
Pt: I was 15 years old.	
Dr: You can just take a guess.	
Pt: I'd say in his 40s, I guess.	
Dr: Do you know how he passed away?	
Pt: He had a heart attack.	
Dr: Did he have any diabetes or high blood pressure?	
Pt: He had high blood.	
Dr: Any strokes?	
Pt: No.	
Dr: How about your mother? How's her health?	
Pt: Fine. She has a—I forget what they call it but it's connected with a hernia.	
Dr: Do you have brothers and sisters?	
Pt: Yes, one brother and one sister.	
Dr: How's their health?	
Pt: Fine.	
Dr: Any brothers or sisters passed away?	
Pt: No.	

Typescript	*Comments*
Dr: Are there any diseases or illnesses that run in your family?	
Pt: No.	
Dr: Heart conditions? High blood pressure? Diabetes?	
Pt: Yeah, my uncle had—he was a diabetic.	
Dr: I'm just going to run through a bunch of questions now. Have you had any headaches recently?	Transition and beginning of formal review of systems.
Pt: No.	
Dr: Blurred or double vision?	
Pt: In one eye. This one jumps. It's the left one. That's been about 3 months now.	
Dr: What do you mean by jumps?	Attempt at establishing precise meaning.
Pt: It gets to quivering. I don't know whether it's nerves. I used to say something's going to happen.	
Dr: Any blind spots in your eyes?	
Pt: No.	
Dr: Do you see double out of that eye?	
Pt: No. Once in a while when I come in from a different room area. Like this one will kind of dart and then it will clear up and my vision gets together.	
Dr: Any difficulty hearing?	
Pt: No.	
Dr: Any bleeding through your nose, mouth, lips, and gums? Difficulty swallowing?	
Pt: No.	
Dr: Shortness of breath or wheezing?	
Pt: Wheezing.	
Dr: When do you have the wheezing?	
Pt: At night when I sleep.	
Dr: Do you take anything for that?	
Pt: No, not really.	
Dr: Do you get up, or does it just go away?	
Pt: Sometimes I'll get up and drink some water and that's it.	
Dr: How often do you get that?	
Pt: Every night during the night.	
Dr: Coughing any blood up at all?	
Pt: No.	
Dr: Any fever, chills, or sweats?	
Pt: No.	
Dr: Belly pain?	
Pt: No.	
Dr: Lumps or bumps anywhere in your breasts or under your arms?	
Pt: No.	

Typescript	Comments
(Interruption at door.)	
Dr: What was I asking you, about belly pains?	
Pt: Yes.	
Dr: No belly pains?	
Pt: No.	
Dr: Diarrhea or constipation?	
Pt: No.	
Dr: Any blood in your stools?	
Pt: No.	
Dr: Any swelling of any joints or joint pains?	
Pr: Just my ankles.	
Dr: Okay, we already talked about that. Any rash anywhere on your body?	
Pt: No.	
Dr: I think that's about all the questions. Do you have any questions for me? Is there anything else?	Inviting the patient to have the last word.
Pt: No.	
Dr: I think we have covered mostly everything.	Closing.

The Write-up

CC (Chief Complaint).   This is the first medical clinic visit for this 31-year-old white mother of four who presents for a physical and "just that I'm overweight."

HPI (History of Present Illness).   Patient states that her weight goes "up and down" but that she's always been big, and is from a family of big people. At age 18, prior to the birth of her first child, she weighed 140 lb and a year ago she weighed 230 lb. Current weight is about 200 lb. Patient believes that weight loss is due to additional activity (dance class and tennis) and avoidance of day-time snacking. The major weight gain was during the second pregnancy, attributed to "nerves" and "marital problems." Patient was sad and feeling "What am I worth?" at times, but has felt better since separating from her husband 3 years ago. Current eating pattern is breakfast and supper with an occasional midday snack. Drinks lots of milk. Used to crave sweets, especially premenstrually, but not lately.

OAP (Other Active Problems). Left, but not right, ankle swells from time to time. Onset 3 months ago. Took water pills. Generally wakes without edema, then notes it as day wears on. Denies orthopnea, PND (paroxysmal nocturnal dyspnea). Has nocturia $\times$ 1.

PMH (Past Medical History)

History of anemia since birth of first child. Rx'd with iron 10 yrs. ago.

Hospitalization: "Bronchitis," 10 yrs. ago.

Operations: tubal ligation, 5 yrs. ago.

Allergies: penicillin—hives.

Medications: none.

Immunizations: (missing data).

SH (Social History). Four healthy children at home, ages 13, 11, 8, and 5 yrs. Separated (? divorced) from husband. Unemployed for past 2 months. Employment Hx includes bus driving, cashier, and maintenance work. Optimistic about future employment, applications pending. Smoking: 1 pk q 2 days, onset age 16. [How many "pack-years"? Did she smoke more? Less?] ETOH (alcohol): None since age 18 when first pregnant. [How much did she drink before that?] No other drug use. [The doctor neglected to take a sexual history. Other missing information includes place of birth, years in this locality, education, and personal interests.]

FH (Family History)

Mother age 60, good health, some kind of "hernia"

Father died in his 40s of "heart attack," hypertension

One brother and one sister in good health

One uncle with diabetes

No other significant family history

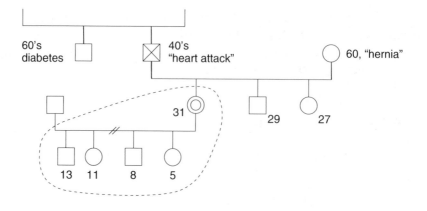

ROS (Review of Systems)

General: good energy level, no fatigue, fever, sweats, chills or swollen glands.

Skin: negative.

HEENT: voice "heavier," left eye "jumps," no headache, no visual changes or diplopia.

Resp: Hx of "bronchitis," daily cough, scant white sputum, smokes 1 pk q 2 days, "wheezes" at night, no dyspnea, no hemoptysis. [There may be enough positive responses here to consider this a problem in the OAP section.]

CV: no heart problems or stroke.

GI: no change in bowel habit, no constipation, no diarrhea, no ulcer history, no abdominal pain, no melena.

GU: no history of kidney trouble.

GYN: no breast lumps. [Menstrual history was not obtained.]

Endo: heat intolerance.

MS: ankle swelling, no pains.

Psychiatric: as noted in HPI.

PE (Physical Examination)

Healthy appearing, obese young woman in no distress

Vital signs: BP 130/78, Pulse 72, Resp 16, Temp 97.5, Weight 207 lb

Skin: clear

HEENT:

> Head. normocephalic and atraumatic
> Tympanic membranes. normal
> Mouth. teeth in good repair
> Throat. tonsils 1+
> Eyes. no redness or swelling, extraocular movements (EOM) intact, pupils equal, regular, react to light and accommodation (PERRLA), funduscopic exam normal

Neck and nodes: negative

Thyroid: palpable, within normal limits

Chest: clear to percussion and auscultation

Cardiac: normal S_1 and S_2, no murmur or other sounds

Breasts: breast self-exam reviewed, no masses, minimal fibrocystic changes noted in the upper outer quadrants bilaterally

Abdomen: no hepatosplenomegaly, no masses, no bruits

Extremities: trace edema over left medial malleolus, none on the right, no cyanosis or clubbing

Rectal and pelvic exam: not done

Neurologic exam: cranial nerves II–XII intact, deep tendon reflexes 2+ throughout, muscular strength and sensation intact

Assessment

1. Health maintenance [or preventive care]
2. Obesity
3. History of anemia ["history" because this condition has not been confirmed by objective testing]
4. Smoker with history of "bronchitis," daily cough, and "wheezing" [grouped as one problem because they are all likely to be related]

Plan

1. Inquire at next visit re: menstrual history, gyn care, most recent Pap smear, immunizations, and lifestyle.
2. Diet diary ×2 wks. Nutrition consult. Blood work—lipids and glucose.
3. Blood work—CBC.
4. Patient education—quit smoking contract, consider nicotine gum. Check "bronchitis" record, consider pulmonary function tests.

PART 2
Advanced Techniques

CHAPTER 8

Adapting the Medical Interview: The Pediatric, Elderly, and Ambulatory Patient

> A human being sheds its leaves like a tree. Sickness prunes it down; and it no longer offers the same silhouette to the eyes which loved it, to the people to whom it afforded shade and comfort.
>
> Edmond and Jules deGoncourt, *Journal July 22, 1862*

In the first six chapters, we presented basic skills of medical interviewing and the "generic" version of a medical history. In clinical practice, you often have to adapt the diagnostic interview to meet the needs of particular groups of patients or specific patient care situations. The brief and highly focused history given by a trauma patient in the emergency room is very different in both style and content from the multifaceted history obtained from a patient being evaluated for chronic illness. In this chapter, we consider how to adapt your interview to patients in three broad categories—children, older persons, and ambulatory patients—that present special problems and challenges in diagnostic interviewing.

THE PEDIATRIC PATIENT*

Why devote a separate section to pediatric interviewing? Are the medical histories of children so different from those of

---

*The pediatric section was coauthored by Kenneth Schuitt, MD.

adults? In the following pages, we take the perspective that children and adolescents are not merely "miniature adults." The style of a pediatric interview is not only different from the medical history elicited from an adult, but the style of the pediatric interview also varies dynamically from one developmental stage of childhood to the next.

Children versus Grown-ups: Similarities and Differences

There are, of course, many similarities in pediatric and adult medical interviews. For example, the basic organization of a clinical history is the same for patients of all ages: chief complaint, history of present illness, past medical history, family history, patient profile, and review of systems (see Chaps. 3, 4, and 5). Similarly, attitudes and values that facilitate good adult doctor-patient interactions are equally important in pediatrics: empathy, respect, privacy, and confidentiality (see Chap. 2).

The two most important differences between the adult and pediatric interview are the individuals who participate in the conversation and the topics that are emphasized at a particular stage of development. For example, with regard to the participants, parents and/or other family members must often provide information instead of or in addition to the patient. Although this need is obvious in the case of a preverbal child, this need introduces potential problems in gathering information, and the precise point at which a verbal child has the skill to contribute his or her own history is not always easy to determine. With regard to topics, the prenatal history, for example, is vitally important in the case of a neonate but not so in the case of an adolescent. And the achievement of developmental milestones, while critical to the assessment of a 6-month-old, is of minimal significance in the evaluation of a "straight A's" second grader who presents with a sore throat.

Setting the Stage for Effective Communication

Even the most precise, empathic historian needs a private and comfortable environment. If the patient is in a hospital room that contains several beds, the neighbor's television is playing, visitors are chatting, and medical personnel are performing procedures, then families will feel uncomfortable even talking about mundane historical items, much less giving thoughtful observations of behavior or potentially embarrassing details. Before starting, you should insist that the television and radio be turned off. If possible, roommates may be taken elsewhere by their parents or by staff members. Otherwise, curtains should be drawn around the child's bed to provide at least the illusion of privacy. Similarly, you should see that a neonate is comfortable and quiet before expecting his or her parents to be relaxed enough to provide you with detailed information. In the case of a preschool child, offering the patient a toy to occupy his or her attention may well improve the efficiency of an interview. Spend a few moments at the beginning of an interview with a newborn's parents to admire the baby, with a 2-year-old's mother to charm the toddler, or with a school child to query him or her about a favorite television show or hobby. With children it is often easier to *establish rapport indirectly* by admiring a toy or a pair of new shoes as opposed to an (overly) enthusiastic greeting to the child himself. Then, spend a few moments talking to the parent or guardian to *give the child time to size you up.*

You should make no assumptions—and certainly no judgments—about the relationship of the caretaking adults to the child patient. The parents of an infant may not necessarily bear the same married name. Thus, the term "his father" rather than "your husband" or "the baby's mother" rather than "your wife" might be more appropriate until the parental relationship is better understood. Similarly, an infant and his or her parent may not carry the same surname. A brief glance at the registration form might reveal that the infant's name is Doe, while the mother's and father's name is Smith. Because you need to understand the relationship for the benefit of the child, it is best to ask simply, and nonjudgmentally, "I notice that your name is Smith and William's name is Doe. Can you explain the relationship to me?"

Finally, try to tailor your vocabulary to the level of understanding of the family members with whom you are speaking. Discernment of their sophistication is subject to bias and may at times be difficult. One senior pediatric faculty member who frequently berated his students for ignoring education and background when talking to parents, was asked to see a child whose mother and father were plainly dressed and who came from a rural part of the state. Following his own admonition, he began speaking very slowly and trying to use a quite simple vocabulary, only to discover that the father himself was a physician and the mother a nurse!

Talking with Patients of Different Ages

The style and content of and the participants in medical interviews vary enormously with the child's maturation. The questions you ask new parents will be very different from those you ask a teenager. The content of the medical history changes with age just as the style and dynamics change. Topics that are obviously important in the prenatal visit or in the newborn interview become distinctly less important as the child matures and, indeed, may not be mentioned at all in the medical conversation with an adolescent. For convenience, we distinguish four types of pediatric medical history: prenatal visit, infant and toddler, school-aged child, and, finally, the adolescent.

THE PRENATAL VISIT

Ideally, the person who will be responsible for the medical care of a newborn should meet with prospective parents. The prenatal visit allows the care giver to obtain important medical information, while the visit also establishes a partnership of mutual trust and respect. The diminished role of extended, multigenerational families means that in many cases the emotional and educational support for new parents may come from a physician or nurse, rather than from grandparents and siblings. A brief informal meeting can initiate such a support system and dispel myths and preconceptions that the potential parents might have. The information you acquire during this prenatal visit includes:

- A detailed family history;
- Plans for feeding the baby (breast versus bottle);
- Circumcision (yes or no); and
- The parent's knowledge about child care.

At this time, practical issues like the schedule for well child office visits, medical fees, and telephone access also can be presented.

During your meeting with prospective parents, you should

obtain important information about the family history: familial disease, previous histories of birth defects, and perinatal deaths. The purpose of a detailed family history is twofold:

1. To alert you to possible genetic disease in the infant; and
2. To reassure or inform parents concerned about implications for their child of certain familial illnesses or tendencies.

Listen especially for details of miscarriages and neonatal or childhood illness or death. The parents' health and their past medical history should be outlined in some detail, especially with respect to disease states that might endanger the life of or have adverse health effects on the fetus during pregnancy. You should pay some attention to the physical, social, and emotional environment into which the child will be born. Parents' discussion of their plans for feeding the baby and their knowledge of child care will direct your educational efforts.

This prenatal interaction also provides an opportunity to give some anticipatory guidance to parents. Your role as a clinician is not only to obtain historical information but also to anticipate and educate. For example, you should take the opportunity to discuss issues such as:

1. The changes that will occur in parents' and siblings' lives with the newborn's arrival;
2. Identification of support persons for the mother and father when the infant goes home;
3. Information about safety for the infant at home and in the automobile; and
4. Preparation of siblings for the new addition to their family.

THE INFANT AND TODDLER

During infancy and the preschool years, the patient is the reason for the visit and the *focus* of the interview, but not usually a *participant* in the interview. Although the patient may add little to the actual conversation, pediatric medicine is certainly not "akin to veterinary medicine" as some cynics would suggest! In most situations, you should conduct the interview with the infant or toddler present for several reasons. First, this small but important person serves as a catalyst to aid parents' recall of historical details. Second, parents are likely to be more comfortable if they are with their sick child, and certainly children will be more comfortable with their parents. Finally, in the case of preschool children, when the child sees you interacting with the mother or father, the child is more likely to (very tentatively) develop a feeling of trust.

If the infant is fussy or clearly in pain, he or she will only serve to distract both you and the parents. The situation might require a pacifier or bottle for the neonate, or giving a familiar toy to the toddler. It is useful to carry around a colorful item or two to interest your preschool patients. Sometimes inexperienced clinicians will either ignore the patient completely (to the consternation of parents) or try to become instant "buddies" with the child, forgetting that usually by 1 year of age a child has become quite wary or even frightened of strangers. Moreover, illness may make the toddler irritable, and the clinical setting may be terrifying. A good compromise is to begin the encounter with a simple friendly greeting, followed by the enthusiastic but brief examination of one of the child's own toys rather than of the child himself or herself.

The medical history here must include information about the *perinatal period:* complications and problems during the pregnancy, duration and complications of labor, and problems during the infant's first days of life. If a *family history* has not already been obtained, you should take a careful family history as well. Crying, sleeping, and bowel and bladder function should be discussed. A careful review of *developmental stages* must be obtained, focusing on different milestones depending on the age of the child. Ascertain the child's *immunization status* with regard to diphtheria-pertussis-tetanus (DPT), polio, measles, rubella, and mumps, including reactions to the immunizations. *Nutrition* questions are also of importance in your clinical history. Three screening questions often suffice:

1. "How many ounces of formula (or for older children, milk) does your baby take each day?" For breast-fed babies, "How many times does the baby nurse in 24 hours?" and "What's the longest he or she goes between feedings?"

2. For older infants and toddlers, "Are there any foods your child refuses to eat?"
3. "Does your child get much in the way of sweets and junk food?"

Because anticipatory guidance plays an important role in every patient-family-doctor interaction in this age group, the clinician should obtain enough information so that he or she can later discuss accident prevention, feeding, toilet training, and such developmental issues as teething and acquisition of normal speech patterns.

The content of the interview varies with the reason for the visit: well child care, an office visit for illness, or a very sick child or a child about to have a surgical procedure. The child's demeanor and the parents' level of anxiety and ability to provide precise information about the child's illness will vary. Parents may be very focused on whether they have cared for their child correctly or have done anything to provoke or worsen an illness. They may require frequent reassurance that they are good parents and have acted properly. Sometimes, especially early in the interview, you may be unable to provide such reassurance and may need to say:

> I understand your concern about whether you should have given Molly that cold medicine, but I'd like to leave that aside for the moment and get back to how she's been acting over the last few days. When did you first notice that she wasn't her usual self?

Once you have established the history, you will be able to reassure the parents that they have not hurt their child or, alternatively, educate them in the proper care of a sick child.

The symptoms of pediatric illness, particularly in the preverbal child, are often nonspecific and tell us more about how sick the child is than precisely what the illness is. A 15-month-old cannot tell us that his left ear hurts; rather, he will cry, be irritable, have a fever and possibly a loss of appetite or even vomiting and diarrhea. If we are lucky, he may tug at his left ear, but many children with healthy ears do that as well. We have to rely on our physical examination to make the diagnosis of left otitis media. But if he is exceedingly irritable, refuses to play, and refuses liquids, we may need to rule out meningitis as well with additional

TABLE 8–1. Content of Infant and Toddler Interview

Reason for Visit	Topics Discussed
Well child visit	Parental concerns
	Dates of prior immunizations. Is child current?
	Prenatal and birth history
	Developmental milestones achieved
	Eruption of teeth
	Habits: sleeping, crying, and bowel and bladder function
	Intercurrent illness and other illnesses
	Nutrition history
	Cultural and family practices (feeding, taping umbilical hernias, keeping face covered to prevent colic, etc.)
Sick visit or admission to hospital	All of the topics discussed in a well child visit
	Same as history of present illness (Chap. 3) with special emphasis on time of onset, initial symptoms, and subsequent symptoms
	Difficulty feeding—too slow, not at all, refusal of liquids, refusal of solids, or preference for water or juice as opposed to milk or formula
	State of hydration
	Does the infant or child seem himself or herself?
	As playful, alert, and pleasant as usual?
	Acting sick?
	Temperature taken? at home? rectal? axillary?
	Medications (including over-the-counter medications) already given and dosages?
	What concerns the parents most?
	What do they think is causing illness?
	History of recent similar illnesses in patient or family?

diagnostic studies. Table 8–1 lists the key information required in the infant and toddler interview.

THE SCHOOL-AGED CHILD

When a child reaches the age of 5 or 6 years, the interactive balance in the interview begins to change. Children are now more able to contribute substantially to the collection of data, but their reports are usually broad and sometimes difficult to interpret. Thus, you must turn to parents to provide accuracy and precision while always trying to confirm the data insofar as is possible with the patient himself or herself. An enormous maturational range is found in elementary school-aged children. You can expect to find behaviors ranging from the shy, sullen, and silent child to the garrulous child who cannot be stopped! Thus, as a sensitive historian, you must take your cues from observing the patient before deciding whether and how much to involve the child in actual history taking.

In general, the school-aged child is a healthy child. In addition to obtaining historical information concerning immunizations, development, and nutrition, the *psychosocial aspects* of a child's history become more important during these years. Knowledge of the child's *school performance* and *friends* is necessary for the global understanding of a school-aged child's well being. Anticipatory guidance at this age emphasizes accident prevention, both in the home and at school, and good nutrition. Special aspects of the content of the interview of the school-aged child are indicated in Table 8–2.

TABLE 8–2. Content of School-Aged Child Interview

Reason for Visit	*Topics Discussed*
Well child visit	Parental concerns
	School progress, school readiness, relationships with peers
	Developmental milestones achieved? At what age?
	Habits (eating, sleeping, and continence)
	Age-appropriate play?
	Similarities to and differences from peers
	Significant past and birth history
	Illnesses since last visit
	Dates of prior immunizations
	Nutrition
Sick visit or admission to hospital	All of the topics discussed in well child visit
	Same as history of present illness (Chap. 3) with special emphasis on parent's observations
	Child's descriptions of symptoms
	Medications (including over-the-counter medication) already tried
	Similar illnesses in household or peer group

THE ADOLESCENT

Your interactions with teenagers are potentially the most complicated and difficult of any interviews you will conduct. The adolescent person is frequently ambivalent or confused by his or her own feelings and resists talking about them. Moreover, during the adolescent years, patients take an increasingly active role in their own health care, while their parents move progressively into the background. This is a change that many mothers and fathers, as well as their teenage children, find difficult.

You may initiate the interview with an unfamiliar teenager with a direct, unaffected introduction:

> Hi, I'm Dr. Smith and I'm glad to meet you. Tell me what made you decide to come to see me or (as is often the case) what made your parents bring you?

Remember that initially you are a stranger and must establish a basis for trust. Many physicians try to become instant friends with teenagers, succeeding only in confusing or antagonizing them. It is appropriate to talk with adolescents alone for part of the interview, if not for the whole interaction. Most parents are cooperative and will leave the room without difficulty when you explain:

> You know how important it is for you to feel that you have a private and confidential relationship with your doctor, and most of my young patients feel the same way. So I'm going to ask you to leave while I talk with Jamie. Is there anything you'd like to tell me before you go?

When speaking with an adolescent, establish that your conversation is confidential. Whether the information is potentially embarrassing or not, build trust by assuring the patient:

> I always want to make it clear to all my patients that what they tell me is private. I will not repeat anything you say unless you give me permission to do so. But you know, your Mom cares about you and may have some concerns about what we do today. If she asks me anything, in order to protect your privacy, I'm going to tell her that she has to ask you. So you might want to think about what you'd like to tell her, and we can talk about that some more at the end of our visit.

This kind of statement not only respects the adolescent's desire for autonomy but at the same time acknowledges the parents' rightful interest in their child who has not yet achieved full adult status. It also implies that parents and their children should talk about important things, even those that are difficult, such as sexuality. The sexual history is a particularly difficult topic for adolescents. As with patients in any other age group, you should employ clear language that the patient understands and proceed from less intimate questions ("Tell me about your family and friends." "Do you have any special friends?" "How about boyfriends or girlfriends?") to more intimate ones ("Do your friends go on dates?" "How do they feel about having sex?" "How do you feel?" "Are you sexually active now?").

One problem, of course, is making sure that when you use a term such as "sexually active," that you are sure the patient understands what you mean. Young teenagers vary widely in their sexual knowledge and experience; among 14-year-old girls, you will find those who have already been pregnant and others who will look wide eyed and disbelieving that you could even think of asking such questions. For this reason, questions about their peer group as well as questions that do not imply any right answer or particular level of experience are useful. For example:

> Dr: Some girls your age who are late with their period will worry that they may have gotten pregnant. Have you had any worries like that?
> Pt: No, because I know I can't be.
> Dr: You can't be. Tell me more.
> Pt: Well, I didn't have sex. I don't even go with boys; none of my friends do.

Sometimes the conversation takes a different turn:

> Dr: Some girls your age who are late with their period will worry that they may have gotten pregnant. Have you had any worries like that?
> Pt: Well, I thought about it.
> Dr: Tell me more.
> Pt: Well, I don't really think I can be.
> Dr: Did he touch you or did he put his penis near you or inside you?

Notice the need to be simple and precise in your language so you can be sure that you are obtaining accurate information.

Important information to obtain from the teenager centers around the teenager's interaction with his or her environment and social world. Tactfully posed questions dealing with *drugs and alcohol, sexuality, contraception,* and *sexually transmitted diseases* are an important part of a medical history in this age group. But even the most tactful interviewer often has difficulty breaking through the outward reserve that many adolescents show. If this is the case, posing sensitive questions in the past tense is sometimes helpful. For example, rather than asking, "Do you smoke cigarettes?" you might ask, "Were you smoking cigarettes 6 months ago?" This avoids direct confrontation. Here is another example of how you might "open up" a silent—and possibly angry—adolescent interview:

> I'm sorry that your father dragged you in here against your will. I know if I were in your shoes I'd be pretty angry. But since we have this time together do you think we could talk about some of the things that have been going on in your life? None of this is any of my business unless it's okay with you for me to get to know you better. I'd like to hear more about how you've been feeling.

Other important issues to discover during the interview are:

1. School performance;
2. The presence or absence of close friends; and
3. Behavioral difficulties both at home and at school.

Ideally, most of this information should be obtained directly from the adolescent rather than from a parent or guardian.

THE ELDERLY PATIENT

In this section, we consider some of the special sensitivities and skills required for effective interviewing of older or geriatric patients. Who are these "older" patients? Here is the opening exchange of a woman seeing her physician in the office for follow-up of hypertension and chronic diarrhea:

> Dr: So how are you?
> Pt: Okay, I guess. I guess it's just old age.
> Dr: What about old age?

When does old age begin? This patient was 88 years old; but what if she had been only 78, 68, or 58? Although you should have special concerns if a 58-year-old woman or man complains of "old age," you will find it difficult to have any hard and fast rules about when an "older person" has become "old." The 68-year-old chief executive with neither health problems nor plans to retire is certainly not the same kind of older person as the 68-year-old retired mill worker with oxygen-dependent chronic lung disease and recent memory loss. The former would find questions about his ability to perform routine activities of daily living insulting if not bizarre; the latter would find such questions very relevant to his overall management. So the approach to older persons must be individualized and *geared to the patient's stage of life,* as opposed to making rigid classifications based on *chronologic age.*

Special aspects of history taking in this group include the style and content of the interview, mental status testing, and the problem of the "third party" in caring for elderly patients.

Style

The short vignette presented above illustrates the way in which many elderly patients attribute their symptoms to normal aging and may require open-ended prompting ("What do you mean by 'old age'?") to discuss symptoms that could indicate a specific disease process as opposed to senescence. Patients, for example, may attribute nocturia or joint pains to aging, even though these symptoms may, in fact, be indicative of specific diseases, such as heart failure or tendinitis. Moreover, vague symptoms may have special implications in the elderly, as in the case of a 90-year-old man with pneumonia who experiences loss of appetite and feelings of malaise rather than a more typical presentation with fever and cough. Likewise, chronic symptoms must be distinguished from acute or unstable symptoms. For example, the sudden onset of urinary incontinence requires a different approach than a report of incontinence of many years' duration. You also will notice that the pace of the interview is often slower and that the elderly are likely to infuse their medical stories with a lifetime of experience that demands and informs our respect. These are just some of the stylistic changes that you will note as you interview the geriatric patient.

Content

In addition to changes in style, the geriatric history emphasizes somewhat different content areas as well. For example, remote events, such as childhood history, are not usually relevant and may be obtained with a minimum amount of detail, like "Any unusual illnesses when you were a child?" The family history may assume less importance as well because most familial diseases will have expressed themselves by the time a person reaches old age. The family history also takes on a different twist since you look not only at the preceding generation but query the elderly about their children and grandchildren as well. For example, an older woman whose daughter has breast cancer may herself be at increased risk of the disease and may not know that, in fact, it was breast cancer that took the life of her mother 40 years ago. Moreover, elderly persons may worry about the health of their children and grandchildren, and your interest in their families provides an opportunity to explore those concerns.

Perhaps the most striking difference in the history of the elderly patient is the need to assess their functional status in terms of everyday activities and their abilities to do those things necessary to sustain and enjoy life. The social history (or patient profile, see Chap. 5) includes most basic activities of daily living. Among these are the older person's ability to eat (chew and swallow), sleep, bathe, dress, walk or move about unaided, and maintain continence. Ability to cook and to perform simple household chores also must be assessed. Several useful rating scales are available for measuring functional status or activities of daily living.[38,48]

Try to determine if the person is able to maintain a normal sleep-wake cycle; one useful question is "Are you able to sleep when you want to sleep and not sleep when you don't want to?" If bowel or bladder incontinence is a problem, you will need to get additional details such as the location of the bathroom and the patient's ease in getting there. Details about diet include the ability to afford, shop for, and prepare food, as well as some consideration of specific nutrients such as calcium (which may be needed to prevent osteoporosis) and fiber (which may help prevent constipation and treat diverticular disease or hemorrhoids).

You should also assess sexual feelings and function, but this must be done sensitively and in context. Frail, sick, or widowed elderly patients may find questions like, "Are you sexually active?" or "Are you having any sexual problems?" surprising if not downright inappropriate. It is better to give the patient plenty of room to answer, based on his or her own situation. For example, "As people get older they sometimes find that their marriage changes. How has it been for you?" and then "Has anything changed in your sexual relationship?" Change in sexual function also may be related to specific illness, rather than to age per se. For example, "I can see that you're having problems with the circulation in your legs. Sometimes when men have this problem they also notice problems getting an erection. Have you noticed anything like that?"

Another content area of special importance in elderly persons is the detailed review of all medications, including over-the-counter as well as prescription drugs. This is best accomplished by asking patients to bring all their pill containers with them, even those they no longer take. Finally, immunization status, including diphtheria-tetanus, influenza, and pneumococcal vaccines, and any adverse reactions to these immunizations are an important part of the geriatric history that frequently is not given sufficient attention.

Mental Status Assessment

The interviewer must facilitate a technically competent interview with patients who may be frail, hard of hearing, visually impaired, or suffering from memory loss. You should quickly and inconspicuously assess cognitive function in the opening moments of the interview, usually without a formal mental status examination. The purpose of this informal assessment is to determine whether the patient is competent to give his or her own history, and what assistance might be needed to help ensure accuracy and precision of medical data. How is this informal assessment accomplished? *First*, certain clues about mental status arise even prior to the examination as you observe the interaction between patient and family members or caretakers.

- Does the patient himself or herself call to make an appointment or to report symptoms?
- Does he or she arrive in the office alone, having driven a car or taken a bus or taxi?

- Does the patient forget an appointment even when reminded with a postcard or phone call?

Patients who are unable to remember having made appointments also may be unable to remember medications, and while these patients may experience symptoms, they may be unable to recall them and report them precisely to their physicians.

Next, as you enter the examining room or the patient's hospital room, you should pay careful attention to the patient's *level of alertness* (awake or drowsy). The patient sedated with a narcotic to alleviate renal colic may not be able to tell you very much (other than that he or she is feeling better now) until the medication wears off. Is the patient alert enough to focus attention on you and follow you from one question or statement to the next? Problems with alertness are common in hospitals and are probably underrecognized. You should also notice the patient's *general appearance and behavior.* Does he or she appear socially appropriate? Is the patient clean and quiet, or disheveled and agitated? Is the patient physically active or slow and retarded? As you begin the interview, you next assess the patient's *verbal output or speech.* Is it relevant or irrelevant? rambling or reticent? repetitious or almost mute? coherent or incoherent? These characteristics, in turn, tell you a great deal about the patient's *thought process and content.* Is the pattern of thought logical or tangential? Is the patient preoccupied with thoughts of death? Does he or she have an obvious delusional system?

Here is an example of the opening moments of a follow-up visit with a 76-year-old woman who was brought in by her family because of weight loss and abdominal pain:

Dr: You said you've been feeling sad.
Pt: Yeah, my mother died before the baby was born and I just started talking to the women about it and all of a sudden I said I couldn't. It's just sad. Well, I raised a boy, his name was Andy, and he stayed in Europe and he couldn't get out there and he was about 10 years or something like that. And then my sister you know wanted to come back and I went to look for the money we were trying to collect for. So I went up and you

> know how it is, and on a Sunday I went over there and the baby was born.

How would you describe this patient's thought process? While her statement does seem vaguely related to the issue of sadness, it is difficult to follow the thread of this story, and it is certainly not a response to the question. We would describe it as rambling, tangential, and incoherent. It is typical of this patient who could not really remember how she had been feeling. This is dementia, not psychosis.

In observing the patient, you will also certainly notice *mood and affect.* Is the patient flat or sad? anxious or inappropriately gay? cooperative or combative? While *orientation to time, place, and person* may be obvious in the opening moments of your interview as you engage in social "chitchat" with your patient, be aware that many mildly and even moderately demented older persons retain excellent social skills that belie their cognitive deficit. We are reminded of two elderly women, both 93 years of age who came to the office one day for back-to-back appointments. The nursing and reception staff commented, "Aren't they doing well!" But, in reality, one was and one was not. Both exhibited the social amenities of saying hello, observing how much she liked her doctor, and commenting on the weather. One then went on to give a detailed account of her arthritic symptoms over the past month; the other, despite enthusiastically greeting her doctor whom she had seen many times before, replied as follows:

> Pt: It's so very nice to see you. You're such a grand person.
> Dr: Why thank you. It's nice to see you, too. Do you remember who I am?
> Pt: Well, you look very familiar. What's your name again?

The patient's *ability to remember* becomes readily apparent as the history proceeds and you try to gather precise information about symptoms. The elderly gentleman who repeats items in his history at different parts of a brief interview may not remember that he has already told you these details. The patient who says he has been feeling fine despite his family's concern about his repeated complaints of chest pain may not remember these episodes of pain. Indeed, sometimes you encounter obvious factual contradictions, such as a patient who states that she never had surgery but who has surgical scars on her abdomen.

Formal Mental Status Testing

As summarized in the preceding paragraphs, much of the information required for formal mental status testing is readily obtainable during a careful medical interview. Usually, this is sufficient to assess your patient's reliability, and rule out a significant organic mental problem, such as delirium or dementia. Sometimes it is important to perform a more complete mental status evaluation that includes specific descriptions of the following:

- Appearance and behavior;
- Attention and alertness;
- Speech and language;
- Mood and affect;
- Memory and orientation;
- Thought process and content;
- Judgment and insight; and
- Abstract thinking, knowledge, and calculation.

One semiquantitative tool that is often useful in this respect is the *Mini-Mental Status Exam*.[48] While this questionnaire does not cover all the attributes of a complete mental status examination, it does give a relatively rapid and reliable numerical score estimating cognitive function. In the hospital, the Mini-Mental Status Exam can be used to follow patients with fluctuating mental status by administering it at various times, for example, in the morning and evening. In the outpatient setting, it can be used to evaluate and follow patients who have problems with cognitive function over the course of months or years.

The Folstein Mini-Mental Status Exam is shown in Table 8–3. A score of 20 or greater is considered normal, while a score less than 20 is suggestive of neuropsychiatric or neurologic disorder such as delirium, dementia, or the pseudodementia of severe depression. Changing scores are also significant even if they remain more than 20. For example, a patient who scores 30 in the morning and then 22 later that day definitely has a problem with cognition that demands the physician's attention. False-positive results may occur in patients who are not able to concentrate because of extreme anxiety or thought disorder. In highly intelligent patients, the test may not be very sensitive and, thus, false-negative results may occur. Such problems should be noted during the test; when in doubt, more complete cognitive testing (beyond the scope of this chapter) should be done.

Clinicians are often reluctant to do mental status testing and find it awkward to incorporate these tests into their interview format. Indeed, the data obtained are not really part of the medical history as such, but, more correctly, part of the objective database, akin to the physical examination. Patients also may find specific questions about memory or cognition stressful. To ease these tensions, it is best to introduce mental status testing after the history part of your interaction, either just before or just following your physical examination. By this time, you will already have developed a relationship with your patient as well as an understanding of what some of his or her problems are. Such knowledge gives you a way to introduce this part of your evaluation in a straightforward and natural way. For example:

Dr: I've noticed that as we've been talking there are some things you have trouble remembering. Would it be all right if I test your memory?
Pt: How do you do that?
Dr: Well, I will ask you questions, some of which will seem silly to you and easy, and others may be hard for you. Would that be okay?

or

Dr: Do you ever forget to take your medication?
Pt: No, I never do.
Dr: How do you remember?
Pt: That's the first thing I do every day. But sometimes my memory is not so good. Sometimes I forget things I'm going to say.
Dr: Is that a new problem for you?
Pt: No, it has been for some time. I guess at 88, what can you expect?

TABLE 8–3. The Folstein Mini-Mental Status Exam

	Score	Maximum Score
Orientation		
What is the (year)——(season)——(month)——(date)——(day)——?	( )	5
Where are we (state)——(county)——(town)——(hosp.)——(floor)——?	( )	5
Registration		
I am going to name three objects and I want you to repeat them after me. (Interviewer, give one point for each correct answer. Repeat the objects until the patient can name them all–six trials maximum.) Number of trials ( ).	( )	3
Attention and Calculation		
I am going to ask you to do some subtraction. Think of the number 7. I want you to subtract 7 from 100. Now subtract 7 from that and keep on going. 100,——,——,——,—— Stop. Alternative: Spell "world" backwards.	( )	5
Recall		
Please name the three objects that I had you repeat after me just a short while ago. (Interviewer, give one point for each correct answer.)	( )	3

Language

Please name these for me. (Show patient a watch and a pencil.)	( )	2
Now, please repeat the following: "no ifs, ands, or buts."	( )	1
Now I am going to ask you to do something for me. "Take a paper in your right hand, fold it in half, and put it on the floor."	( )	3
Now I want you to read this and do what it says. (Interviewer, hand the patient a card that says "Close your eyes.")	( )	1
Now, please write a sentence for me on this blank piece of paper. (Interviewer, give the patient a blank piece of paper and ask him or her to write a sentence for you. Do not dictate a sentence; it must be written spontaneously. It must contain a subject and verb and be sensible. Correct grammar and punctuation are not necessary.)	( )	1

Visual–Motor Integrity

Please copy this design. (Interviewer, on a clean piece of paper, draws intersecting pentagons, each side about 1 inch, and ask him or her to copy it exactly as it is. All 10 angles must be present and 2 must intersect to score 1 point.)	( )	1
TOTAL SCORE	( )	30

INTERVIEWER: Assesses patient's level of consciousness along continuum.

Alert	Drowsy	Stupor	Coma

Source: From Folstein et al,[48] with permission.

> Dr: At 88 I think you're doing fine. Would it be okay for me to test your memory so we can get an idea of how much of a problem it is?

During the examination, patients will be more relaxed if you provide support and encouragement, especially when they struggle with finding the correct answers. For example:

> Dr: Please name this for me (interviewer shows patient a pencil).
> Pt: Well, it's something for something to say in, I don't know.
> Dr: Would you know how to use it?
> Pt: No, I don't think so. I couldn't even write my name anymore.
> Dr: You couldn't write your name anymore? Do you know what you could use this for?
> Pt: I have no idea.
> Dr: Okay, well it's a pencil.
> Pt: A pencil.
> Dr: You can write with it, you just do like this and you can write with it. I see that you wrote your name pretty well here.

Notice in this case how the physician provides information and positive reinforcement to the patient (an 82-year-old man with multi-infarct dementia) who, in fact, made a connection with the object ("I couldn't even write my name anymore.") but was unable actually to name it or describe its use.

The Third Party

No discussion of interviewing elderly patients would be complete without mentioning the issue of autonomy and the role of concerned family members or caretakers. Difficulties arise when the patient and "concerned others" disagree on the extent of disability caused by dementia or other illness, or when the patient and family disagree about the value of some proposed plan of treatment. In the case of a failing or frail octogenarian with mild dementia, it is often difficult to evaluate competence for medical decision making or to assess the legitimate interests of family or caretakers. Within the interview, we may hear different histories: The family of an 80-year-old woman reports that she leaves the stove untended and soils herself, but the patient denies these problems. Family members may want to see the doctor in private, out of the patient's earshot, then they forbid the physician to discuss their concerns with the patient. Or a daughter brings her mother to the office pretty much against the patient's will. How do you respect the concerns of family members and at the same time nurture the patient's autonomy?

The preceding sentence contains two words that summarize the last paragraph (and indeed this entire section on interviewing elderly patients): *respect* and *autonomy. First, you should approach your elderly patient with the same respect and concern that you have for any other patient.* Your contract as a clinician includes honesty, privacy, and confidentiality, as discussed fully in Chapter 15. Consequently, while being sensitive to the family's concerns about what grandma should or should not be told about her condition, it is important for you to stress her right to know and the fact that most elderly patients respond well to being fully apprised of their situation. Moreover, you should be sensitive to the patient's feelings about privacy and minimize the involvement of a third party in the interview if the patient so wishes. Respect for other family members demands that you make them aware at the outset of your clinican-patient contract: You will not collude with them to withhold information or to "help" the patient against his or her competent wishes.

Second, insofar as it is possible, you should nourish the patient's autonomy. Some elderly patients will have deficits that render them temporarily or permanently incompetent to make medical decisions. Standards for clinical evaluation of competence are presented in Chapter 15. However, even if your patient is judged incompetent, you continue to have an obligation to respect his or her interests. Sometimes you may disagree with family members about just what the patient's best interest is. For example, optimal medical treatment of an elderly, mildly demented man with heart disease might require a low-salt, cholesterol-lowering diet. This diet may eliminate most of the foods that he has enjoyed eating all his life. The patient's daughter might insist on sticking to "the letter of the law," cooking him only bland food that he doesn't like. Perhaps she believes this is in "dad's best interest." "He doesn't know what's good for him," she tells the doctor. Doesn't he? It might be far more beneficial to the patient as a person to enjoy life and enjoy eating, than at age 75 years to have a small reduction in his cholesterol level. In this case, the clinician's obligation (nourishing autonomy) might be to counsel the daughter to provide a more enjoyable—though perhaps less medically "correct"—diet for her father.

THE AMBULATORY PATIENT

We end this chapter with some consideration of the medical interview in ambulatory practice. In fact, most medical care takes place in the office or clinic, rather than in the general hospital. Yet most of us first learn to interview in an inpatient setting, assuming that patients have all the time in the world and that we can return to their rooms if we forget something and later wish to get more information. This "complete history" perspective ignores practical concerns that confront most clinicians, such as a reception area full of waiting patients. If hospitalized patients do not quite see the relevance of our asking about chickenpox in childhood, at least they are likely to bear with us because they are not concerned about the meter running out, a bus to catch, or a job to get back to. The ambulatory setting presents us with two priorities that seem to conflict with one another. *First,* because of time constraints and the sometimes minor nature of the medical conditions we encounter, we must learn to be efficient in interviewing and taking care of patients. *Second,* the wide array of problems that patients bring to their physicians, combined with another wide spectrum of beliefs about illness and expectations about medical care, demand that we invest a great deal of time "sorting things out" with most every patient we see. Can we be efficient while remaining sensitive to patients' needs and agendas? This section presents some suggestions about how to adapt the interview to serve both of these objectives in ambulatory practice. Here we focus on the ambulatory interview as a history-taking tool. The additional skills of contracting and negotiation are of critical importance to office or clinic practice, and are considered in detail in Chapter 14.

Letting Patients Have Their Say

Sometimes a desire for efficiency tempts us to abandon an open-ended interviewing style in favor of more focused questioning; we think that if we ask only the "right" questions or follow an algorithm, we will save time. If the patient has chest pain, we should ask "chest pain questions." If the patient has dysuria, we should immediately branch to a set of "cystitis questions." Another temptation is to cut the patient off before he or she finishes the opening statement, or perhaps even the chief complaint.[10] It might be difficult to imagine a medical history without a chief complaint, but here are some examples.

Example 1
Dr: Hello. You're here because of back pain?
Pt: Yes, I have lower back pain. And . . .
Dr: How long have you had it?

Example 2
Dr: Hi, how you been? I had you come back today to see how your depression is doing.
Pt: That part's okay. But . . .
Dr: How many pills are you up to now?

Notice it is the physician, not the patient, who states the "chief complaint" in these examples. The physican has closed the inquiry to other problems or symptoms by indicating what topics he or she wants to discuss. Beckman and Frankel[10] found in their study of internal medicine residents in an ambulatory clinic that the average time a patient was allowed to speak before being interrupted was only 18 seconds! Patients who are initially cut off and over controlled are likely to be dissatisfied and try to return again and again to "their" issue; perhaps worse, the clinician will work with inadequate data.

Paradoxically, *you often save time by remaining quiet and allowing the patient to talk.* Open-ended questions allow you to generate hypotheses quickly without relying on the patient's hypotheses about his condition. Although questions such as, "How's your diabetes?" or "How's your chest pain?" also may be necessary, they should be delayed until later in the interview.

Here are some examples of better ways to begin with office patients:

Example 1
Dr: Hi Mrs. Jones, I'm Dr. Walker. Nice to meet you.
Pt: Same here.

Dr: What brings you here today?
Pt: I'm having a problem with my back. It's still bothering me. And for the past 10 years, I've had a chronic problem with phlebitis in the legs, and I have some problem with my feet swelling at times and therefore circulation in both legs. But right now I'm having a devastating problem with my lower back. It's been going on ever since about the 20th of October. And I would like to see if I can get into a diet program.
Dr: A diet program?
Pt: Uh huh.
Dr: First, why don't you tell me about your back.

Example 2
Dr: What brings you here today?
Pt: Well, I have lumps on my head and they are itchy. I have had a stiff neck and a sharp pain. Since I am here, I might as well have it checked.
Dr: Okay. Have you had any other medical problems recently?

These physicians begin with open-ended questions that permit the patient to state a chief complaint and elaborate a bit on other concerns. In the following examples, the physicians go even farther to encourage the patients to state their problems.

Example 3
Dr: Tell me why you came today.
Pt: Well, I haven't had physicals on a regular basis. I'm feeling like I'm getting to a point where I ought to do that.
Dr: So you need a good physical.
Pt: Right.
Dr: You sure it's not a specific problem you noticed?
Pt: Not really.
Dr: Okay. But if you think of something while we're talking don't hesitate to mention it. How has your health been?

Example 4 (adapted from Beckman and Frankel[10])
Dr: How you been doing?
Pt: Oh well, I been doing okay, except for Saturday, well

Sunday night. You know I been kinda nervous off and on, but I had a little incident at my house Saturday and it kinda shook me up a little bit.

Dr: Okay.

Pt: And my ulcer, it's been burning me off and on like when I eat something if it don't agree, then I'll find out about it.

Dr: Right, okay.

Pt: But lately I've been getting this funny . . . like I'll lay down on my back, and my heart'll go "brrr," you know like that. Like it's skipping a beat or something, and then it'll just start . . . it'll just start beating boom-bom-bom and it'll just go back to its normal beat.

Dr: Okay.

Pt: Is that normal?

Dr: That's a lot of things. Anything else bothering you?

Pt: No.

In the third example, the physician notices the patient's hedge ("Not really," as opposed to something like "No, not at all.") and reassures him that he is welcome to bring up symptoms as the interview progresses. In the last transcript, the physician listens to each response, and continues to encourage the patient to state problem after problem until it is clear that there are no more. If you were seeing this last patient, would you be feeling just a little anxious that the list of concerns might never end? Beckman and Frankel[10] found in their study that no completed statement of concerns required more than 150 seconds. These two and a half minutes (usually much less) may be the most critical time of the interview, avoiding frustration and anger on the part of both physician and patient, preventing the "hands-on-doorknob" (see Chap. 3) phenomenon and ensuring that the patient's "hidden" agenda does not remain hidden.

In ambulatory care, the patient's needs may dictate that your interview lead to one of many different kinds of "history." In one case, the history might be a database on an asymptomatic person seeking guidance with regard to health risk factors or, in another case, a complex story of a patient with multiple severe symptoms who feels terrible and has little interest at the moment in his or her cholesterol levels. Other outpatients seek care for chronic illnesses that are influenced by both medical and psychosocial factors. Others being followed for chronic diseases may present with acute, perhaps unrelated, problems. Here is an example of a woman scheduled for a routine follow-up visit for two chronic conditions, who also had developed a new symptom and some "nonmedical" concerns. In the write-up, the first-year resident describes the "subjective" data (see Chap. 7) as follows (we have annotated the text to indicate the different types of problems):

> L.B. is a 50-year-old black female whom I am seeing in follow-up for newly diagnosed diabetes mellitus and hypertension. [chronic diseases] She has been on oral hypoglycemics and her concerns for this visit are that about 1 week ago she experienced a dramatic change in her visual acuity. [acute problem] She states that even with her glasses she is still unable to read as she had before. She can't see, her vision is blurry. She denies headaches or eye pain. She denies any other neurologic deficit. No numbness or tingling, no swelling of her extremities. Ms. B's other concern is that the Department of Labor states that if she has been ill, she is unable to collect unemployment benefits. [psychosocial concern] She requests a notification stating that she is medically cleared to continue seeking work and, therefore, eligible for unemployment benefits. [need for preemployment exam] Currently she states that she does have an appointment for an ophthalmologist, and she is going to follow up with that. She denies abdominal pain, nausea or vomiting, dysuria, and frequency or vaginal discharge.

Given this complexity, you frequently cannot attend to all the issues in one visit. Fortunately, you do not have to. For experienced clinicians, the complete database develops and evolves, extending and changing over the lifetime of the relationship with the patient. The database changes not only because the data may change but also because there is always more relevant data to know about the person.

Setting the Agenda

But what if the patient offers more complaints than you can handle in the time allotted? The answer lies in the opening moments of the visit during which you should not only demonstrate openness but also set the agenda for this visit. When the patient presents several concerns, you must establish priorities. What has to be attended to today? Next week? Next month? What is of most concern to the patient? To the physician? When there is disagreement between doctor and patient about these priorities, it is the physician's responsibility to take the lead in negotiating a resolution of the conflict (see Chap. 14).

In Example 4, notice how the interviewer obtains a little information about each problem in the opening seconds of the interview through the repeated use of minimal facilitators and open-ended questions. This initial phase establishes the range of problems and their breadth, but not their depth. It may be likened to the overture of a musical score in which each theme is briefly introduced but then dropped, only later to be developed more fully. In music, certain conventions and the composer's artistry determine the order in which the themes or melodies may be developed; in medical interviewing, the clinician and the patient decide how to proceed. When one problem is not clearly more urgent than another, the patient may be the one to decide how to use the limited time. However, when there is an urgent problem that the patient does not recognize or if the patient is not competent, the physician may play a more direct role in setting the agenda.

Failure to address the agenda issue early in the interview is likely to lead to "new" concerns popping up as you are ready to conclude the encounter. As you escort the patient to the door, he or she says, "By the way, I have this crushing substernal chest pain." What do you say at that point? Unrevealed agendas lead to *missed diagnoses* (some of them life threatening) not to mention *angry patients* (who know that they did not get what they came for) and *frustrated physicians* (who get telephone calls later that same day from patients who have just been seen and now have "new" complaints).

When there is more than one problem and none is clearly more urgent than another, a summary statement followed by a question and an explanation of your strategy may help:

> You've mentioned three concerns—your weight, this pain in your foot, and the premenstrual symptoms. Since our time is limited, which one would you like to focus on today? (or "first")

Or, if you notice an urgent problem that the patient has somehow overlooked:

> I can see that you're really bothered by this itching (summary statement and interchangeable response). But I noticed that your

weight is up about 10 pounds and you seem a little short of breath. Since our time is limited, is it okay if we check out your heart and lungs first?

It is easy to overlook new problems when a patient is scheduled for what looks like a routine follow-up visit and you start the interview off with, "How's the diabetes doing?" (open-ended but restricted to the diabetes) as opposed to, "How have things been going?" (totally unrestricted and may even invite nonmedical responses such as, "My health is great, but my job is driving me crazy.") "How has your health been?" or "How have your medical problems been doing?" are intermediate queries restricted to whatever concerns the patient perceives as health related. "What can I do for you today?" is a good beginning, especially for those clinicians with direct patient responsibilities; it is open-ended yet indicates the desire to focus on "today."

Here is an example of how you might begin an interim history for a patient with a number of chronic health problems:

Dr: Tell me why you came in today.
Pt: Just my regular visit. Dr. Smith said I had to come back for a checkup.
Dr: A checkup?
Pt: Yeah, he said I needed to have my blood sugar rechecked after he changed the medication.
Dr: Okay, fine. We can certainly take care of that. Anything else I should know about or that we should discuss before we get to that? Are you having any other problems?
Pt: Well, since my last visit I have noticed some trouble with my breathing.

Notice how the physician makes sure nothing else is going on. The blood sugar may not be a priority if the patient has since developed paroxysmal nocturnal dyspnea suggesting congestive heart failure. This search for *other active problems* (OAP, see Chap. 4) is an essential part of every initial or follow-up outpatient interview. In contrast to the complete database on a hospitalized patient, where the discussion of OAP tends to occur after the complete development of the history of the present illness, in the ambulatory setting, particularly for those with chronic disease, the discussion of OAP occurs early. The search for OAP is essential in setting the agenda to make the most efficient use of your brief time with the patient. In this context, the OAP pretty much replaces the complete ROS, which neither the physician nor the patient has the tolerance to repeat on each and every visit. Remember, if there is a new problem, the patient knows. Ask. Then give the patient time to respond.

We close this section with one final example. This is the opening segment of an interview with a 60-year-old woman who scheduled an appointment because she had been having chest pain. Notice the physician's confusion as she states her chief complaint:

Dr: How are you feeling today?

Pt: Oh, not too good. I still have that goofy headache.

Dr: You still have the headache?

Pt: And it's, I could say, one side, just sick. It's on the right side, and it starts here and it goes to the top of my head.

Dr: Have you ever had a headache like this before?

Pt: Oh, I've had headaches ever since 1950. I would take attacks and my blood pressure was very high and the doctor gave me medication.

Dr: I see. Is there anything different about this headache that you have right now compared to your other headaches that you've had? [search for iatrotropic stimulus, see Chap. 3]

Pt: Compared to the other headaches, this one is not quite as bad. But um, I've had it several days and it started about Sunday, and I'm worried about my blood pressure. Then I started having those chest pains.

Dr: And you've been having chest pains? Tell me about them. [search for other active problems]

Pt: Well, they're right here. (Patient points to right pectoral area and then reaches around to her back.) It's right up in here and down around in there. Sharp. Like I went to pick up something off the dresser and it just grabbed me.

Dr: Okay. And you're also worried about your pressure? [other active problems]

Pt: When I went to the store, they were taking it, it was a hundred and ninety something.

Dr: Okay. Uh, what, what would you say is the thing that's worrying you the most right now?

Notice that the physician has established both the range of problems (there are at least three) as well as their urgency (none are particularly urgent—the headaches are old and no worse, the chest pain is probably musculoskeletal, and the blood pressure has been taken and is 140/90). Given the limited time available, the physician now turns the agenda over to the patient who will dictate which problem to deal with at this visit. (By the way, this is the patient we met in Chap. 5 who responded that her big worry was "how to get those bills paid." So the agenda in this case was, indeed, hidden until the clinician "opened" the interview and permitted the patient to decide how best to use the visit.)

CHAPTER 9

The Difficult Interview:
Process and Topical Problems

... Seal up the mouth of outrage for a while
Till we can clear these ambiguities
And know their spring, their head, their true descent ...

The Prince, *Romeo and Juliet*, Act V, Scene 3

In our interactive model of the medical interview, both the doctor and patient play an active role in generating data that are as accurate and precise as possible. Sometimes even a novice interviewer finds it easy: The patient is alert, helpful, concise, and spontaneous; the problem itself is relatively straightforward; and there are no awkward elements such as a sexual problem. Sometimes, however, the interviewer—and usually the patient also—becomes aware that things are not going well. We label particular patients or specific situations as "difficult" when they present problems for us. These problems might arise from the patient, from the doctor, from the topic under consideration, or from extraneous events. We have argued earlier in this book that *observer bias* and *instrument precision* play a part in any medical observation, such as gallium scans, auscultation of heart murmurs, or generation of a medical history. There are ways of improving the quality of each of these observations even in the presence of adverse circumstances. For example, the interviewer can close the window so as to better hear the heart murmur or jiggle the ear pieces of the stethoscope to improve the air conduction component in order to perceive a murmur. The same is true with the difficult patient situation; remedial actions can improve the outcome.

There are many ways of classifying barriers to effective patient-doctor communication. Quill,[83] for example, presents a comprehensive taxonomy that includes environmental, physical, psychological, sociocultural, and interpersonal factors that can lead to failures in communication. Billings and Stoeckle[13] present a less extensive list that places more emphasis on physician emotional response and patient somatization. We prefer a simple taxonomy that focuses on certain difficulties that regularly arise during the course of medical interactions (Table 9–1).

These problems can happen to any physician and any patient, and are neither an indication of failure nor cause for despair; in fact, overcoming these problems can be an exhilarating experience for both patient and physician. At times, however, when the difficulty is more than a matter of one interview, i.e., the diffi-

TABLE 9–1. Difficult Patient-Doctor Interactions

1. Process problems
    a. Technical impairments
        (1) Organic (delirium or dementia)
        (2) Language barrier
    b. Style impairments
        (1) Reticence
        (2) Rambling
        (3) Vagueness
2. Topical problems
    a. Drugs, alcohol, diet, and smoking
    b. Sexual functioning
    c. Positive review of systems
3. Personality styles°
    a. Dependent, demanding patient
    b. Orderly, controlled patient
    c. Dramatizing, manipulative patient
    d. Long suffering, masochistic patient
    e. Guarded, paranoid patient
    f. Superior patient
4. Difficult feelings and defenses
    a. The patient's feelings and defenses
        (1) Anxiety
        (2) Anger
        (3) Depression
        (4) Denial
        (5) Manipulation and seductiveness
    b. The doctor's feelings and defenses
5. Somatization and somatoform disorders

Source: Adapted From Kahana and Bibring.[60]

culty pervades the entire doctor-patient relationship, it may be helpful to seek the advice of a colleague or suggest that a colleague assume the patient's care. We find it useful to categorize difficult patient interactions into five general types, even though there is frequently overlap between them (see Table 9–1). This taxonomy does not include *environmental* factors such as lack of privacy or noise level in the room. These are discussed in Chapter 3. Likewise, it does not deal with *sociocultural* and *health belief* issues that fit more appropriately into our discussion of negotiation (see Chap. 14). In this chapter, we discuss *process* and *topical* problems that can arise in the interview. In Chapter 10 we deal with *personality styles* and *difficult feelings and defenses*, while in Chapter 11 we cover the topic of *somatization.*

DIFFICULT PROCESS

Technical Problems

One type of difficult interview occurs when there are technical problems with obtaining information from the patient. Some obvious examples are: The patient speaks another language or the patient is comatose or semicomatose, delirious, psychotic, or demented. The patient simply lacks the cognitive or language skills to give good historical information that the physician can understand. Two examples of technical problems follow; the first is a non-English-speaking patient and the second is a demented patient.

In this interview with an Iranian woman everything was proceeding well until the physician asked the patient if she had any allergies:

> Dr: And do you have cough? (Demonstrates)
> Pt: No, no cough.
> Dr: Fever? Hot? (Touches forehead)
> Pt: Yes, yes I feel hot.
> Dr: Uh, allergy to medicine? Pill give you rash? Reaction? (Points all over skin, scratching to get at idea of itchy rash)
> Pt: (Looking confused) I don't know.
> Dr: Excuse me, I'll get your brother to help us speak.

In the following encounter with an elderly, demented patient, the patient simply cannot remember the symptoms he has been experiencing; rather, he is only aware of how he feels at present:

Dr: Do you know who I am?
Pt: Well, I don't know, no.
Dr: I'm Dr. Smith.
Pt: Oh.
Dr: I'm glad to see you today. How have you been feeling?
Pt: Oh, I don't know, just all poured out.
Dr: Weak, are you weak?
Pt: I imagine to a certain extent, but it seems just that nothing just seems to be right.
Dr: (Taking pulse) Your pulse feels good today.
Pt: I'm glad there's something good about me.
Dr: Do you feel there's not much good about you?
Pt: Oh well, I guess I'm just average.
Dr: How's your heart been treating you?
Pt: Oh, it never did bother me.
Dr: How are you sleeping at night?
Pt: No trouble at all.
Dr: How's your appetite?
Pt: Always with me.

We do not ordinarily label these situations "difficult" because we quickly dismiss the possibility of a useful interview and seek information elsewhere. In our examples, the physician got an interpreter for the Iranian woman and interviewed a family member of the demented patient. In fact, the elderly gentleman's wife stated that his appetite was poor, that he was having trouble sleeping, and that he was frequently short of breath. (Notice how the physician lapsed into a series of closed-ended questions that produced little in the way of useful information.)

There are other situations, however, that present problems of a more subtle and more frustrating nature. The profoundly depressed patient may not have enough energy to give a detailed, logical story of his problem, while the anxious and talkative patient may embellish her story with unnecessary details. Some patients are so reticent that you find yourself asking closed question after closed question until the interview comes to a distressing stop. Other patients seem to have so much to say that you feel as though you are losing control and getting confused about the nature of the diagnosis. You are worried that when the time is up, you may know a lot about the patient but very little about the illness. Let us look at ways to handle some of these problems; in particular, we will look at reticent, rambling, and vague patients. In each instance we will try to define the problem, give examples, and suggest possible remedies.

Style Impairments

THE RETICENT PATIENT

The Problem. The reticent patient does not say enough. Sometimes this is not a problem and may even be desirable: examples include the young person with a simple complaint like a sore throat in which only a limited amount of information is needed to develop a diagnostic strategy or therapeutic plan, or the patient with uncomplicated acute trauma such as a laceration. There are other times, however, when the lack of detail in a history creates serious problems in establishing the etiology of a symptom. An example is the patient with chest pain in whom a detailed and unambiguous history is essential for making the diagnosis. Such a patient may be very willing to answer "Yes" or "No," and you soon find yourself asking question after question in very tedious fashion and then running out of questions before gaining any idea as to what is going on.

The Remedy. The trick is to guide the reticent patient without asking leading questions; sometimes one way of asking an open-ended question works where another way does not. Consider this example:

> Dr: Can you tell me what the problem is?
> Pt: Uh, that's what I came to see you about, Doc.
> Dr: What have your symptoms been?
> Pt: Tired, awful tired.

It almost appears as though the interview will come to an end with the first question, but the interviewer simply asks another open-ended question that, this time around, elicits the chief complaint.

Another trick is to use a menu. This interview went on:

> Dr: Can you tell me more about it?
> Pt: No, just tired.
> Dr: When you say tired do you mean a feeling of not being rested or a feeling of weakness in your muscles? Or do you have trouble doing things you used to do because you get short of breath?
> Pt: That's it Doc, just not rested.

The physician uses a menu or "laundry list" to clarify further the symptom without leading the patient. Notice the difference between asking the patient to make a choice of a response and asking the same questions in sequence in yes/no fashion. If you find yourself asking many yes/no questions, you should question the worth of the response. The data are better when patients volunteer information than when the information has to be elicited, because in the latter instance, you can never be sure that these patients are not simply being agreeable or saying what they think they should say.

There are many reasons why some patients do not say much. Some of the more common ones are depression, dementia (the patient simply cannot remember his or her symptoms), anxiety, denial, a taciturn personality style, or cultural distance from the physician. Some patients expect to be interrogated like witnesses and must learn that we value their own selection and sequence of responses. These persons may have trouble with a directive such as "Tell me what happened." These individuals do better with "Tell me what happened first" and then "What happened next?" and even better with frequent reminders demonstrating your open, relaxed attitude, such as "It is important for me to know exactly how you felt when that happened—tell me as best you can."

THE PATIENT WHO RAMBLES

The Problem.   Some patients embellish their problems with numerous details that seem unrelated to the reason they came to see the doctor. In other settings such patients might be considered exquisite storytellers, but you may have a limited amount of time in which to get the story and you do not wish to be entertained. Sometimes the details seem connected to the story; at other times it is difficult to see any connection at all. At times the details are related to the medical history but are unnecessary, such as the patient who has an attack of diarrhea and describes in great detail his or her attempt to find a bathroom.

The Remedy. The trick is to direct the patient who rambles back to the task at hand without appearing to be rude or uninterested. One way to do this is to acknowledge your own confusion and feeling of being lost in the details, as well as your need to accomplish the task in a limited period of time. Most patients accept this kind of direction very well. For example, you might say to the patient with diarrhea:

> Dr: It certainly sounds as though you had a hard time with that episode; since our time is limited, perhaps you can tell me more about the diarrhea itself. Tell me what it was like.

In this instance the physician uses a summary statement (" . . . sounds as though you had a hard time . . .") and a reminder of time constraints, followed by a question that directs the interview back to the diarrhea; all the while the physician is making it clear that he or she is interested in what the patient has to say.

Here is an example, presented earlier in Chapter 3, of an open-ended question that leads to a deluge of disconnected information that would leave most students and many physicians feeling totally bewildered:

> Dr: Now what can I do for you, Mrs. P?
> Pt: Well, first of all, I'm here mainly because I've been experiencing that tired, worn out feeling, most of the time. I can go to bed say 9:00 in the evening and get up at 8:00 or even later and I still feel very tired. And, I don't know, maybe that's due, I've been still experiencing hot flashes and sometimes, now it's not I don't experience them as often as I used to but I still do and especially towards the evening or at night, and it awakens me when I do experience something like that. Maybe that's part of the reason why I feel so tired, I

> don't know. Anyways, now in the evening when I experience this kind of a hot feeling I just get that craving I want to eat, you know, or sometimes it works just the opposite where I feel kind of nervous, I get that nervous feeling, and now last week I had headaches just about every day on arising . . .

Although this patient may have just stated most of her medical history, it is hard to sort out the data. The fear most of us have of asking open-ended questions is that we may receive precisely this kind of rambling response. In reality such responses occur infrequently. The best thing to do is to acknowledge your confusion and try to direct the patient to one topic at a time. One possible reply might be:

> Dr: Okay, I'm getting a bit confused. Let's see if we can take one problem at a time. You mentioned tiredness even though you seem to get a lot of sleep. Other than the hot flashes is there anything else that seems to wake you up at night?

Either during or after the interview, you will have a chance to think about why the patient talks this way. There are many possible etiologies, among them anxiety, loneliness, histrionic personality style, thought disorder, or an unusual set of beliefs about how symptoms and events are related. Sometimes this kind of response is simply the person's conversational style, which is less appropriate in the context of a professional relationship than it is in a social interaction. Sometimes the associations are so bizarre that you must consider psychiatric illness as the cause.

THE VAGUE PATIENT

The Problem. With the vague patient, the interviewer cannot figure out exactly what the patient is describing. You may wonder whether it is the symptom that is vague or the patient's description that is vague. Some sensations are rather difficult to describe, e.g., dizziness or poorly localized abdominal pain. This is particularly frustrating when the diagnosis rests principally on an unambiguous history, as in the case of migraine or vertigo. When you know the patient, it is easier to know whether the problem is with the patient's description or with the symptom itself; the patient who has always given a precise history and is unable to describe a symptom precisely is probably experiencing a vague symptom, whereas a patient who has always given a vague history may well have a precise symptom that simply requires more work to translate into medically useful words.

The Remedy.   The technique for the vague patient is to provide a choice of useful descriptors without leading the patient. For example, you might use a menu such as, "Was the pain sharp or dull?" and "Was it all over, in one place, or did it move from place to place?" Alternatively, you can ask if it is anything like a symptom with which both the patient and physician are familiar, such as (for lower abdominal or pelvic pain in a woman) "Does it feel anything like menstrual cramps?" Another approach is to ask the patient if he or she has ever felt anything like this particular symptom before, and then to ask, "What's different about it this time?" To find the location of a vague symptom, you can point to various parts of the patient's body, especially while doing the physical examination, and ask, "Is this where it hurts?"

The following two examples illustrate vague openings. In the first example, the doctor simply indicates that vague terminology such as "cold or flu" (". . . tell me more about what you mean.") is unacceptable, and the patient begins to describe the symptoms in more detail. The patient in the second example does not respond to simple requests for more precision. Here is the first example, in which the doctor helps the patient to be more precise:

Dr: What can I do for you?
Pt: (Clearing throat) I think I've got, um, a cold or flu or something . . . yesterday I felt terrible, so I feel I just need some kind of a prescription. . . .
Dr: OK. Tell me, you say you have a cold; tell me more about what you mean.
Pt: Um (Clearing throat) fatigue is the most. . . .
Dr: Fatigue?
Pt: Just kind of drained.

Dr: Aha.

Pt: Kind of scratchy throat, not really sore. Ah, a lot of drainage. . . .

Dr: Coughing?

Pt: A little bit, but not getting anything up.

Dr: Just sort of dry?

Pt: Dry coughing, I don't feel as though there's anything collected down there yet. And, that's another thing that worries me, having had a history of asthma, I have a fear of bronchitis.

Here is the second example in which the patient remains vague:

Pt: Well, doctor, well, I got the dizziness, I'm getting more, looks like I'm, looks like I'm getting tired and more tired, I go up the steps and I just, just like dizziness, I, I go like this, I just go dark, I, and I can't see.

Dr: What do you mean by dizziness?

Pt: When I go up the steps and when I get up in the morning, I got that dizziness again, I'm just falling back.

Dr: What happens to you when you're dizzy?

Pt: Well, when, when I drink water, if I drink cold water, that's when I get it, then I start having chills, I get real cold, just like I'm shaking.

Dr: But how do you feel when you're dizzy?

Pt: I just go back, like this, and then sometimes I, I can't see, I, I have to close my eyes like that and then open my eyes up like that and I still can't just like. . . .

We are still left wondering whether the patient's description is vague or the symptom is vague. Dizziness is often hard for patients (even "precise" patients) to define. The physician in our last example above could have also tried to get more information by asking: "Tell me what you mean, but try not to use the word 'dizzy.'" Another remedy is to provide a menu:

Dr: When you say dizziness, is it a feeling that you may pass out or that you may lose your balance?

Pt: No, not exactly.

Dr: Could you describe it as a spinning sensation as though you or the room is moving, or is it more of a lightheadedness?

Pt: That's it lightheaded, just lightheaded.

While it would have been better for the patient to volunteer this information, you can be fairly safe in assuming that the patient does not have vertigo or presyncope.

Storytelling

All patients—whether reticent, verbose, rambling, or vague—are being asked for a story. You want a story that is clear, internally consistent, logical, and not fictional. Most patients desire these features as well but may not necessarily share with the physician the same criteria for judging them as such. Your first approach is to clarify and educate, teach, or demonstrate the kind of story that will be helpful. If this approach does not work, you are probably faced with one or more of three issues:

1. The patient's basic personality style, perhaps stressed by the illness, interferes with telling an adequate story.
2. Some strong emotion or affect gets in the way of the patient's telling a clear, logical story.
3. The patient's beliefs are both different from yours and unspoken, so a story that appears incoherent is actually quite logical once you understand the basic premises from which the patient reasons.

We examine these issues in Chapters 10 and 14. However, first we consider the second category in our taxonomy, topical problems in the interview.

DIFFICULT TOPICS IN THE INTERVIEW

At times, it is not so much that there is a technical impediment that prevents communicating with the patient, but rather there is a specific topic that is difficult to talk about. In this section we discuss three such topics because they are frequently troublesome in medical history taking:

Dieting, smoking, and drug and alcohol use;

Sexual functioning; and

The "positive" review of systems (ROS).

Each of these items is difficult for different reasons. A discussion of a history of drug or alcohol abuse requires the patient to be truthful about something that he or she may wish to hide, while a discussion of sexual history may violate certain societal taboos of what constitutes proper material for conversation. The "positive" review of systems is tedious and overwhelming for both patient and physician.

Dieting, Smoking, and Drug and Alcohol Use

You will encounter issues of patient motivation and intent when obtaining certain types of histories. Is the patient telling the truth? How do you judge intent? While physicians sometimes doubt the accuracy of patients' reports, in most cases these doubts are inappropriate because the patients are usually the best witnesses of their own symptoms. The situation is different, however, with self-reports about certain kinds of behavior. Assessing truthfulness is a common problem when trying to elicit dietary, smoking, drug, and alcohol histories. These are loaded topics, and most people (patients and physicians) feel that there are "right" and "wrong" answers to questions about them. For example, when asked "How much do you smoke?" many smokers reply "Too much." There is no quantification in this answer. The reply is colored by the patient's awareness that it is "wrong" to smoke. It may be easier for such patients to talk more neutrally about what age they started to smoke or how many times they have tried to quit.

Here is a smoking history obtained from a 40-year-old man presenting with shortness of breath. The physician tries to find out exactly how much is "not too much" and also tries to determine whether the patient's current respiratory symptoms caused him to cut down and whether the cumulative smoking history is sufficient to cause respiratory problems, such as chronic bronchitis or carcinoma of the lung:

Dr: Okay. How much do you smoke?
Pt: Oh, not too much.

Dr: How much is not too much?
Pt: Oh, umm, not half a pack a day.
Dr: Is that as much as you've always smoked? Have you ever smoked more than that?
Pt: Uh, when I was barbering, I would smoke more, sometimes a pack. You know, but they would burn out. You know, because when I was doin' a customer or something, they'd burn out, so I'd just light up another one.
Dr: Uh hmm. How old were you when you started?
Pt: Thirteen.

Similarly, a dependence on drugs or alcohol is seen by most patients as a habit of which the physician will disapprove. Some will deny the use of these substances, particularly if asked a yes or no question. Here is an example of a physician (who can smell alcohol on the patient's breath) trying to elicit the history of alcohol use in a 28-year-old woman presenting for evaluation of hypertension:

Dr: . . . You are using some aspirin and Tylenol?
Pt: Every once in a while. It's not regular but that's the only drugs I take.
Dr: And are you a pretty steady drinker?
Pt: I have one or two drinks at work, you know. After work I . . .
Dr: . . . Okay. Do you have any more than that?
Pt: Sometimes it's more than that but basically . . .
Dr: Is that something that would be hard for you to give up?
Pt: Well, it's a very social type thing for me, I guess . . . so . . . ye, yeah, I'd have to think about it, ha ha.

Often in this situation it is not so much what the patient says but how she says it. This patient paused and looked away when asked about how much she drinks, and she began to use phrases such as "you know" and hedges such as "basically." She also displayed some nervous laughter. These are often clues that the patient is saying something less than the truth. There may be pauses (time to censor material), shifts in position, eye aversion, and hedges in the verbalization, such as "not really" instead of "no." In this example, the physician does not gain much quantitative data about how much the patient actually drinks. The most revealing question is the indirect one ("Is that something that would be hard for you to give up?"), to which the patient's answer ranges from denial ("Well it's a very social type thing . . .") to agreement ("I guess so, yeah . . .") to ambivalence ("I'd have to think about it"). It is rarely useful to state to the patient that you doubt the accuracy of a story, especially when you have not already built a relationship with that person. You should, however, make a mental note of the behavior in the hope that at some time in the future, you will be able to use the information to help the patient.

Illicit drug use and narcotic addiction, particularly when the doctor is potentially the patient's source of drugs, is an even more difficult situation. Perhaps the best illustration we can give is the following story, written by a drug abuser for the express purpose of helping medical students and physicians understand and avoid pitfalls in the interview:

> I must convince this doctor that I *need* a narcotic, he thought, not that I *want* it. The peculiar logic practiced by doctors says that if I *needed* a narcotic, I wouldn't *want* it. And vice versa.
>
> Likely doctor's questions move through his mind and he rehearses his answers. He sees the coming scene as a confrontation of sorts. One which will have a winner and a loser. The doctor settles back in his chair. "What seems to be the problem?"
>
> Ernst's face shows pain. "There doesn't *seem* to be a problem, Doctor. There *is* a problem." Slowly and carefully he shifts his weight in the chair. "It's pain, and you wouldn't believe how it's ruining my life." He takes a breath. "I can't sleep at night; my boss is about to fire me; my wife's always in a bad mood now; my sex life's evaporated, I . . ."
>
> The doctor holds up a hand. "Just where," he asks, "is the pain located?"
>
> With a forbearing grimace, Ernst leans slowly forward in his chair. "My back. My lower back." He raises his eyebrows and looks the doctor in the eye. "I hurt it at the warehouse where I work. I do a lot of heavy lifting." He feels a sudden thrill of fear and thinks: Am I losing him? "Here," grunts Ernst, turning around and presenting his back.
>
> Ernst summons a mental image. He thinks: imagine his hands are tremendously hot. Fingers are red hot pokers. When they touch my skin, it'll burn like hell.
>
> The doctor probes with his fingers; Ernst, periodically hissing

through clenched teeth, twitches and jerks. The doctor makes note of "involuntary spasms."

"My dad had back trouble most of his life," states Ernst. "Something to do with herniated discs."

The doctor returns to his chair behind the desk. "What's your job at the warehouse?"

"Oh, a little of everything," Ernst replies.

The doctor frowns. "Perhaps you should find another type of work, something more suited to your problem."

"That'd be great—but who'd feed the kids in the meantime?" Ernst says, picking at the blank emblem on the breast of his blue workman's uniform.

The doctor opens a drawer in the desk. "There's a few questions I need to ask before we go on." He brings out the prescription pad. "Are you allergic to any drugs?"

Eyeing the prescription pad, Ernst says no and hurriedly clears his throat. "Ah, last week, when the pain was pretty bad, my wife gave me these pain pills she had left over. They worked just fine. I put in a good day's work."

"Do you know the name of them?"

"Perk, something."

"Percodan?"

"Well, she had two kinds. Both were Perk-something. One kind—they were yellow—gave me heartburn; the other—they were white—really helped."

The Doctor begins to write. "Perco*cet* is what you mean." Pleased with himself, Ernst thinks: Perco*cet* is *exactly* what I mean!

This story was written while the patient was in remission. It was designed not to make physicians skeptical of all such requests for pain medication but rather to illustrate the importance of a careful history and clinical evaluation. Sadly, the patient subsequently relapsed and died of an overdose.

Sexual Functioning

This is an important part of the medical history. Depression, anxiety, and anger may relate to underlying sexual problems; conversely, many physical symptoms or diseases may lead to sexual dysfunction. Asking even a few questions about sexual functioning sends the message that the physician is willing and available to discuss sexual concerns if the patient wishes.

As with any other part of the medical interview, how much you need to know depends on the situation. There is no requirement to get a complete sexual history from every patient, just as there is no need to get a complete cardiorespiratory history from a 20-year-old woman who jogs 6 miles a day and has come for a pre-employment examination. Sometimes one question ("Are you having any sexual problems?") suffices. If the patient answers in the negative, no more need be said at that point; you have, however, indicated that sexual problems are legitimate fare for discussion to which the patient may return later (either in that visit or in a subsequent one). Of course, some patients will answer a simple screening question about sexual concerns in the affirmative, or sometimes the patient's constellation of symptoms leads you to inquire more thoroughly about sexual behavior and functioning. Then it is your job to be skillful and appear comfortable (even if you are not) in discussing sexuality.

A discussion of sexual matters may not feel routine to the patient and may be unexpected, especially if the patient is used to physicians who do not ask about sex or if he or she feels that the presenting complaint is unrelated to sexual functioning. For example, the young man presenting with severe sore throat may be very surprised at your interest in his sexual activity, unless you explain that his negative streptococcal culture, negative test for mononucleosis, and failure to improve raise the question of gonorrhea pharyngitis.

Unless they relate to the presenting complaint, it is best not to jump right in with sexual questions early in the interview. In fact, knowing something about the patient as a person facilitates asking such difficult questions. For example, once you know whether the patient is married or is living with someone, it is easier to ask about sexual preference and activity. When in doubt, you should use the term "partner" rather than a gender-specific terms such as "boyfriend" or "wife." If you ask only about opposite-sex partners, the patient may infer that you would be shocked by a report of homosexual activity. The homosexual patient may, therefore, avoid relating his or her actual sexual preference. On the other hand, the happily married 65-year-old may well be offended by the use of the term "partner." There is no easy way to ask about sexual preference, but it is almost always necessary to know; the more you know about the patient's lifestyle, the easier it is to ask such intimate questions.

Delaying this part of the history until later in the interview will also make it easier to use words that the patient can understand, as you become more familiar with the patient's language style. As with other intimate bodily functions (voiding and defecating), patients may describe their sexual functioning with words conditioned by their age, level of education, and cultural background. Some other descriptions may be idiosyncratic and obscure. What do the words "relationship," "birth control," or "careful" mean? Open-ended questions permit the patient to use his or her own words. In your follow-up questions, you can use the patient's words, thereby ensuring a common language, once you know precisely what the patient's words mean.

The sexual history can be included in a nonthreatening way as part of the ROS, for example, while dealing with menstrual or obstetric issues in women or with genitourinary issues in men. The focus is always on the patient's own perception of whether there is a sexual problem, not a voyeuristic account of frequency and techniques. As in any other intimate matter, you should not probe if the patient does not wish to discuss the matter. You may continue with questions about other aspects of the health history, at the same time building rapport, and return to the sexual history, if necessary, when more trust exists.

Here are some examples of useful questions to initiate a discussion of sexuality:

- "Are you having any sexual problems?"
- "Do you have any questions or concerns about sexuality or sexual functioning?"
- "Many people who are ill experience a change in their sexual function. Have you noticed any change?"
- "Has your interest in sex changed recently? Since you've been ill? Since you've been on the new medicine for your blood pressure?"

An introductory statement followed by a question often puts patients at ease:

- "A lot of men have sexual problems when they take Inderal. Have you noticed any problems?"
- "It sounds as though your marriage has been a good one. How about your sexual relationship?"

- "Many girls your age have questions about sex and birth control. How about you?"
- "Many people these days worry about AIDS. Do you have any concerns about possibly being at risk for AIDS?"

If the patient indicates problem areas, then proceed with more detailed questioning. Sexual dysfunction may result from any combination of physical, pharmacological, or emotional problems. Physicians should explore the medical reasons that may account for or contribute to dysfunction, as well as assess the emotional component.

The sexual history, like any other part of the medical interview, should be tailored to the situation. The history should be more extensive, for example, when a patient requests birth control, fears a sexually transmitted disease, or has a sexual problem as a presenting complaint. Consider this example:

Dr: You don't look as tired as you were before.
Pt: I'm not as tired since I've been taking the iron pills.
Dr: That's helped, huh. Well, do you have another problem?
Pt: Yeah, with my stomach. When I have sex, my stomach hurts right here. After, that, it doesn't bother me.
Dr: When you have sex? Otherwise you feel good?
Pt: Uh huh.
Dr: Okay. When did all this start?
Pt: About a month ago.
Dr: And has it gotten any better since that time?
Pt: Uh uh, it's the same.
Dr: Has it gotten any worse?
Pt: Sometimes it gets worse.
Dr: When you're not having sex you feel fine?
Pt: Uh huh. But sometimes, when I walk I get this real sore pain and then I get real bad.
Dr: When you have the pain during intercourse, is it all the time during intercourse or at the beginning or at the end? Or, only when he is thrusting inside?
Pt: Right here.
Dr: Only on that side. Does it hurt anywhere else?
Pt: Uh uh.

Dr: Have you ever had this problem before?
Pt: It always did that.
Dr: So you've had this a long time.
Pt: Ah ha.
Dr: What made you think now it might be serious even though it didn't get worse.
Pt: It gets worse sometimes. But I just get . . . but I just thought it was nothing.
Dr: Can you think of any reason why you want to get it checked now?

Pain on intercourse can be a sign of pelvic abnormality (pelvic inflammatory disease or endometriosis), underlying depression, or problems in the particular relationship. The physician in our example above follows simple rules of good history taking, asking open-ended questions ("Do you have another problem?") and then the basic when ("When did all this start?"), where ("Does it hurt anywhere else?"), why, and why now questions ("Can you think of any reason why you want to get it checked now?"). The physician also uses more specific questions to obtain precise details of the problem ("When you have the pain during intercourse, is it all the time during intercourse or at the beginning or at the end? Or only when he is thrusting inside?") Because many patients have difficulty discussing such details, in part because they are unsure of what words are acceptable, the physician gives the patient a number of choices from which to choose her answer. This reticent patient has difficulty even with these choices and, instead, answers the question by pointing to the location of the pain. The physician obtains the useful information that the pain is limited to one side, but still does not know at what part of intercourse it occurs.

In this example, because the symptom relates directly to sexual activity, there is much more that we need to know. It would be helpful to know if the patient's desire—libido—has changed ("Do you feel like making love—having sex—more or less than you used to?") or if her ability to enjoy sex has changed ("Do you feel satisfied when you make love?"). Choose words that you are comfortable with and that the patient can understand. If you are not sure you are being understood, ask ("Do you understand what I am asking?"). As much as possible, you should ask questions that permit patients to answer from their own point of view and in their own way ("Do you feel satisfied?" as opposed to "Do you have an orgasm?").

When you suspect a sexually transmitted disease, it may be necessary to know about sexual preference as well as number and regularity of sexual partners, and to ask if the partners have had any sexually transmitted disease symptoms. These are difficult questions to ask because a sexually transmitted disease may be embarrassing for the patient and he or she may not want to acknowledge that a partner may have gone outside the relationship. Patients may feel anger and guilt and perceive the physician as accusatory.

Skill is required to express your questions in the same neutral way that you talk about illnesses or infections. "Are you concerned that you might have gotten this from someone?" or "Is there any chance that you have been exposed to someone with a similar infection?" Such questions often help the patient talk about the situation more easily with responses such as "I don't see how I could have gotten this from my boyfriend unless he's not playing straight, while I am," or "My lover did go to the doctor because he had a drip, but he never told me to get checked or anything." Sometimes it helps to introduce a difficult question with a statement, such as "I think you may have an infection that is acquired only during sexual intercourse, but I don't want to make any assumptions about your sexual relationships. Is it possible that you've been with someone who has this?" If the patient says "That's impossible," you must accept that statement as representing the patient's belief at that moment. The doctor can still prescribe the appropriate treatment and add, "If you do know anybody who might have this, it would be good if you could tell them to get checked." Do not argue with the patient. If the diagnosis is uncertain, say so and outline the plan for making the diagnosis clear. In the case of reportable venereal diseases for which health departments do case finding, the doctor can say, "By law, I am required to report this illness, and there may be someone from the health department who will talk to you about who else might have it."

Another difficult situation arises with teenagers (see Chap. 8). Sexually active teenagers are at risk for sexually transmitted disease and females, of course, are at risk for pregnancy. In evaluating any genitourinary or pelvic problem, it is therefore necessary to ask about sexual activity. You should do so, however, without implying either approval or disapproval of the patient's having intercourse. Some 13-year-old girls have been pregnant, while others have little knowledge of sexuality at all. It is helpful to begin with the patient's interest in school, social activities, then "boys?" (or "girls?"), and finally "sex." Some helpful questions are:

- "Do you have any questions about your body? About sex? About how not to get pregnant?"
- "Do you have any need for birth control?"
- "Are your friends or the kids at school into having sex yet? How about you?"
- "Some girls (boys) your age get pretty serious about boys (girls) and start having sex. How about you?"

Patients should be allowed to answer in their own way, with your assurance that the information will be confidential. Males should be questioned about their risk of getting someone pregnant as much as females should be asked about their risk of pregnancy.

Here is an example of the kind of sexual problem that arises frequently in medical patients. You should determine if the problem is the result of medication side effects or of difficulties in the relationship or some combination of factors.

Dr: ... Are you living at home now? Living with your boyfriend?

Pt: He's like 16 years older than me and we've been together for about 15 years, but see there's a, a little bit of a problem when we have to, 'cause see since I've been on those steroids, you know it messes with your sex life, too. I don't have any.

Dr: You don't have any desire?

Pt: No, and uh, that creates a problem. I just have no desire. It was like if he put his hands on me, I might get real evil, you know, like get your hands off of me, you know.

Dr: I see. How are things between you and him otherwise? Are things strained in general?

Pt: I wish he would get out of my life.

One final note will be discussed here. The sexual history may be that part of the interview in which patients are most likely to ask how you personally feel about something, in this case sexual matters, perhaps because sex is a common experience about which most people have opinions and beliefs. Many people also want to know what is "normal" and discern whether they fit the normal standard. Do not confuse being genuine with giving personal details of your own life that you are not comfortable discussing. You are not having a conversation with a friend. You are a professional trying to obtain information essential to the diagnosis and management of a patient. Some questions that patients may put to you are clearly inappropriate ("What would you do? Would you have an abortion?" or "Did you have sex before you got married?" or "Don't you think homosexuality is a sin?"), and it is best to answer (no matter what you think) in a polite and straightforward manner, "Well, we're not here to discuss what I think. I'm more interested in finding out how you feel about this pregnancy (or about learning that your daughter is gay)." In this way, you will help the patient explore his or her own feelings and symptoms as opposed to yours, which are not the focus of the interview.

The Positive ROS

Some patients give a very literal interpretation to the questions in an ROS, answering "yes" to almost every question. When this happens the task seems to become interminably tedious, and the interviewer fears that the history will never end. Sometimes, in addition to being positive, the answers are also given in great detail about relatively trivial matters. For example, while you may want to know if the patient wears glasses, you may have little interest in the fine details of how the patient's refractive error has changed in the past 5 years or what the patient feels about his or her optometrist. A difficult ROS might begin this way:

Dr: Now I'd like to ask you a series of questions just to make sure we haven't missed anything important, Okay?
Pt: Fine.
Dr: I'll start with your head, and we'll work our way down. Do you get headaches?

Pt: Oh, I'm used to terrific headaches all through my life,
and one doctor said it was high blood pressure though
I didn't know it at the time.

We seem to be off to a bad start as we do not expect or desire
a severe chronic problem to surface for the first time in the ROS;
now, instead of zipping down the list of questions, the interviewer has to stop and ask the details about the headaches. When
this happens, usually one of two things is going on: Either the
physician has failed to inquire in an empathic way about other
active problems and significant past medical history or the
patient "overinterprets" the question and is describing in detail
a problem that is neither active nor significant.

The best way to deal with this situation is to prevent it in the
first place by asking about other active problems and significant
past medical problems soon after the questions concerning the
present illness. Not only does this maneuver uncover such problems early in the interview, but it also facilitates seeing connections between these problems and the present illness. If this
technique fails or if one forgets to use it, however, there are a
number of other approaches.

First, you may try to bring the patient back to the present
with a reminder that the primary interest is those symptoms
that are a problem now.

Second, you may make the questions very general—"Have
you ever had any stomach or bowel trouble?"—and ask for
further details only when the initial screening is positive.

Third, you may encourage the patient to filter out the
unnecessary details by reminding the patient of the time
limitations or by asking him or her to pick out the most
important symptoms.

Fourth, you may undertake the ROS while performing the
physical examination and save time in that way.

CHAPTER 10

The Difficult Interview: Personality Styles and Feelings

> When you've once said a thing, that fixes it, and you must take the consequences.
>
> The Red Queen *in Lewis Carroll's Through the Looking Glass*

PERSONALITY STYLES

Another difficulty in medical interviewing arises when the patient's personality style interferes with obtaining objective and precise data. This, of course, is a matter of degree; everyone has a personality style, and under stress, such as that which accompanies illness, distinct coping behaviors identified with certain personalities may become exaggerated. Sometimes identifying a particular style gives you important information: how patients perceive their illness, how they "filter" historic data, and how they generally interact with other people. For example, many patients have a difficult time coping with the hospital schedule and milieu. The hospitalized patient whose nurse did not bring the bedpan promptly and who is generally being treated with a lack of compassion has good reason for fury; this patient may generalize that anger to other personnel, including the medical student or resident who is trying to get a history. The interviewer is confronted with real anger arising out of a real situation, but the anger is not of his or her own making. The best thing to do in this situation is to acknowledge the anger and the patient's right to be angry and to accept the patient's good reasons even if you do not personally agree with them. Allowing the patient time to ventilate his or her feelings in a controlled way permits most interviews to proceed and reinforces your interest in the patient.

Kahana and Bibring[60] present some useful observations on personality styles and suggest ways of coping with them during the interview in order to maximize your ability to obtain accurate data. The styles are:

1. The dependent, demanding patient;
2. The orderly, controlled patient;
3. The dramatizing, manipulative patient;
4. The long-suffering, masochistic patient;
5. The guarded, paranoid patient; and
6. The superior patient.

This is a useful classification to orient our discussion, although we rarely see people who exhibit a truly "pure" style.

The Dependent, Demanding Patient

This type of person strives to impress the physician with the urgent quality of all of his or her requests. The patient needs special attention, great reassurance, and constant advice. The doctor may first see an optimistic, compliant, and "good" patient, but soon finds that the patient expects a limitless amount of attention and care. Groves[53] described this type of person as one of his "hateful patients" and used the term *dependent clinger.* When the patient's need for "boundless interest and abundant care" is unmet, he or she may become depressed or withdrawn, or blame the doctor in a complaining or vengeful way. The physician who tries to meet every demand risks exhaustion.

In many acutely ill patients, dependent tendencies temporarily come to the fore and should be met with active, empathic, and generous care directed toward the patient's physical and emotional comfort. However, when this pattern becomes exaggerated or chronic, the doctor must set limits by stating specific follow-up appointments, specific written instructions, and a clear understanding of the patient's responsibility. It is important for the beginning physician to learn to "protect the patient from promises that cannot be kept and from illusions that are bound to shatter."[53] This is not the patient for whom you should arrange special appointment times, permit repeated phone calls after hours for nonemergency problems, or make the repeated calls to the pharmacy for prescriptions that all seem to run out on different days.

Similarly, within the interview itself, the goal is to set limits for the patient so that the basic task at hand, that of obtaining accurate historic data, can be accomplished. This means that the patient must understand the limits of the "contract" (e.g., you are a student, albeit an interested one, doing a medical history), as well as the need to discuss specific types of information in order for you to understand the patient's problems. Useful techniques include the following:

1. Suspect this problem in new patients who make you feel that you are the only one who has ever cared about them or understood their illness.
2. Avoid making promises that you cannot keep, such as solving a medication or nursing problem.
3. Give the patient responsibility with a statement such as "Perhaps you can talk with the nurses about your pain medication."
4. Remind the patient that your time is limited, despite the fact that you are interested in his or her story. Try a statement such as "You certainly have a lot of important problems, but since my time is so short, I'd like to get back to the reason you came into the hospital."
5. Do not take credit for remission in the patient's symptoms, as you will be likely blamed for a relapse, which is sure to follow. Give responsibility to the patient with a statement such as "You're the one who did what was necessary to get better."

The Orderly and Controlled Patient

These patients, when under stress, cope by gaining as much knowledge as possible about their situation, not only to deal with their problem rationally but also to handle their anxiety. These patients are punctual for appointments, conscientious in taking medications, and preoccupied with the right way and the wrong way of carrying out your instructions. Sickness threatens these patients with loss of control. They find the scientific medical approach congenial to their way of thinking and respond well to the professional, systematic sequence of history taking, physical diagnosis, laboratory studies, and therapy. They may present with a list of carefully thought-out questions or a precise diary of their symptoms.

Since this type of patient is often on the same "wavelength" as their doctor, it would not appear to present a difficult situation. However, the doctor must be careful to explain the problem thoroughly and describe carefully any laboratory tests or procedures. Pausing a little longer over auscultation of the heart or inquiring into an area of history seemingly unrelated to the patient's problem may cause excessive anxiety in these patients unless the physician takes care to explain why he or she is doing these things. These patients must be permitted to take charge of their own medical care and be given positive feedback about their efforts and abilities.

Within the interview, this type of patient finds it helpful if the physician has an orderly and systematic approach, with frequent explanations as to what is happening. Summarizing what you have heard reassures this patient that you are listening and that you are not missing any of the details the patient considers vital to making the diagnosis. This patient will be reassured by note taking (he or she does not want you to forget anything important) but will be alarmed if you suddenly write something down when you have not been writing all along. If you are asked why you are pursuing a particular line of questioning, make it clear that the purpose is routine or that you want to clarify an item; do not alarm the patient by revealing the diagnostic hypotheses that may be running around in your head and that led to a particular question. Here is an example:

Dr: How have you been?
Pt: I was trying to remember if I was supposed to call you. I think, I don't remember when I called last and now I couldn't remember if I was supposed to call you again or not.
Dr: Well, that's fine. I just was hoping that you hadn't tried and not gotten through or something like that. I understand you got new glasses. Has that helped?
Pt: I don't see the slightest difference.
Dr: You're not happy because you're having trouble seeing?

> Pt: I'm not happy because I don't see as well as I would like to see. I can't see numbers well.
> Dr: Does the eye doctor give you an explanation?
> Pt: Well, he keeps talking. He talks to me, referring, speaking to me as "your cataract" and I said to him plainly, I said you referred to my cataract many times. You have never told me I have a cataract. Do I? And he said everyone over 30 years old has a cataract. So that's . . .
> Dr: So that's really not an answer. So you don't know whether it's the cataract, whether you have it in both eyes, or whether there's some other problem.
> Pt: I don't know and I can't get a straight answer.

And later in the interview,

> Pt: I wanted to tell you about that and I'm trying to think if there is anything else I should tell you. I don't remember anything. Of course, some of the problems are getting worse but I don't consider that something that wasn't expected. I assume that's what we should expect. Everything else is pretty much under control.

Notice how carefully this patient uses her words. When the physician says, "You're having trouble seeing?" she "corrects" this wording with "I don't see as well as I would like to see." She does not say, "There isn't anything else I should tell you," she says instead, "I don't remember anything" (and this is interesting, because she is elderly and knows she has a little trouble with her recent memory). Notice her concern with doing the right thing, being compliant—"I was trying to remember if I was supposed to call you.") Consider the importance to her of explanations and how disquieted she is by the ophthalmologist's evasiveness—"I can't get a straight answer.") Despite the fact that "some of the problems are getting worse," she tolerates that because "I don't consider that something that wasn't expected." What is good is that "everything else is pretty much under control." Note how the physician is able to clarify her concerns while avoiding explanations about a problem with which he is unfamiliar (i.e., her eye problem for which she sees someone else).

The Dramatizing, Manipulative Personality

This type of patient may first present as interesting and charming, even when he or she dramatizes and makes global statements about symptoms: The pain is "the worst pain I have ever had . . . it's with me all the time, day and night, nothing seems to help . . . I haven't been able to sleep in weeks. . . ." This type of person may have a great need to be at stage center and may resent the doctor's interest in other duties and other patients. "To the dramatizing emotionally involved kind of person, sickness may feel like a personal defect; it means being weak and unattractive, unappreciated, and unsuccessful."[60] These patients are frequently characterized as manipulative and sometimes, particularly when dealing with a doctor of the opposite sex, as seductive.

We have emphasized the importance of allowing the patient to tell the story in his or her own words with some direction from the interviewer but without the high control style that produces poor data. However, there are times when the issue of control is central to the interview process; the patient wants too much control, and you are unable to obtain the information you need. Sometimes the problem permeates the entire history. At other times, the problem is limited to a particular part of the history, e.g., the patient with a drug problem steers the discussion into other areas every time you approach the question of substance abuse.

Sometimes the patient wants to control you and engages in a type of behavior not usually appropriate to a professional relationship, such as noticing your new watch or hairstyle, complimenting you on your good taste, or asking personal questions about your social relationships or sexual preference, or asking whether you have ever had an abortion. Here are some guidelines for dealing with this type of behavior in the interview:

1. Listen and observe the patient as he or she demonstrates this type of behavior. Think: What does the patient gain by this behavior?
2. Control the urge to engage in open warfare for control of the interview by feeding back what you hear and clarifying points.
3. Remain calm, gentle, and firm, using frequent summaries to regain or stay in control.

4. Remain descriptive, not judgmental or evaluative; focus on the how, not the why. For example, "I've noticed that when I try to ask you about drug use you tend to change the subject," *not* "Why don't you answer my question?"

5. Identify the strengths of the patient and feed them back by establishing a profile of the premorbid person, as well as of the patient you are currently interviewing.

6. Remember that if the patient with chronic pain has been suffering for months, or years, he or she will survive suffering one more minute, hour, day, week, month.

7. Try reflecting back to the patient with a statement such as "Well, we're really not here to talk about my opinion . . . I'm interested in hearing more about you. How did *you* handle that?" if the patient asks you a personal question or one you are uncomfortable about answering.

8. Reframe seductive behavior positively as one of the patient's many possible moves toward attaining goals in his or her life. For example, you can say, "I see that you enjoy being an attractive person and you enjoy being with a man and being noticed by him and taken care of by him. How do you meet those needs in your life?" or "So you are a widower, how has that been for you?"

A thorough history in a respectful atmosphere where you demonstrate you are in charge is the best way to build a solid relationship with the patient and to establish a treatment plan that will be acceptable.

The Long-Suffering, Masochistic Patient

Groves[53] describes this group of patients as *help rejectors.* They give a history of continual suffering from disease, disappointment, and other adversity. They see their lives as a sequence of bad luck. Often they disregard their own needs in order to do things for other people. Despite apparent humility, these patients may have a tendency to be exhibitionist about their long-suffering fate. With regard to medical care, they feel that no treatment will help; when one symptom goes away, another appears in its place.

The physician must understand that simple reassurance of optimism will not be "bought" by the masochistic patient. He or she will be better able to cooperate in a medical history or a medical treatment if it is seen in the context of adding to his or her "burden," rather than for personal relief. "The physician may have to present the recovery to the patient as a special additional task, if possible for the benefit of others."[60] The doctor might have to share the patient's pessimism rather than try to talk it away.

Within the interview it is important to avoid talking the patient out of the severe nature of his or her suffering. Similarly, it is helpful to avoid overly optimistic or patronizing remarks, such as "I'm sure your doctor will have you feeling better in no time." While this patient may not regard talking to a medical student as therapeutic, he or she may like the idea of helping *you* by permitting you to do a history and physical. Accept the patient's pessimism with a statement such as "It sounds as though you don't think there is much hope of you getting better."

Consider the following interchange with an 82-year-old woman who is experiencing failing abilities and is trying to care single-handedly for her severely demented 89-year-old spouse:

Dr: How have things been going for you?
Pt: Well, not much different. Same as usual. Same problems, same lack of solutions. I'm not saying that anyone would give me a different answer, but I still don't have to like it.
Dr: Yeah, you feel that you've gotten that answer to a lot of problems.
Pt: I feel that I've gotten that answer everywhere. Everything that I have problems with. Everything, that is, except Dr. Jackson who wants to operate on my throat . . .
Dr: Which you don't want.
Pt: No. Pretty hopeless, isn't it.
Dr: Well, I think you're doing about as well as anyone could do.
Pt: Well, I don't know, maybe I am. Again I say it's not good enough, but I don't suppose there's any good enough in a situation like that.
Dr: How do you feel about the medication right now? Do you think it's helped your spirits at all?
Pt: I like to believe it does. I can't be real sure because I

> don't know how I'd be feeling without it, but I try to imagine it soothes me some.
>
> Dr: Good.
>
> Pt: I don't think it's doing me any harm.
>
> Dr: Good. What about getting some extra help at home. Have you made any progress with that?
>
> Pt: I don't know. The reason I have resisted is because I had a sister-in-law who could not live alone and she had an endless succession of people that I know stole from her and robbed her.
>
> Dr: The best thing is to get either someone that you know well or a person that is recommended by someone you trust.
>
> Pt: That's true but I don't think that person exists.
>
> Dr: I wish there were something I could do to help.
>
> Pt: I don't expect you to have solutions. It's just how things are. Nothing can change.

This kind of interchange is enough to make any physician feel pretty hopeless as well. Note the patient's repeated return to the theme of no solutions. The most (and it is not much) optimistic she gets is "I like to believe" that the antidepressant she has been taking is helpful, at least "I don't think it's doing me any harm." The physician finally gives up making suggestions and begins to share the patient's pessimism—"I wish there were something I could do to help." (The patient, in turn, paradoxically reassures the physician—"I don't expect you to have solutions.")

The Guarded, Paranoid Patient

These patients are inclined to be suspicious of the doctor and the medical care establishment. They may present a long list of slights from other doctors and openly point out how the illness was mishandled; or they will blame others for their illness. During stress, the patient may become "even more fearful, guarded, suspicious, quarrelsome and controlling of others."[60] The doctor may find himself or herself always feeling "on guard" during the interview, as if to avoid being "caught" in some sort of competitive relationship.

It is important to give this patient clear explanations of your strategy for diagnosis and treatment. If you are a medical student or house officer, you must pay particular attention to identifying your role and clarifying its limitations. These patients may make provocative statements, but arguing with them or ignoring the suspicious attitudes does not help. The best approach is to maintain a friendly and courteous attitude, while acknowledging the patient's beliefs; it is not necessary to agree with these patients, but there is no hope of dissuading them.

Within the interview, a frequent problem you will encounter with these patients is their stated disgust with those caring for them, namely doctors and nurses. The patient may say with great exasperation, "All I want to know is, if I've had a heart attack . . . why doesn't my doctor tell me yes or no?" If you were to analyze this request, several issues would have to be resolved: Does the doctor know and is not telling, or does he or she simply not know yet and therefore cannot tell? And is there some reason the patient expects to know now as opposed to tomorrow? It is rarely useful to try to unravel such a situation, in part because the answers may not be there and in part because the patient may think that you are taking sides either with or against him or her. It is better to acknowledge and accept the patient's suspicions and frustrations with a statement such as "It must be terribly frustrating, not knowing." Then try to proceed with a history by reminding the patient that while there is nothing you can do to help with that particular problem, you are interested in hearing more about the symptoms that brought him or her to the hospital.

The Superior Patient

These patients have strong self-confidence and may appear smug, vain, or grandiose. Their behavior in the medical care situation is often that identified by Groves[53] as the *entitled demander*. They may demand the most senior physician or the most well-known subspecialist, and be very condescending or arrogant toward house officers and students. They may attempt to control the physician by making many demands and sometimes by threatening litigation. As Groves[53] writes, "entitlement serves for some persons the functions that faith and hope serve in better adjusted ones." Often, this patient may react to situations that occur in the hospital with anger and hostility; anger that can impinge upon you as the medical student or house officer. Some suggestions for dealing with anger are presented later in this chapter and are appropriate for this type of patient.

Sometimes a patient makes demands on the physician that he or she would not ordinarily make. Consider this example of a young actor who had never had any difficult interactions with his physician until he developed a "cold or flu or something which normally I would just wait until it went away except I'm involved in a show right now." The dialogue continues:

> Pt: And it's the leading role in a rather important production and we open this Thursday (clears throat) and I went into this cold.
> Dr: You open this coming Thursday.
> Pt: And I went into a cold; it feels like it's been in my system for about 2 weeks, but then on about Thursday it started clearing up. Then because of an audition Friday morning I got like 6 hours of sleep. Friday I started to feel coldish, Saturday I felt terrible, yesterday I felt terrible, so I feel I just need some kind of prescription . . . to be able to deal with it.

So this patient who would "normally just wait" suddenly feels entitled to treatment for a problem that is self-limited and that has no definitive therapy. It is as though the patient is saying, "I know there is no cure for a cold, but since I'm the lead in an important production you must make an exception and cure me." This sounds paradoxical and illogical. In such a situation, the physician might respond:

> Dr: There's no cure for the common cold! Actors are no different from anyone else!
> Pt: If you won't help me I'll find someone who will.

But things go better if the doctor says:

> Dr: I can understand your concern what with this production and all. As you know, there's no cure for the common cold. But why don't I take a look at you and maybe

> I can recommend something to get the symptoms under
> control so you'll feel in better form.
> Pt:　Okay. I sure hope there's something you can do.

DIFFICULT FEELINGS AND DEFENSES IN
MEDICAL INTERVIEWING

Sometimes the patient's behavior or affect interfere with transmitting adequate information of the kind you need for a precise and accurate history: An angry patient may not wish to speak with you at all, a depressed patient may say too little, and a denying patient may be unable to reveal the very symptoms that are so terrifying to him or her. Such situations are likely to make you have several conflicting feelings at once: You may be frustrated at the difficulty in obtaining the history yet feel sorry for the depressed patient, concerned about maintaining a "professional" attitude yet feel defensive or outraged at the angry patient, or pleased at the gratitude shown by the seductive patient yet upset at being manipulated. It is also likely that when you sense strong emotions occurring in the interview, you will either have some fear about your ability to handle the situation and may, therefore, try to ignore it, or feel that it is really not your job as a medical student or a medical doctor to deal with the patient's emotions.

While it may not be your job to manage or treat the cancer patient's depression or the multiple sclerosis patient's denial, it is your job to get an accurate history. When such feelings get in the way of a good history, the feelings will need to be acknowledged in the course of the interview so that the history taking can proceed efficiently and accurately. Experienced clinicians find that an empathic response that acknowledges emotional content not only helps the patient feel understood but also actually facilitates the interview, from the point of view of both time (it takes *less* time) and accuracy (the patient gives better data). While your fear of being overwhelmed by the patient's emotions is a legitimate one, most patients are eager to talk about how they feel and will actually reduce your fear by revealing how they cope with their own personal tragedies.

When feelings interfere with obtaining the history, you should observe carefully the basics of any good interview, which we recapitulate here:

1. Make sure you have the patient's permission to do the interview and that he or she understands the "contract" with you, the student. While this is important for all patients, it is particularly important for the angry patient. Helpful techniques include:

   a. Empathize with the patient's position; stopping short of "accusing" him or her of being angry, you might begin with "I know many doctors have already come in and bothered you. . . ."
   b. Elicit the patient's permission, perhaps with a question such as "Is it all right?" If the patient says yes, show your appreciation of his or her cooperation. If the patient says no, accept his or her noncooperation and ask for the patient's reasons in a noncombative way, recognizing his or her right to refuse.
   c. Inform the patient gently of your obligation to do the interview, without attempting to convince or control him or her. Give control to the patient by indicating your willingness to compromise within your limits, e.g., "Would it help if I came back in an hour? If I rearranged your pillows? If I talked softer (louder), faster (slower)? If I stood (sat)?"

2. Give the patient **time** to respond, particularly when the subject under discussion is hard for the patient to talk about. Specific techniques include:

   a. Wait for the patient to finish his or her thought or sentence even if the patient hesitates or stumbles over words.
   b. Ask open-ended questions and observe the total communication, including words, gestures, facial expressions, and voice quality.

3. Summarize periodically both the symptom content and the feeling content. Specific uses of summaries include:

   a. To regain control if the patient has wandered off the topic or you are feeling confused. For example, "You are telling me a lot about yourself. Let me tell you what I understand so far, because I will want to ask you a specific question."

b. To prepare the way for a potentially threatening question. For example, "You have had a lot of back pain, and from what you tell me, it has also made you quite depressed. . . . Has it affected your marriage? Your sex life?"

c. To clarify and remain "in sync" with the patient, particularly when you notice that the patient feels upset or misunderstood. For example, "Just now as you were describing your pain, you got a very worried look on your face. . . . Did I say something that upset you?"

4. Use the interchangeable empathic response to show that you "understand exactly." Try to describe precisely in your own words the patient's symptoms as well as the intensity of emotions being expressed. Look to the patient for confirmation of your statement and acknowledge any corrections. For example:

> Dr: So as I understand it, you've been having this pain in your chest for the past 2 to 3 months and you notice it when you go jogging, and you're a little worried about what's causing it (doctor looks up at patient)?
>
> Pt: Well, it's not pain exactly, more a discomfort. And actually I'm more than a little worried. My father dropped dead of a heart attack when he was 43 and I'm 42.
>
> Dr: I see. So you're worried that the same thing might happen to you?
>
> Pt: Yeah, I'd really like you to take a cardiogram on me, doc.

5. If you feel lost, acknowledge it as a fact, not as a criticism of the patient. Then proceed to ask the patient to help you, such as "I'm confused about this, can you help me?" or "I did not quite understand this point, would you help me?"

We now consider patient anxiety, anger, depression, and denial and, in each case, suggest specific approaches to supplement those we have already discussed.

Anxiety

Every illness produces a mixture of fear and anxiety in the patient. The most common sources of anxiety are feelings of helplessness, fear of dependence, inability to accept warmth or tenderness, and fear of expressing anger. The usual indication that a patient is becoming very anxious is an intensification of his or her customary ways of coping with the world. For example, a compulsive patient will become *more* compulsive, while a paranoid patient will become *more* paranoid. The signs of anxiety that you may observe in the interview include facial flushing, sweating, rapid speech, cold hands, fidgeting, or even trembling. The anxious patient may be difficult to interview until the anxiety has been discussed.

All patients are anxious and to some extent fearful about their encounter with a physician. Some ways you can help the anxious patient are:

1. Be unhurried and calm in your manner.
2. Sympathize, but remember that too much sympathy may magnify the patient's fears.
3. Be very specific as to what you expect of the patient: what clothing the patient should remove or what position the patient should assume and where.
4. Tell the patient that some anxiety is normal and appropriate: Most patients feel this way and it is OK.
5. Some patients express their anxiety by asking what you think is causing their symptoms. When this happens, it is appropriate to remind the patient that you are a student or that you have not completed your evaluation. In addition, you can explore the patient's concerns by asking "Have you asked your doctor? Why not?" or "What do *you* think is going on?"

Consider this case example. A 57-year-old woman saw her family doctor for an annual examination. Doctors made her nervous and the thought of a visit, even on this day when she had no particular worrisome symptoms, made her nervous. Her red lipstick was coated with antacid as she entered the office; she was so distraught that her stomach felt queasy. It was clear (in retrospect) that just showing up for the examination was a major effort for her. Everything, fortunately, was in order. The physician had only one prescription for her:

> Dr: Everything is fine. I have only one recommendation and that is that I'd like you to get a mammogram.
> Pt: Oh my God! You mean I've got cancer? Not my breast!
> Dr: No, no, of course not. No, I recommend a mammogram for all my patients over the age of 50. It's routine.

And, as though the physician were not leveling with her:

> Pt: I couldn't stand to lose a breast; chemotherapy is awful. I already have thinning hair, you know, chemotherapy makes that worse. No, I won't do that, I can't.

In retrospect this patient's fragile adaptation to her encounter with a physician was shattered by one suggestion of a routine test, the purpose of which is to screen for cancer. She seemed to believe that the recommendation was particular, not routine, despite her doctor's protests to the contrary. If we look back at how the doctor introduced the idea we notice what may have seemed to be a contradiction to the patient: "Everything is fine . . . get a mammogram." For this anxiety-ridden patient if "everything is fine," why do I need a mammogram? The physician may have been able to achieve the aim of getting her to take a mammogram (which, by the way, she never agreed to) by saying:

> Dr: Everything's fine. Your exam is completely normal. Just like you come for a Pap test because you know that's routine in all women, so we now routinely recommend a mammogram for all women your age. Do you know what that is? Have you ever had one done?

In this instance, the physician is more reassuring because the physician is specific about what is "fine" ("Your exam is completely normal."), frames the "routine" nature of the mammogram in a concrete way to which the patient can relate (i.e., by comparing it to the "routine" Pap test), and anticipates the patient's worry by explaining the reason for the test *before* the patient can spin a fantasy of calamity.

Anger

While anxiety may facilitate our feeling sympathetic toward the patient, many physicians find anger more difficult to handle. Patients may behave in a hostile manner for many different reasons. Most of the time the reasons have nothing to do with you personally; rather, they relate to the patient's own situation, such as inconsiderate care by hospital staff, failure of the patient's physician to communicate, or the patient's unique response to his or her illness, disability, or prognosis. What makes one patient depressed may make another patient angry. Some ways to handle anger include:

1. Recognize and acknowledge anger with a statement, such as "I can see (hear or feel) you are angry and frustrated" or "Waiting so long makes people angry." If you are not sure that what you are hearing is anger, ask, "Are you feeling angry?"
2. Accept the anger by continuing to *listen to the patient* while explaining the situation in a neutral fashion even though a logical explanation will not necessarily change the patient's feelings. Do not take sides.
3. Explore the contributing factors and identify the underlying feelings, such as fear, hurt, disappointment, or powerlessness. Accept the patient's reason even if you do not personally agree with it. Remember, *there is always a reason*, although it may not be immediately evident.
4. If the patient's anger is justifiably directed at you, acknowledge your mistake. You are learning, mistakes are unavoidable; you can learn from them and correct them. If the patient's anger is not directed at you, help the patient recognize ways he or she can deal with the anger-provoking situations. For example:

Pt: You're just as insensitive as the rest of 'em.
Dr: I guess that was a foolish question to ask. Now that I understand you a little better, do you think we could start over?

This next patient regretted being interviewed in front of a group of residents at a psychiatric case conference. She is talking to her physician following the conference.

> Pt: I now know what it's like to be poor. I never would
> have been at that conference if I had my own private
> doctor. I know what it's like to be a guinea pig. That
> doctor asked about my early childhood when what I
> needed was someone to find out what's been going on
> over the last 10 years and how tough life has been for
> me so that he could help me. I thought he would be
> able to give me something to help my nerves right now,
> not just talk about my grandmother.

While this patient reminds us of the entitled demander, and indeed may be one, she is clear, if we listen, about what is upsetting her. She is focused on how she feels at present and is looking for relief from feelings that are unpleasant. Talking about what seemed to her to be ancient history confused and frustrated her. The conference ended apparently without a prescription or clear plan of action, and although the physician was trying to remedy the situation, the patient may not have known that. Here an explanation and an acknowledgement of her feelings are in order:

> Dr: It certainly must seem strange to talk about old things
> when you feel so bad now and want relief. I can cer-
> tainly understand your frustration. Actually, the reason
> I wanted to talk with you is to discuss what to do next
> to get you to feel better. Because Dr. Smith had some
> good ideas which I think we should try. In fact, he sug-
> gested some medication which he thinks will be help-
> ful, and I think so, too.

The other aspect of her anger was a sense of being on display or of being experimented with (perhaps two sides of the same coin). She may have been surprised by the conference format, requiring her to sit in front of a room full of strange doctors who she had never met before. If she was not prepared for what was to occur, as she should have been by someone, her physician can only apologize:

> Dr: I'm sorry, I guess I didn't really explain very well what
> was supposed to happen to you. I'm sorry you felt

uncomfortable. But I did learn a lot about you which I
think will help me to take better care of you.
Pt: Okay. What I really need is to feel better.

Depression

Depression may be a manifestation of a diagnosable psychiatric
disorder, a response to recent tragedy (such as death of a
spouse), an expression of a general pessimistic approach to life,
or a more transient feeling state. Major depressive disorder may
be the underlying problem in a substantial percent of those
patients who complain to their physicians of fatigue, weakness,
lack of energy, insomnia, backache, or headache, but depression
as a *response to illness* is also common. Depressive characteristics
include feelings of worthlessness, hopelessness, apathy, and
guilt, together with a profoundly empty and lonely feeling.
These are manifest in the patient's manner, tone of voice, posture, and speech; thinking is slow, speech is sparse, and voice
volume is low. The patient may speak softly, looking down or
away from you and may be tearful. Sometimes a statement such
as "You look sad" gives the patient an opportunity to talk about
depressed feelings and thereby facilitates other more "medical"
aspects of the history.

Some patients have endured such tragic events that you fear
being overwhelmed with the sadness of it all. In such instances,
it is appropriate to say that you, too, find the situation sad; in this
way you make it clear to the patient that you are a fellow human
being with feelings. However, in addition to this commonality
you are also a professional, and your feelings should be used in a
constructive way to help the patient. Here is an example that has
both a feeling focus and a constructive focus. The patient is a 57-
year-old woman who had coronary bypass surgery at the age of
53, followed 2 years later by a left radical mastectomy for aggressive carcinoma of the breast. She is now suffering from metastatic
disease and is about to lose her health insurance coverage
because her husband's business is failing and they can no longer
afford the coverage.

Dr: A lot of bad things have happened to you. You must be
a pretty strong person to have endured all this . . . How
have you managed?

> Pt: Well, I have my faith . . . and my family has been just
>   wonderful to me.

Notice how the physician acknowledges the feeling content, but instead of getting deep into the tragedy, allows the patient to express her strength and her coping style. This technique serves the dual purpose of keeping both patient and physician from being overwhelmed.

Some useful questions to assess the depth of depression, particularly assessment of suicide risk, are:

- Do you get pretty discouraged (or blue)?
- What do you see for yourself in the future? How do you see the future?
- Do you ever feel that life isn't worth living? Or that you'd just as soon be dead? Or that you just can't go on?

If answers to the above question indicate a risk of suicide, you should pursue the question of suicide:

- Have you ever thought of doing away with yourself? Ending your life? Of suicide? Are you having any thoughts of killing yourself?
- Did you ever think about how you would do it?
- What would happen to your family (parents, spouse, and so on) after you were dead?

It is important to give the patient time to answer these questions. Most patients are relieved to talk about feelings of suicide; such discussion does not put the idea of suicide into their heads. Often the best follow-up questions are simple statements such as "Tell me more about these feelings" or "Tell me more about it" or the use of simple prompters and facilitators such as "Mm hmm" followed by silence to allow the patient to continue. Often this technique uncovers information vital to the diagnostic process:

> Dr: You look sad. Is it about this chest pain you're having
>   or something else?
> Pt: I guess I am sad. My chest has been hurting all week.
>   Well . . . see . . . I don't know if I can say it . . . I get all

> choked up . . . excuse me (trying to hold back tears).
> My mother died on Monday. Every time I think about
> her I get this choked up feeling in here and it starts to
> hurt like my angina down into my arm.

Here the physician discovers the crucial connection between an
exacerbation of the patient's angina and the recent death of the
patient's mother. Shea[94] has said, "If ever there was a moment of
critical importance in interviewing, it is the moment when one
listens for the harbinger of death." Here is an example of an
assessment of suicide risk in a patient who is seeing an internist
for follow-up of abdominal pain and asthma:

> Dr: Last I talked to you, you were feeling pretty bad.
> Pt: You know, sometimes I scare myself.
> Dr: You mean . . . , have you ever tried to kill yourself?
> Pt: Yeah.
> Dr: How did you do it? How did you try?
> Pt: Uh, I turned on the gas once.
> Dr: What happened?
> Pt: Somebody, they smelled the gas.
> Dr: When was that?
> Pt: That's not the first time I tried to kill myself. One time
> I climbed up on the bridge.
> Dr: Uh hmm. What stopped you?
> Pt: I don't know.
> Dr: I'm glad you did. How are you feeling right now?

It is not uncommon that the need to assess suicide risk arises
within the context of routine care for ordinary medical problems.
Notice how this physician does not shy away from asking specific
questions about past and current suicide intent. The physician
also reaches out to the patient by sharing genuine happiness ("I'm
glad you did") that the patient is still alive.

Denial

Denial is a common response to illness that most patients have,
at least to some degree. It is the feeling that "This isn't really
happening to me," "I can't believe it," or "That wasn't blood I
saw in my bowel movement—at least, I don't think it was." In

some patients the denial is strong enough that they either ignore it or do not remember symptoms. Alternatively, patients may play down a worrisome symptom and report it as a trivial event—"I had a little pain in my chest, but it only lasted an hour." Only later do you find out that the pain was not only severe but associated with nausea and sweating and a feeling of impending doom. While some patients play down the symptoms, others deny the emotional impact of a particular diagnosis or prognosis. At times, it is hard to tell the difference between optimism and denial, e.g., the patient with a potentially lethal disease who smiles and says, "I know I can beat it." When patients accept bad news with apparent equanimity, it is difficult to know whether they are "handling it well" or denying some or all of the meaning of the diagnosis or prognosis. While denial can lead to serious delays in seeking care, it is also a useful mechanism by which many patients cope with bad news. The clinician, therefore, should handle denial with circumspection and respect, while trying to assess the patient's understanding of what is happening. Some useful techniques for doing this include:

1. Accept denial as the patient's unique and current experience.
2. Inform the patient gently and calmly that many people feel differently, including you. For example, you can say, "Most people feel very sad when they hear they have a serious illness" or "I guess I would be worried."
3. Drop the subject if the patient is silent. The patient may come back to it, tentatively saying that once or twice he or she has felt as you described.

Consider this example of a young woman who came to the doctor for a "checkup." This was her first visit to this physician. On palpating the abdomen, the physician found a large mass which, on pelvic examination and subsequent ultrasound proved to be an enormous uterine fibroid. The patient seemed unaware of its presence, despite the fact that the mass was the size of a 5-month pregnancy. When she was told that a hysterectomy might be necessary, she seemed unconcerned. The physician needed to find out if this 30-year-old woman who had not yet had children understood what a hysterectomy would mean to her and was accepting that, or simply did not understand the implications of the surgery. (The physician's concern was, perhaps, heightened by the fact that the patient seemed to have denied the presence of a large abdominal mass.)

Dr: You don't seem very concerned at the idea of a hysterectomy.

Pt: Well, if I have to have it, that's it.

Dr: Do you know what a hysterectomy is?

Pt: Well, I guess that's when they take everything out.

Dr: Well, actually, it means the removal of the uterus or womb, that's where this fibroid is. Now this tumor is an overgrowth in the muscle, but even though it's not cancer, it may be impossible to remove without removing the uterus. Now your ovaries, which are the glands next to the uterus that make female hormones like estrogen—you've heard of estrogen? Okay, the ovaries would not be removed. (Draws picture) They would stay, so your hormones would still work right.

Pt: But I still couldn't have babies.

Dr: That's right, you couldn't have babies. What do you think about that?

Pt: I don't know. I guess I never thought much about it, not being married and all, but I guess it hasn't really hit me yet. I'm more worried about the operation itself.

Notice how the physician gently probes the patient's knowledge and offers a clear explanation as to what will happen. The patient is not denying the outcome of the surgery but is, perhaps, delaying dealing with it pending resolution of her more immediate fears about the operation itself.

Patients' and Physicians' Feelings About Each Other

The interaction between physician and patient may be highly charged with emotion. This relationship may bring out attitudes and behaviors reflecting previous relationships that either patient or doctor have had. The sicker the patient, and the more helpless and dependent he or she is, the more likely it is that the patient's attitude toward the doctor will reflect a great deal of previously learned attitudes and experiences. Sometimes these attitudes are manifest in ways that appear totally irrational to the interviewer. For example, a patient who has had an angry, competitive relationship with his father, perceiving the male physician as a powerful authority, may become antagonistic, sarcastic, and competitive even though the physician has done nothing that would ordinarily elicit such a response. Similarly, female physicians may encounter seemingly irrational responses based on the patient's early experiences with being mothered. Although you may not be able to figure it out at the time, there is always a reason for what looks like irrational behavior. You can only maintain a respectful attitude toward the patient and use the techniques outlined above to establish rapport and obtain the history.

Your interaction with the patient is, or course, two sided; thus, while patients have feelings about you, you will most certainly have feelings about your patients. You may try to hide these feelings or even wonder if it is appropriate to have them. You will like some patients a lot and others less so; there may be some that you actively dislike. Some will make you angry, and others you will dread. Some will make you laugh, and you will wonder whether it is "professional" to do so. You may even feel sexually attracted to certain patients and feel embarrassed or behave awkwardly. The best approach to such feelings is first to identify and acknowledge them, at least to yourself. Think: How is the patient making me uncomfortable? And why? The answer to the "how" questions will allow you to identify behaviors in the patient that are helpful in your assessment. For example, ask yourself, do you dread seeing this patient because the individual makes too many demands on me? If so, the patient may be an entitled demander that we spoke of earlier and will require particular attention during your interview. Alternatively, perhaps you are uncomfortable with another patient who is depressed or dying, and you are afraid that there is nothing you can do for the individual. Remember, this is your problem, not the patient's. You may want to share such feelings with helpful colleagues, and, finally, as you become comfortable with these feelings, you will be able to share them with the patient and so improve his or her self-understanding. The opportunity to create a real connection with your patient can be the basis for a professional intimacy as you learn more about each other over time.

CHAPTER 11

The Difficult Interview: Somatization

> A bodily disease, which we look upon as whole and entire within itself, may, after all, be but a symptom of some ailment in the spiritual part.
>
> Nathaniel Hawthorne, *The Scarlet Letter*

You will encounter one group of medical patients whose symptoms are legion but in whom, despite considerable investigation, no "organic" etiology for these symptoms can be identified. Some of these patients have relatively acute functional somatic problems that resolve over time. Some have recurrent and multiple physical complaints that span many years, many doctors, and many diagnostic workups, yet you cannot make any pathophysiologic sense out of the story as a whole. Sometimes the patient will tell you that "doctors have never been able to find anything" and that "they said it was all in my head." Other patients in this group will have been provided a series of diagnoses and treatments: gallbladder disease followed by cholecystectomy, uterine fibroids followed by a hysterectomy, degenerative disc disease followed by a laminectomy, or abdominal adhesions (from previous surgery) followed by yet another operation for lysis of adhesions. Despite these diagnosed disorders to which they ascribe their symptoms, the patients only improve partially and temporarily when treated, and they soon develop a new set of symptoms. Such patients, often identified as "crocks" or "turkeys," suffer real pain and often develop real disability, even though their problems appear to resist the ordinary disease categories.

These patients are "somatizers." Somatization is a process whereby people experience and express emotional discomfort or psychosocial stress in the language of physical symptoms. The somatizing patient attributes these symptoms to physical disease and seeks medical help for them. This process may occur in the absence of other disorders (primary somatization), or this process may be associated with other medical or psychiatric conditions (secondary somatization). We consider somatization in this book for three reasons:

1. Patients with functional somatic symptoms are frequently encountered in practice, and they often utilize large amounts of interview time.
2. Somatizing patients are difficult to interview.
3. The medical interview and thorough review of the past medical history are critical to the diagnosis of somatoform disorders.

Table 11–1 presents a typology of differential diagnosis of somatization. In the somatoform disorders (hypochondriasis, conversion, psychogenic pain, and somatization disorder) the

TABLE 11–1. Differential Diagnosis of Somatization

1. Occult physical disease
   a. Syndromes of unknown etiology
      (1) Fibromyalgia or fibromyositis
      (2) Chronic fatigue syndrome
      (3) Mitral valve prolapse syndrome
   b. Diseases with subtle, multisystem manifestations (e.g., systemic lupus erythematosus, multiple sclerosis, hyperparathyroidism, and porphyria)
2. Secondary somatization
   a. Secondary to known chronic disease
   b. Secondary to other psychiatric disorders
      (1) Major depression
      (2) Adjustment reactions
      (3) Alcohol or other substance abuse
      (4) Panic and other anxiety disorders
3. Primary somatization
   a. Transient functional somatic symptoms
   b. Somatoform disorders
      (1) Somatization disorder
      (2) Hypochondriasis
      (3) Conversion reaction
      (4) Psychogenic pain disorder
4. Factitious disease

TABLE 11–2. Manifestations of Somatization in Clinical Practice

1. Selective focus on somatic symptoms of a psychiatric disorder (e.g., depression or panic)
2. Amplification of somatic symptoms or organic illness
3. Use of somatic symptoms in absence of demonstrable organic disease to avoid dysphoric affect or intrapsychic conflict, or to manipulate social environment for personal gain
4. Selective focus on psychophysiologic symptoms with denial or minimization of life problems that precipitate or exacerbate the illness
5. Expression of somatic complaints as a culturally sanctioned idiom of distress

Source: Adapted from Katon et al.[62]

process of somatization is a primary feature, and specific diagnostic criteria apply (see below). A larger group of patients suffer functional somatic symptoms but do not meet DSM-IIIR criteria for one of these conditions or for any other psychiatric disorder. These patients may be said to have an "amplifying somatic style." Table 11–2 presents a more general survey of the manifestations of somatization in clinical practice.

How prevalent are functional somatic symptoms? Between 60% and 80% of healthy persons experience some physical symptoms in any given week. About one-third of all primary care patients visit their doctors because of ill-defined symptoms not attributable to physical disease, and 70% of those ultimately found to have a psychiatric disorder present a somatic symptom as the reason for their primary care visit. When broad criteria for somatization are applied in community-based surveys, 4% to 5% of all adults can be considered somatizers. Studies suggest that the prevalence of somatization disorder itself is less than 1% in the community, 5% among primary care outpatients, and 9% among hospitalized medical and surgical patients.[33,34,45] Most patients with somatization disorder are female; this is not true of individuals with hypochondriasis, which characterizes 5% to 10% of medical office patients, both male and female.

Somatization occurs throughout the world but is more prevalent in cultures in which emotional distress tends to be expressed in nonpsychological terms. In the United States, somatization appears to be particularly frequent among Hispanic and Asian populations. Older age, poor education, low socioeconomic status, urban residence, and unmarried state have all been associated with a higher prevalence of somatization. Somatizers utilize more medical services, require more sick leave and disability, and perceive themselves as less healthy than those in comparison groups. Although somatizers are more likely to have negative medical findings, they perceive that their health is significantly worse than the health of medically ill patients. The per capita health care expenditure and physician expenditure of somatizers are 9 times and 14 times, respectively, that of nonsomatizers.

By what mechanisms do such symptoms arise? Some of the theories of somatization etiology are summarized in Table 11–3. It is useful for the physician to have a holistic perspective of somatization that includes:

1. Predisposing characteristics, such as abnormal central nervous system regulation of incoming information;
2. Precipitating factors, such as stressful life events; and
3. Maintaining factors, such as financial rewards and other forms of secondary gain, as well as morbidity that arises from repeated medical procedures or side effects of medications.

Maintaining factors are often of crucial importance in persons with chronic somatization. Their interpersonal relationships, families, and ways of looking at the world are all affected by unending sickliness. Medical care itself provides a positive feedback loop that validates these patients' sickliness, creates new anxiety ("After all, if no one can find out what it is, it must be

TABLE 11–3. Theories of Somatization Etiology

1. **Neurobiologic.** Abnormal central nervous system regulation of incoming sensory information leads to an impairment in attentional processing, resulting in patients who perceive more stimuli as "symptoms."
2. **Psychodynamic.** Somatization is a defense mechanism that serves to replace or disguise emotional conflict with physical symptoms.
3. **Behavioral.** Somatization is a learned pattern of behavior in which environmental reinforcers serve to maintain the patient's abnormal illness behavior.
4. **Sociocultural.** "Correct" ways of dealing with emotions and feelings are culturally determined.

something strange and terrible."), and causes additional suffering.

In one study, the final diagnoses of somatizing patients referred for psychiatric evaluation[62] included major depression (48%), conversion reaction (12%), psychogenic pain disorder (11%), psychological factors associated with physical illness (9%), alcohol abuse (8%), adjustment disorder (7%), somatization disorder (6%), organic brain syndrome (4%), panic disorder (4%), and factitious disease (4%). Patients sometimes had more than one of these diagnoses. Over one-third of the patients had, in addition to their primary diagnosis, a definite personality disorder. Hypochondriasis was not represented, perhaps because it rarely leads to psychiatric referral.

The following pages briefly consider (1) the diagnosis of somatization in the medical interview, (2) special features of somatoform disorders, and (3) somatization as it relates to the doctor-patient relationship.

SOMATIZATION IN THE MEDICAL INTERVIEW

It is important to distinguish among three types of "symptom generation,"all of which may be considered manifestations of somatization:

1. Patients may amplify symptoms of acute or chronic organic disease, or they may preferentially report somatic symptoms (while deemphasizing emotional symptoms) of psychiatric conditions. The latter process results in, for example, masked depression, a condition often poorly diagnosed and treated by medical doctors.[14] Patients with masked depression may visit their doctors with a chief complaint of fatigue and be almost unaware of their low mood. In such cases the interview must be directed toward identifying those "unamplified" or suppressed symptoms that complete the diagnostic pattern. Primary care patients who suffer from major depression usually will, in fact, report their affective symptoms if asked directly.[28]

2. Patients may report psychophysiological disturbances (e.g., headaches, tachycardia, palpitations, or irregular

bowel movements) mediated through autonomic or other known pathophysiological mechanisms. Much of medical practice consists of treating patients with these sorts of problems. Each problem can be diagnosed as a separate syndrome. Examples include irritable bowel syndrome, fibrositis or fibromyalgia, and premenstrual syndrome. However, if you obtain a history of multiple, recurrent, and/or disabling psychophysiological syndromes, you should give specific attention to the process of somatization. It is important not to lose sight of the forest because you are carefully studying every tree.

3. Patients may experience actual conversion symptoms. These symptoms serve a symbolic function in the patient's life (i.e., they actually represent or replace an emotion), rather than being nonspecific responses to conflict or life's stress. Consequently, conversion symptoms do not necessarily correspond to known physiological mechanisms or anatomical distributions. These symptoms often develop acutely (an important historical feature) and simply do not make sense to the doctor. The patient's description of a severe deficit (e.g., complete loss of feeling in the left leg or paralysis of the right arm) does not correspond at all with the physical signs. These symptoms originate in the unconscious; in other words, their symbolic meaning is hidden from the patient.

Persons with recurrent or persistent somatization may experience all three types of symptoms. However, most often you will find amplified or psychophysiological complaints, either separately or in combination. True conversion symptoms, although not rare, are infrequent.

Virtually any specific symptom can be a manifestation of somatization. It need not be a weird, complex, or inexplicable complaint. In fact, when evaluating a patient for somatization, you should concentrate on the pattern, logic, and context of the symptom, rather than trying to decide whether dizziness, for example, is more likely than dysuria to represent somatization. You should look for "positive" features in the medical history that suggest somatization rather than simply taking the "negative" approach of ruling out any conceivable organic disease. Table 11–4 presents nine such positive characteristics. If two or

TABLE 11–4. Characteristics of Patients and Symptoms
Suggestive of Somatization

1. The symptom's description is vague, inconsistent, or bizarre.
2. The symptoms persist despite apparently adequate medical therapy.
3. The illness began in the context of a psychologically meaningful setting,
   e.g., death of relative, conflict with spouse, or job promotion.
4. The patient denies any emotional distress or psychological role of the
   symptoms.
5. The patient has engaged in polydoctoring and/or has had polysurgery.
6. There is evidence of an associated psychiatric disorder.
7. The patient has features suggesting a hysterical personality style.
8. The discussion reveals that the patient attributes an idiosyncratic meaning
   to his or her symptoms.
9. The patient has difficulty describing emotions or inner processes in words.

Source: Adapted and abridged from Lipkin.[71]

three of these are present, you should consider the hypothesis
that the patient's symptoms are (at least, in part) attributable to
somatization. You can test this hypothesis by directing your
interview toward establishing whether additional features are
present. For example, given a vague symptom that persists
despite therapy, you might be particularly careful to explore the
symptom's cognitive or emotional meaning ("What do you think
is causing this?") and to search for evidence of psychiatric
disorders.

With regard to specific symptoms, pain is the most frequent,
present in over 80% of somatizing patients. Three symptom clus-
ters that should lead you to consider somatization (particularly
secondary to depression, anxiety, or panic disorder) are:

1. Nonexertional chest pain, palpitations, tachycardia, and/
   or difficulty catching one's breath ("sighing" or a feeling
   of not being able to take a deep enough breath, not true
   dyspnea);
2. Headache, dizziness, lightheadedness, presyncope, and/
   or paresthesias; and
3. Dyspepsia, heartburn, "gas," flatulence and/or other
   gastrointestinal symptoms.

Globus hystericus, the sensation of a "lump" in the throat that
interferes with swallowing, is a frequent conversion symptom.

SOMATOFORM DISORDERS

Full discussion of these disorders is beyond the scope of this text, but they should be mentioned here because most of the data used in diagnosing them arise from complete and often repeated medical interviews. The first disorder is somatization disorder and is characterized by being found in women (rarely men) who develop multiple chronic but fluctuating physical symptoms that involve several different organ systems (Table 11–5). These symptoms usually begin during adolescence but by definition must begin before the age of 30 years.

Sometimes patients will date their illness (and doctoring) from some major event that occurred when they were older than 30 years:

Pt: I haven't been right since I got banged-up in that car accident, the back, the dizziness, they just never got better . . .

Dr: That, was let's see, 6 years ago? You must have been about 35. And so that was the first . . . you were well before then?

TABLE 11–5. Diagnostic Criteria for Somatization Disorder

1. The individual has a history of many physical complaints or a belief of being sickly that began before the age of 30 and persists for several years.
2. The individual has at least 13 symptoms from the list below. To count a symptom as significant, the following criteria must be met:
   a. No organic pathology or pathophysiological mechanism (e.g., a physical disorder or the effects of injury, medication, drugs, or alcohol) exists to account for the symptom or, when there is related organic pathology, the complaint or resulting social or occupational impairment is grossly in excess of what would be expected from the physical findings.
   b. The symptoms occur, at least occasionally, in the absence of a panic attack.
   c. The symptoms have caused the person to take medicine (other than over-the-counter pain medication), see a doctor, or alter her lifestyle.
3. The symptom list includes:
   a. Gastrointestinal symptoms
      (1) **Vomiting (other than during pregnancy)**°
      (2) Abdominal pain (other than when menstruating)
      (3) Nausea (other than motion sickness)
      (4) Bloating (gassy)

TABLE 11–5. Diagnostic Criteria for Somatization Disorder (*Continued*)

      (5) Diarrhea
      (6) Intolerance of (gets sick from) several different foods
  b. Pain symptoms
      (7) **Pain in extremities**
      (8) Back pain
      (9) Joint pain
    (10) Pain during urination
    (11) Other pain (excluding headaches)
  c. Cardiopulmonary symptoms
    (12) **Shortness of breath when not exerting oneself**
    (13) Palpitations
    (14) Chest pain
    (15) Dizziness
  d. Conversion or pseudoneurologic symptoms
    (16) **Amnesia**
    (17) **Difficulty swallowing**
    (18) Loss of voice
    (19) Deafness
    (20) Double vision
    (21) Blurred vision
    (22) Blindness
    (23) Fainting or loss of consciousness
    (24) Seizure or convulsion
    (25) Trouble walking
    (26) Paralysis or muscle weakness
    (27) Urinary retention or difficulty urinating
  e. Sexual symptoms for the major part of the person's sexual life
    (28) **Burning sensation in sexual organs or rectum (other than during intercourse)**
    (29) Sexual indifference
    (30) Pain during intercourse
    (31) Impotence
  f. Female reproductive symptoms judged by the person to occur more frequently or severely than in most women
    (32) **Painful menstruation**
    (33) Irregular menstrual periods
    (34) Excessive menstrual bleeding
    (35) Vomiting throughout pregnancy

*Note: The seven items in boldface may be used to screen for the disorder. The presence of two or more of these items suggests a high likelihood of the disorder.

Source: From American Psychiatric Association. *Diagnostic and Statistical Manual of Mental Disorder.* 3rd ed. Revised. Washington, DC, American Psychiatric Association, 1987.

> Pt: Yes. No problems. I never had that back pain.
> Dr: But did you have other things, like aches and pains, things you went to the doctor for?

In further discussion, this patient revealed that she had been "sickly all my life" and had two operations (hysterectomy and cholecystectomy) before the age of 30 years. The diagnostic criteria for somatization disorder are quantitative as well as qualitative and require a thorough review of systems for their application. These patients will likely give a positive review of systems (see Chap. 9), but their symptoms are far more persistent and disabling than those of patients who simply have an "amplifying somatic style."[8]

Patients with hypochondriasis consistently misinterpret normal physiological sensations as being indicators of disease (Table 11–6). These patients are sometimes called the "worried well," although hypochondriacs can obviously also suffer from physical disease. Unlike patients with somatization disorder, they are not usually disabled. They often keep returning to a particular worry (e.g., high cholesterol), which is perhaps based on family history or personal experience. Hypochondriasis is more a style than a specific syndrome, and it must be judged by the person's pattern of reactions over time to ordinary aches and pains and to self-limited illness. Although one DSM-IIIR criterion requires that

TABLE 11–6. Diagnostic Criteria for Hypochondriasis

1. Preoccupation with the fear of having, or the belief that one has, a serious disease. This fear or belief is based on the person's interpretation of physical signs or sensations as evidence of physical illness.
2. Appropriate physical evaluation does not support the diagnosis of any physical disorder that can account for the physical signs or sensations or the person's unwarranted interpretation of them. In addition, the symptoms are not just those of panic attacks.
3. Fear of having, or belief that one has, a disease that persists despite medical reassurance.
4. Duration of the disturbance is at least 6 months.
5. Fear or belief in item 1 is not of delusional intensity, as in delusional disorder, somatic type (i.e., the person can acknowledge the possibility that his or her fear or belief of having a serious disease is unfounded).

Source: From APA,[2] with permission.

the patient maintain his or her "unrealistic fear" despite medical reassurance, many such patients can be reassured effectively about a particular symptomatic episode, although they will likely return in a few weeks or months panicked about another episode of the same symptoms or, perhaps, a new set of concerns. In the interview, these patients may ask repeatedly for reassurance or say, "What do you think it is, doc?"

SOMATIZATION AND THE DOCTOR-PATIENT INTERACTION

What can you do for the somatizing patient? This is a broad subject, but consistent application of good listening and responding skills is the basis of any effective therapy. Although difficult, with such patients it is necessary to build a trusting relationship, to validate their suffering as a "medical" problem, to provide a clear explanation of symptoms, and to engage active patient participation in the treatment. The following are a few specific pointers useful in early encounters with somatizing patients:

1. In the initial assessment, obtain a complete patient profile, including functional status and family interactions, even though the patient wants only to discuss his or her symptoms.
2. Likewise, pay particular attention to details of the past medical history. This may require obtaining the names and addresses of numerous doctors and sending for the patient's records. Somatizers often fragment their health care. A patient may not volunteer, because she doesn't think it is relevant, the names of her cardiologist and her dermatologist when she is seeing you for a gastrointestinal complaint. One of the authors sees a patient with somatization disorder who at one time had regular, ongoing relationships with 12 doctors, including 2 gastroenterologists, 2 pain control specialists, and a neurosurgeon, otolaryngologist, cardiologist, urologist, general surgeon, family doctor, general internist, and psychiatrist.
3. Establish goals with the patient. In particular, if there are multiple symptoms expressed in the interview, agree on which one(s) need attention first. If a symptom is

chronic, point out that a long period of treatment may be required before the symptom improves or resolves.

4. Avoid vague references (see Chap. 14). While you may not be sure of a symptom's underlying etiology, you can still explain its operation in physiological terms as well as your plan for treatment.

5. Speak of the body, not the mind. Many of these patients will have been told by other doctors, "It's all in your mind." It is generally not useful (at least, until your relationship with the patient is well established) to explain the symptom as something that originates in the mind. When talking about "stress" or "tension," relate them to the autonomic nervous system.

6. Focus some attention in each encounter on "healthy talk" (e.g., the patient's strengths and activities), rather than concentrating only on symptoms. This will be difficult at first because the patient may find any talk other than "symptom talk" irrelevant and perhaps suspicious. Genuine empathic concern can often "break through" and allow the somatizer to be more open with you.

7. Examine the patient. There are two reasons to repeat selective, but careful, physical examinations of these patients. *First,* you do not want to miss signs of organic disease that may develop. *Second,* since somatizers are focused on their bodies, your attention to the body is evidence that you take their concerns seriously. It helps validate their symptoms and thus helps you develop a healing relationship.

In addition, good care for the somatizing patient requires a management strategy that includes explicit rules and guidelines, regularly scheduled office visits, careful monitoring of health status, supportive discussion or counseling, education, appropriate symptomatic medication, and sometimes consultation with a psychiatrist or psychologist.

What about good care for the doctor? What can you do for yourself? Somatizing patients hit us in two vulnerable places. *First,* they hit us in our finely honed, high tech belief systems. These patients don't fit well into our disease categories, defying the logic of mind-body separation. They present us with the unending conundrum of "when to say when"; after all, there is always the remote possibility that we have, indeed, missed an occult physical explanation for their symptoms. *Second*, somatizing patients hit us in our already stressed emotions. We may see them as stupid, recalcitrant, perverse, frustrating, or futile. One chronic somatizer on the morning's office schedule can sour a doctor's whole day. We deal elsewhere with doctor's feelings and responses to difficult doctor-patient interactions in general (see Chap. 10). Here we emphasize the three C's: control, communication, and colleagues.

1. The physician can better survive repeated encounters with patients who somatize by establishing some *control* over the relationship. Control means setting goals, limits, rules, and guidelines. Empathy and respect go a long way, but they will wear out quickly without some clear-cut framework in which to operate.

2. Every encounter should focus on *communication* and education. In caring for somatizing patients the physician-teacher is more likely to be successful in managing his or her frustrations than the paternalistic physician because there is almost always an opportunity to teach something in an interaction, even though there is rarely an opportunity for cure.

3. A physician who gets in touch with his or her feelings and is able to discuss them with *colleagues* is much more likely to "survive" difficult patient-doctor interactions. The ideal setting in which this can occur is a Balint group, i.e., a type of regular, small-group meeting named after the British psychiatrist, Michael Balint.[4] In such a group, a number of primary care physicians and a psychiatrist or psychologist discuss the care of difficult patients and the difficult feelings such patients engender.

PART 3

Special Aspects of Medical Interviewing

CHAPTER 12

Questionnaires, Case Finding, and Computers*

And if you're the type that gets finicky-finick
at this point you'll try to get out of that clinic.
But they will outwit you as quick as a winick!
The Quiz-Docs will catch you!
They'll start questionnairing!
They'll ask you, point blank, how your parts are all faring.

Dr. Seuss, *You're Only Old Once: A Book for Obsolete Children*

FOCUSED QUESTIONING

In recent years investigators have begun to study how clinicians think and make decisions during the medical interview. How do they decide what questions to ask? How do they generate hypotheses? How do they then test their hypotheses and build cases in favor of a particular diagnosis? Patients potentially have enormous quantities of information to provide about their symptoms and experiences. Although many of these data are potentially relevant to the illness, there may be a "minimal diagnostic pathway"[37] by which a clinician could navigate, eliciting only those data relevant to the particular illness at hand. In real life, clinicians only approximate such an efficient pathway. One of the ways they do so is to utilize *focused questioning*. Such questions may maximize the "expected value" of information obtained while at the same time they are efficient, i.e., small number of hypotheses, relatively few questions, and short time spent. This notion of efficiency is analogous to a cost-benefit ratio, i.e., obtaining the most information with the least effort.

Focused questioning is a style of questioning in which the phy-

---

*This chapter was coauthored by Richard Bankowitz, MD.

sician asks for a specific "yes" or "no" answer. This style is often called "closed ended" because it allows only an either/or option in answering rather than an opportunity for explication. The strength of this approach is its efficiency in obtaining the specific bits of information that the interviewer deems necessary and that might not arise at all, or might be lost in extraneous detail, if only "open ended" questioning were used. The weakness of the focused approach is that it does not allow the patient latitude to generate a description of new problems or characterize the problems further, thereby limiting the potential for developing new hypotheses about the patient's problem.

Nardone[77] reviewed strategies of history taking, contrasting a "breadth" or "cautious" approach with a "depth" or "aggressive" approach.[59,75,77] In the former, the physician seeks a bit of new information to choose among several diagnostic hypotheses (using mostly open-ended questions), while in the latter he or she exhaustively pursues a single hypothesis (using mostly focused questions). However, decision-making strategy does not always correlate with questioning style. The focused style of questioning may be used with either a focused (e.g., hypothesis-driven) or nonfocused intent. In the former, the physician is building a case for a specific diagnosis by seeking confirmatory or disconfirmatory data. In the latter case the physician is using the focused question as a screening tool, as in the review of systems.

Kassirer and Gorry[61] shed some light on the role of focused questioning when they analyzed the behavior of experienced clinicians who were presented with a simulated patient with analgesic nephropathy. Each clinician's interview with the "patient" was taped. Later, during a debriefing, the physicians were asked about their hypotheses and reasoning at various points in the interaction. The authors found that specific diagnostic hypotheses were often generated with very small amounts of data. The clinicians then used various case building strategies to corroborate or discredit these hypotheses. They employed very focused questions to

1. Confirm their impression, i.e., add a crucial bit of data that would effectively clinch the diagnosis;
2. Discriminate among hypotheses, i.e., solicit important cues that would weigh either for or against one of two or three competing hypotheses; and

3. Eliminate possibilities, i.e., obtain a crucial piece of information that would rule out one of the competing hypotheses.

Since this sort of focused questioning is in some ways analogous to a branching protocol, there has recently been much interest in the possibility of using structured questionnaires, computer-generated protocols, and/or artificial intelligence programs to assist in taking the medical history. DeDombal[32] concluded that physicians tend to identify the patient's "main problem" rather well during the first part of the doctor-patient encounter. This phase of the interview involves both "asking the right questions" and "asking the questions right." However, after the main problem is identified, physicians are faced with building the case for or against a specific diagnosis. Structured instruments like questionnaires might be useful in this focused questioning part of the interview.

A few studies have compared the case-building efficiency of physician interviews with that of a structured questionnaire. Hickam et al.[57] for example, studied patients with chest pain admitted to the hospital for elective coronary angiography. They found that internists who interviewed the patients were better able to predict the presence or absence of significant coronary lesions than was a 68-item questionnaire designed specifically for evaluation of chest pain. This suggests that the ability to modify the inquiry as it proceeds leads to more accurate diagnosis than an inflexible, albeit lengthy, questionnaire. Of course, a computer program might be designed to make such modifications as well. This possibility is discussed below. It will suffice to say here that structured questions have not as yet proved to be more accurate than a face-to-face interview.

Questionnaires as Reminders

Questionnaires, then, cannot replace talking with patients as a source of diagnostic information. Carefully selected instruments can, however, supplement the medical interview in two important ways. First, checklists completed by patients can provide useful background information. They can serve as reference points for discussion of past medical history, family history, and review of systems. Some physicians ask new patients to complete such standardized "history forms" before the first appointment. The process of thinking through a series of questions may refresh a patient's memory and focus his or her attention so that, ultimately, the interview yields a more complete history. Likewise, the completed questionnaire allows the physician to "zero in" on particular problems or symptoms, thus making the interview more efficient.

The review of systems is quite adaptable to a checklist approach (see Chap. 4). An extensive checklist would be very sensitive, i.e., it would be unlikely to miss any important symptoms (no false negatives would slip through the net). However, checklists are not very specific; that is, many trivial symptoms that do not indicate a disease will surface. Patients may acknowledge a wide array of symptoms that are mild, intermittent, transient, or unrelated to current disease states, and the form itself may not permit assessment of severity or level of patient concern. Thus, a symptom checklist may yield many false-positive symptoms. The physician, then, must utilize the subsequent interview to explore each positive response, attempting to ascertain its clinical importance.

Case Finding by Questionnaire: The Examples of Depression and Alcohol Abuse

The second important role of questionnaires in medical interviewing is their use as diagnostic aids or case-finding instruments. Some questionnaires have been designed to identify persons at high risk for certain disorders such as depression, e.g., the Beck Depression Inventory and the Zung Self-Rating Depression Scale (SDS), or alcohol abuse, e.g., the Michigan Alcoholism Screening Test (MAST). These are relatively short lists of questions structured so that patients can complete them in a few minutes. Sometimes these instruments are called "screening tests" because, as with a traditional screening test, if a patient scores above a specified cutoff point, the clinician should undertake a more complete diagnostic evaluation.

These questionnaires are not, however, "true" screening tests. Routine blood pressure determination, serum cholesterol, mammography, endocervical smears for cytology, sigmoidoscopy, and stool tests for occult blood are all widely used in primary medical care to screen for asymptomatic disease. One of the requirements for an effective screening test is that it identify patients whose disease is in a preclinical or asymptomatic phase. Thus, early treatment can potentially prevent the full-blown clinical syndrome and its complications. Certain parts of the medical history are actually "screening tests" in this sense. For example, knowledge of cardiac risk factors is important in predicting and attempting to prevent heart disease. Thus, a "risk factor history" is a screening test, analogous to a blood pressure check or a cholesterol determination. The patient's family history of heart disease, smoking habits, and exercise profile are all important screening data. In the same sense, any part of the medical history that relates to the risk of developing a disease or to the detection of an asymptomatic disease, rather than to the presence of an established disease, can be considered a screening test.

Instruments like the SDS rely on the fact that characteristic symptoms are already present. They simply direct the clinician's attention to a possible diagnosis—in this case, depression—by assigning quantitative weight to a cluster of symptoms. This characteristic makes them *case-finding* instruments rather than *screening* instruments.

Such case-finding questionnaires have been developed primarily for psychiatric disorders. This is understandable since most psychiatric disorders are, in fact, defined by a constellation of symptoms and behaviors. Diagnosis relies almost entirely on a thorough interview. Neither scans, blood tests, nor biopsies can serve as "clinchers." These questionnaires can be useful in interviewing medical patients because psychiatric conditions occur frequently in medical patients and physicians often fail to diagnose them correctly. Questionnaire scores might assist physicians in suspecting a condition and then making the proper diagnosis.

Depression is a prime example. Of all patients seen in primary medical care settings, 6% to 9% suffer from a major depressive disorder, while another large group experience other variants of depression. Yet, less than half of all depressed patients are accurately diagnosed and even fewer receive appropriate treatment. Why is this the case? Several factors may contribute. Medical physicians—quite properly—look first to physical illness and consider the possibility of a psychiatric disorder only after somatic disease is thoroughly ruled out. Physicians often do not understand how common depression is and how much morbidity it may cause. They may be unaware that depression usually causes somatic or vegetative symptoms (e.g., fatigue, weight loss, sleep disorder, or difficulty with memory and concentration). Moreover, they may not be familiar with proper methods of treatment for depression. In some cases, doctors may recognize the presence of depression but withhold formal diagnosis because they believe a psychiatric disorder stigmatizes the patient.

Tables 12–1 and 12–2 present two frequently used depression questionnaires. The Center for Epidemiological Studies Depression Scale (CES-D) is a 20-item instrument (see Table 12–1) that, although structured for patient self-administration, can easily be adapted for use by a physician or other health care provider in a medical interview. When used with a cutoff score of 27 to "screen" all medical outpatients, the CES-D has a positive predictive value of between 27% and 42%.[27,29] This means that, if a patient has a score of 27 or above, he or she has about one chance in three (or two in five) of currently suffering from major depressive disorder. Based on this information, the doctor should further question the patient about specific symptoms of major depression which ultimately will lead to a more accurate diagnosis. The SDS (see Table 12–2) when used with a cutoff score of 55 or 60 and the CES-D have similar positive predictive values. Since the predictive value depends in part on *prior probability*, a "positive" CES-D or SDS in a patient with a high risk of depression would have a higher predictive value than a "positive" test in a low-risk patient. Some examples of high-risk patients include persons with chronic disease, those who have unexplained symptoms, and those with a prior history of depression.

Table 12–3 presents the MAST, a 25-item questionnaire that focuses on abnormal drinking behavior as well as its social, legal, and health consequences. A score of 5 indicates a very high probability of alcohol abuse or dependence.[93] While this instrument is fairly long, much of its diagnostic information can be obtained by using small subsets of MAST questions. For example, in one study the two questions, "Have you ever had a drinking problem?" and "Was your last drink within the last 24 hours?," when combined had a positive predictive value for alcoholism of 69% and a negative predictive value of 98%.[31] In other words, if the patient answers both question in the affirmative, there is better than two chances in three that he or she has a drinking problem;

TABLE 12-1. Center for Epidemiological Studies Depression Scale

Name:_____ I.D. No._____

CES-D Scale

Circle the number for each statement which best describes how often you felt or behaved this way—DURING THE PAST WEEK.

During the Past Week	Rarely or None of the Time (Less than 1 day)	Some or a Little of the Time (1–2 days)	Occasionally or a Moderate Amount of the Time (3–4 days)	Most or All of the Time (5–7 days)
1. I was bothered by things that don't bother me	0	1	2	3
2. I did not feel like eating; my appetite was poor	0	1	2	3
3. I felt that I could not shake off the blues even with help from my family or friends	0	1	2	3
4. I felt that I was as good as other people	3	2	1	0
5. I had trouble keeping my mind on what I was doing	0	1	2	3
6. I felt depressed	0	1	2	3
7. I felt that everything I did was an effort	0	1	2	3
8. I felt hopeful about the future	3	2	1	0
9. I thought my life had been a failure	0	1	2	3
10. I felt fearful	0	1	2	3
11. My sleep was restless	0	1	2	3
12. I was happy	3	2	1	3
13. I talked less than usual	0	1	2	3
14. I felt lonely	0	1	2	3
15. People were unfriendly	0	1	2	3
16. I enjoyed life	3	2	1	0
17. I had crying spells	0	1	2	3
18. I felt sad	0	1	2	3
19. I felt that people disliked me	0	1	2	3
20. I could not get "going"	0	1	2	3

Source: From Radloff,[84] with permission.

273

TABLE 12–2. Self-Rating Depression Scale

Below are twenty statements. Please rate each using the following scale: 1 = some or a little of the time; 2 = some of the time; 3 = good part of the time; 4 = most or all of the time.

Please record your rating in the space to the left of each item.

_____   1. I feel down-hearted, blue, and sad.
_____   2. Morning is when I feel the best.
_____   3. I have crying spells or feel like it.
_____   4. I have trouble sleeping through the night.
_____   5. I eat as much as I used to.
_____   6. I enjoy looking at, talking to, and being with attractive women/men.
_____   7. I notice that I am losing weight.
_____   8. I have trouble with constipation.
_____   9. My heart beats faster than usual.
_____ 10. I get tired for no reason.
_____ 11. My mind is as clear as it used to be.
_____ 12. I find it easy to do the things I used to.
_____ 13. I am restless and can't keep still.
_____ 14. I feel hopeful about the future.
_____ 15. I am more irritable than usual.
_____ 16. I find it easy to make decisions.
_____ 17. I feel that I am useful and needed.
_____ 18. My life is pretty full.
_____ 19. I feel that others would be better off if I were dead.
_____ 20. I still enjoy the things I used to do.

Source: From Zung WK. A self-rating depression scale. *Arch Gen Psychiatry.* 1965; 12: 63–70. Copyright 1965, American Medical Association.

TABLE 12–3. Michigan Alcoholism Screening Test Questionnaire

Question	Points
1. Do you feel you are a normal drinker?	2
2. Have you ever awakened the morning after some drinking the night before and found that you could not remember a part of the evening before?	2
3. Does your spouse (or parents) ever worry or complain about your drinking?	1
4. Can you stop drinking without a struggle after one or two drinks?	2

TABLE 12–3. Michigan Alcoholism Screening Test Questionnaire (*Continued*)

Question	Points
5. Do you ever feel bad about your drinking?	1
6. Do friends or relatives think you are a normal drinker?	1
7. Do you ever try to limit your drinking to certain times of the day or to certain places?	0
8. Are you always able to stop drinking when you want to?	2
9. Have you ever attended a meeting of Alcoholics Anonymous (AA)?	5
10. Have you gotten into fights when drinking?	1
11. Has drinking ever created problems with you and your spouse?	2
12. Has your spouse (or other family member) ever gone to anyone for help about your drinking?	2
13. Have you ever lost friends or girlfriends or boyfriends because of drinking?	2
14. Have you ever gotten into trouble at work because of drinking?	2
15. Have you ever lost a job because of drinking?	2
16. Have you ever neglected your obligations, your family, or your work for two or more days in a row because you were drinking?	2
17. Do you ever drink before noon?	1
18. Have you ever been told you have liver trouble? Cirrhosis?	2
19. Have you ever had delirium tremens (DTs), severe shaking, heard voices, or seen things that were not there after heavy drinking?	2
20. Have you ever gone to anyone for help about your drinking?	5
21. Have you ever been in a hospital because of drinking?	5
22. Have you ever been a patient in a psychiatric hospital or on a psychiatric ward of a general hospital where drinking was part of the problem?	2
23. Have you ever been seen at a psychiatric or mental health clinic or gone to a doctor, social worker, or clergyman for help with an emotional problem in which drinking played a part?	2
24. Have you ever been arrested, even for a few hours, because of drunk behavior?	2
25. Have you ever been arrested for drunk driving or driving after drinking?	2

Score points for negative answers to questions 1, 4, 6, and 8 and positive answers to all other questions. A score of 5 or more points is highly suggestive of alcohol abuse.

Source: From Selzer ML. The Michigan alcoholism screening test: The quest for a new diagnostic instrument. *Am J Psychiatry,* 127, 1653–1658, 1971. Copyright 1971, the American Psychiatric Association. Reprinted by permission.

those who answer both questions in the negative have almost no chance of having a drinking problem.

Four questions from the MAST instrument have been widely used in the primary care setting to help identify patients with alcohol problems. These are the so-called CAGE questions:

- Have you ever felt you ought to Cut down on your drinking?
- Have people Annoyed you by criticizing your drinking?
- Have you ever felt bad or Guilty about your drinking?
- Have you ever had a drink first thing in the morning (Eye opener) to steady your nerves or get rid of a hangover?

If all answers are negative, alcohol abuse or dependence can be ruled out. If one or more is positive, the physician should be sensitized to explore further the role of alcohol in the patient's life. A third questionnaire is also useful in assessing the probability of alcohol abuse (Table 12–4), especially when interviewing patients in an emergency room setting. This set of questions is based on the fact that alcoholic patients are susceptible to frequent episodes of trauma.

In summary, several questionnaires are available to assist in identifying depression, alcohol abuse, and other psychiatric disorders. Some of these instruments can be self-administered. Any of them can be incorporated as focused questioning into your basic medical interview. They yield quantitative data (scores) that can be compared with general guidelines or standards, but they are not in themselves diagnostic of the different conditions.

TABLE 12–4. Trauma Scale

Since your eighteenth birthday
  1. Have you had any fractures or dislocations of bones or joints?
  2. Have you been injured in an automobile accident?
  3. Have you injured your head?
  4. Have you been injured in an assault or fight? (Excluding sports.)
  5. Have you been injured after drinking?

One point for each positive response. A score of 2 or more suggests alcohol abuse.

Source: Adapted from Skinner et al.[98]

Such questionnaires should be used to enhance your ability to assess these clinical entities that are difficult to detect.

COMPUTER-ASSISTED HISTORY TAKING

The term "computer-assisted history taking" refers to a number of related applications that use computers to improve the collection and interpretation of patient history data. For example, a computer might be used to process and store information collected from multi-item questionnaires completed by patients prior to the physician encounter. A computer can be used to elicit potentially embarrassing information from the patient in a less threatening manner. The computer might be used interactively by a patient or by a health care team intermediary as a supplement to or replacement for a face-to-face interview. You might use a computer to aid you in the construction of a differential diagnoses list. In more sophisticated applications, a computer might generate diagnostic possibilities and then implicitly, or in some cases explicitly, prompt physicians to seek further history and physical data from the patient in order to investigate these possibilities. In addition to obtaining information *from* the patient, the computer might provide educational information or lifestyle modification instructions *to* the patient. Finally, the computer might be used as an aid in teaching students interviewing skills.

Acquisition of Patient Data

Computers have been employed, with varying degrees of sophistication, to assist the physician in acquiring patient data. Though not considered part of the traditional medical history, patient billing data are often collected or stored by computer. Many physicians ask new patients to complete a general health survey before coming in for the initial examination; this data may then be entered into a computerized database by clerical assistants or by electronic means, e.g., by using an optical scanner. Indeed, this use of computers was the earliest attempt at mechanizing the process of history taking,[15,24] and, though not sophisticated, is still a useful technique. In addition to providing a database of patient information, programs that use this technique can generate printed summaries that prepare the physician for a patient encounter, allowing the physician to focus more efficiently on the patient's complaints. Such questionnaires, however, are often time-consuming for the patient to complete and may be time-consuming to enter into the computer if an electronic scanner is not used. Additionally, this technique fails to take advantage of the interactive power of the computer.

Interactive computer-assisted history programs, in which the patient directly enters information, can utilize patient time and energy more efficiently through the use of branching algorithms.[99] With such a technique, if a patient answers no to a general question, the program will bypass the related, more specific questions much as you might do in a face-to-face interview. Thus, pertinent areas can be explored in some detail without needlessly boring or annoying the user with a long list of irrelevant questions. Such an algorithm could also be used to give a patient pertinent lifestyle modification suggestions without subjecting him or her to superfluous information.

Other programs take advantage of stored medical knowledge to obtain information in a more intelligent manner. The Present Illness Program (PIP), for example, used stored knowledge of renal disease states to generate questions that modeled the information-gathering process of a physician encountering a patient with edema.[79] The original intent of this program was not to provide a clinical tool; rather the program was written to model the problem-solving process. Using a slightly different technique, one computer-based questionnaire presented a baseline list of 50 questions to patients and then used statistical information on sensitivity and specificity of symptoms to ask the questions most likely to be helpful in arriving at a diagnosis.[104] This process was recently refined to collect data from patients with pulmonary disease. Another program was developed that obtained data from patients in a cyclical fashion by using tools already available in HELP,[81] a sophisticated hospital information system. Responses to an initial set of questions were used to activate several "disease frames." Information contained in these frames could then be used to request the most useful subsequent information. When the program was tested, the number of questions presented to the patient was reduced (from 182 using a paper questionnaire to a mean of 50.7, using the computer-assisted questionnaire) with no loss of diagnostic accuracy.[55a]

Advantages

There are several advantages to using computer-assisted history collection. Patients generally find the technique acceptable,[18,19,70] and some reports indicate that the practice may result in the recording of more complete information.[70] By collecting some data ahead of time, the physician might be able to focus more efficiently on selected areas. Additionally, some studies indicate that patients may be more willing to disclose information on sensitive topics (such as alcohol use or details of their sexual history) to a computer, rather than to a physician.[73] As an additional benefit, interactive computer sessions may be used to provide educational information.

Problems

Useful as the technique may be, computer-assisted history taking does suffer from some limitations that make it unlikely to ever replace the physician-patient interview. Patients' responses to a computerized questionnaire are limited to yes/no or, at best, to categorical answers. The tendency to ask closed-ended questions may be enhanced when the history is obtained by an intermediary using the computer for assistance.[19] Use of such closed-ended questions may inhibit exploration of areas not specifically included in the questionnaire. Also, it is not unusual for the use of computers to increase (rather than decrease) the amount of time spent obtaining the history. Perhaps most importantly, clinicians know that important information is obtained not only from the patient responses per se but also from the manner in which the patient replies and from subtle, nonverbal cues that can never be captured by a computer-assisted questionnaire. One study found that although the computerized patient interview contained more data, physicians felt that the traditionally obtained medical history better expressed the chief complaints.[82]

Interactive computer programs also suffer one limitation that simpler, batch-mode questionnaires do not. The programs require that the patient complete the questionnaire at the computer in the physician's office. This, in turn, requires the physician to have available a suitable computer that is dedicated almost exclusively to this purpose and is located in a reasonably private area to ensure patient confidentiality. The use of computers also necessitates more sophistication on the part of the patient and may require that office personnel provide instruction. Now that the prices of microcomputers have fallen dramatically and many programs are "user friendly," the option of having available a dedicated computer for interactive history taking is becoming increasingly attractive. Nonetheless, computer-obtained histories are best viewed as an adjunct to, rather than as a substitute for, traditionally obtained histories.

Experimental Programs and Available Applications

Experimentally, computers have been used to facilitate history taking in a variety of medical fields. Computers have been used by midwives to help obtain a history on the first antenatal visit.[19] An interactive computer system was also used successfully to obtain histories in an infertility clinic.[70] The technique has also been applied to obtaining urological histories,[49] histories from patients with low back pain,[101] and histories from patients suffering from other ailments. Recently, a computer was employed to generate genograms containing important family history information.[39]

Currently, a variety of commercial programs are available to assist in history taking. These programs cover a number of areas from general health surveys to preventive medicine to geriatric screening. They range in complexity from questionnaires that provide yes/no prompts and then subsequently produce a printed summary to integrated systems that store patient history in a relational database for later analysis by the clinician.[74]

Computer-Assisted Medical Diagnosis

The types of programs discussed above are designed to accept historical input and then organize it as an aid to the physician's history taking. Systems are now available that can go several steps beyond this—they are designed to accept history, physical, and laboratory input and then suggest plausible diagnoses to the physician. A full discussion of medical expert systems and computer-assisted medical diagnosis is beyond the scope of this chapter; several good general reviews are available.[92,95,96] Here we consider these programs in the context of medical history taking because some are designed to help with the task of data collection.

The Quick Medical Reference Program (QMR) is a microcomputer-based system that provides diagnostic support in the broad field of internal medicine.[76] It was developed at the University of Pittsburgh and uses an extension of the INTERNIST-I knowledge base, which contains information on more than 4100 manifestations and 600 diseases in the domain of internal medicine.[75] The program functions on several levels. In its most sophisticated mode, the program is designed to accept history and physical and laboratory findings and then to generate a differential diagnoses list based on patient-specific information. The program can also be used at that point to generate a list of potentially discriminating history, physical, or laboratory data that can be sought from the patient to help narrow the differential diagnoses further. When used in this mode as part of a consultation service, the program was found to be accurate and led the housestaff to modify their differential diagnoses in the majority of cases.[5]

DXplain is a computer-based system that offers diagnostic support to physicians.[6] The system is available to the general public through AMA/NET, a telecommunication service sponsored by the AMA. In addition to providing a differential diagnoses list based upon patient-specific data, the program can function in an interactive mode by suggesting useful potentially discriminating history, as well as physical and laboratory information.

ILIAD is a microcomputer-based system that is designed as an educational tool to teach differential diagnosis.[104] The program can function in an expert system or "consultation" mode and offer a second opinion about a case. The program can then prompt the student for the "next best" piece of information to acquire from the patient.

All these programs provide diagnostic support to the user based upon patient-specific history and physical and laboratory data. The resulting differential diagnoses lists can themselves prompt the physician to seek more specific history items. Additionally, they all have features that explicitly prompt the user for specific, potentially helpful items. In addition to their use as diagnostic assistants, two of these programs (QMR and ILIAD) are capable of generating simulated cases to teach students problem-solving skills. Both programs have been introduced into the formal medical school curriculum.

SUMMARY

Computers can be useful aids to the process of medical history taking. Available systems vary in level of sophistication from rigid questionnaires to questionnaires that change depending on the patient's responses to programs that suggest diagnoses to the physician. Regardless of level of sophistication, none is likely to replace the physician as data gatherer or diagnostician.

CHAPTER 13

Clinical Judgment in the Medical Interview

> . . . To Ivan Ilych only one question was important: was his case
> serious or not? But the doctor ignored that inappropriate ques-
> tion. From his point of view it was not the one under considera-
> tion, the real question was to decide between a floating kidney,
> chronic catarrh or appendicitis. It was not a question of life or
> death, but one between a floating kidney and appendicitis.
>
> Tolstoy, *The Death of Ivan Ilych*

Throughout this text we have emphasized the use of the medical interview as a method of obtaining objective and precise
data. Our main focus is the medical history as a diagnostic tool,
but most interactions between doctors and patients are not
purely diagnostic in nature. The data you obtain may be used to
delineate other problems (not strictly defined as diseases) bearing on your patient's illness. The data may serve as a starting
point for patient education or for assessing your patient's progress or the outcome of therapy. We argue that most of the information you need to make diagnoses and to take care of your
patients come from your one-to-one interactions with the
patient, the interview, and the physical examination. In one
sense, we stress completeness—the complete delineation and
clarification of symptoms and dysfunction. However, there is
another sense of "completeness" that is unattainable in a medical interview, a physical examination, or in any patient care situation, no matter how many diagnostic tests you use. *There is no
such entity as a complete history and physical examination.*

Clinicians never have all the data that may be relevant to a
given illness or disease situation or a given patient. There is
always something left out, and all diagnostic and therapeutic
decisions are made in the context of some uncertainty. We use

various devices to minimize uncertainty, but in the long run, a physician usually acts to help his or her patient before the data are complete. We make assumptions without knowing "for sure." For example, we assume, based on past experience and on our knowledge of the incidence of disease, that the 30-year-old man without gastrointestinal (GI) symptoms does not need a sigmoidoscopy. Can we say with 100% certainty that no abnormality would be found were we to do one? No. However, a good history is the most effective and efficient way to ensure that our assumption is correct. If we uncover an episode of rectal bleeding or a family history of intestinal polyposis, then any outcome is possible. As Alvan Feinstein[46] put it, all our diagnostic and therapeutic decisions are, in a sense, experiments. We formulate a hypothesis, change variables, and see what happens. We weigh probabilities, risks, benefits, experience, knowledge of pathophysiology, and opinions of our peers, but we are still left with hypotheses—perhaps well supported ones or perhaps questionable ones—that have to be tested. Unfortunately, the experiments are complex ones that involve humans in whom it is impossible to change one variable while keeping all the others constant. Is this disease really causing the symptoms? Will this medication really help the patient? Learning to accept and work within this uncertainty is a major part of the physician's professional education. Sound *clinical judgment* is simply the logical and empathic approach to decision making within this uncertain environment.

Figure 13–1 illustrates the feedback loop of clinical judgment as it occurs during a medical interview. Elements of process or technique allow the physician to obtain certain data (content), which ultimately must be organized into the traditional sections of a medical history (for instance, present illness or patient profile). However, even the initial fragmentary content stimulates the clinician to formulate hypotheses that then influence the continuing process of data collection. Figure 13–1 lists four different types of hypotheses that might be generated, as suggested by Platt and McMath.[80] Naturally, the overt concern of clinical practice is *differential diagnosis*, hypotheses about the disease that is causing the patient to suffer. But differential diagnoses depend on more basic or preliminary hypotheses about the story itself: How does it fit together? Did X happen before or after Y? The effective clinician should, at the same time, be generating

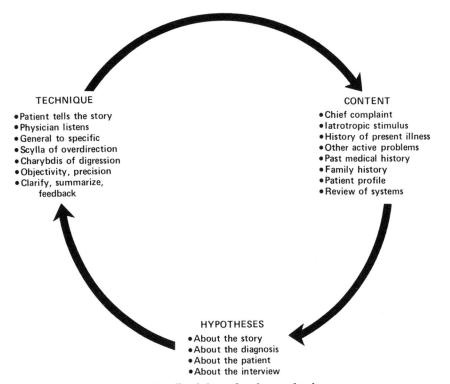

FIGURE 13-1. Feedback loop for the medical interview.

hypotheses about the patient's personality: What sort of coping style does he or she have? What might we expect in terms of compliance or behavior change? Finally, there are hypotheses about the process of the interview itself: What is going wrong? Why do I feel so frustrated or uncomfortable? Chapters 9, 10, and 11 consider hypotheses about the types of interviewing problems that arise when caring for "difficult" patients.

We consider in this chapter some topics raised by the uncertainty of doctor-patient interactions. *First,* we discuss briefly the different types of errors you will make in medicine and their relationship to the elusive "completeness" of our clinical activities such as interviewing. *Second,* we consider what you are thinking about as you conduct the interview. What drives your inquiries? Does the interview simply grow by accretion, or does it change shape and move purposefully as it goes along and you test hypotheses? We review some psychological biases that make it difficult to think logically about the real probability of a given problem or diagnosis. *Finally,* we list some heuristics for good problem solving in clinical interactions, with particular emphasis on problem solving within the medical interview. These are pragmatic guidelines, but the most significant one is the rule that all guidelines have exceptions.

TYPES OF ERRORS

As medical students we make many errors in evaluating patients (Table 13–1); we continue to make errors as house officers and throughout our lives as practicing physicians. Some of these errors are avoidable and some are not. *The first kind of mistake* arises from your own lack of knowledge of what is known, or culpable ignorance. While it is impossible to have a command of all medical knowledge, we each become thoroughly familiar with our medical specialty and continue to keep that knowledge up to date. However, regardless of how well informed you are, you will make some factual errors sometimes—because you are too busy with too many patients or because you are distracted by some other problem, and so forth. For example, you may be preoccupied with a dying patient with whom you have just had a difficult discussion about his or her desire for termination of life support. Your next patient has a relatively simple illness, a sore throat. You do a culture, and because you suspect streptococcus, you write out a prescription for penicillin for the patient to take pending the outcome of the culture. The patient informs you of an allergy to penicillin. You forgot to ask. So one kind of uncertainty in clinical interactions arises from your not knowing what you should know or forgetting it.

A *second error* arises from the "state of the science." We treated enlarged thymus glands with irradiation in the 1940s, threatened abortions with diethylstilbestrol in the 1950s, and treated upper respiratory infections with chloramphenicol in the

TABLE 13–1. Types of Errors in Medical Decisions

The clinician lacks knowledge of the subject matter.
The current state of medical knowledge is inadequate.
Biological events are by nature probabilistic.
The clinician breaches the patient's trust.
The clinician uses faulty logic (an intellectual error).

1960s. Each of these therapies was mistaken and actually posed a health risk that outweighed the benefits. Undoubtedly, we are making similar kinds of mistakes today that will only become clear to us when our medical knowledge improves. In the interview we may emphasize the relationship of certain patient activities to the development, prevention, or treatment of disease, e.g., diet as a treatment for coronary artery disease or the effect of minimal maternal alcohol consumption on fetal development. Yet each of these associations is controversial and will undoubtedly be clarified in the future.

A *third error* is a result of the probabilistic nature of events in medicine and biological variability. For example, since drugs affect different people differently, the best we can do is to say that we expect a high rate of cure or a low rate of side effects in a certain situation. But even when the probabilities clearly indicate that a decision is correct, the improbable may in fact occur, leading to an adverse effect. The natural history of a person's unique illness is not rigidly determined by factors we understand. The second and third types of errors may well be related: With greater medical knowledge, fewer biological events will appear to be probabilistic and more events will be clearly determined by known factors. Whether probabilistic error is ultimately reducible, state-of-the-science error is a philosophic question beyond the range of our discussion.

Breach of trust is a *fourth error* that occurs when we fail to obtain informed consent or break the obligation requiring confidentiality. We are guilty of breach of trust when we lie to our patients or mislead them, or when we blithely accept our version of their best interest without appropriate respect for their own wishes. While this type of error is appropriate subject matter for medical ethics studies, you make "ethical decisions" repeatedly in the interview. You avoid breach of trust in the interview by actively eliciting and listening to your patient's ideas and values regarding the illness and its management. Although there has been little critical study of precisely how one goes about the difficult task of discussing anticipated risks and benefits with patients, a good first step is listening.

The *fifth mistake* is a breakdown in thinking—intellectual error or faulty logic. Investigators concerned with decision making in medicine have focused primarily on the making and testing of hypotheses in the process of formulating a diagnosis. Did you see the facts correctly? Did you judge what is probable as well as what is possible in a given situation? For example, if a patient complains of tarry stools, you must logically use this fact to guide the interview and elicit other GI symptoms that would help substantiate or rule out upper GI bleeding as the cause.

Good interviewing skills help eliminate these errors in logic as you interact with patients. As you learn the basic knowledge and skills of how to conduct an adequate interview, you also learn to devise your interview strategy to move in a logical direction. The more open ended the interview, the less likely that you will miss both facts and values.

ERRORS IN CONDUCTING THE INTERVIEW

Platt and McMath[80] identified five "syndromes" of hypocompetence that they observed during 300 doctor-patient interviews conducted by medical house officers. They labeled their syndromes as

1. Low therapeutic content;
2. Flawed database;
3. Defective hypothesis generation;
4. Failure to demand primary data; and
5. Inappropriately high control style.

Voytovich and coworkers[103] identified four categories of error in diagnostic reasoning:

1. Omission;
2. Premature closure;
3. Wrong synthesis; and
4. Inadequate synthesis.

It is useful to consider how these syndromes and categories of error relate to interviewing style. Table 13–2 illustrates how errors in communication skills during a medical interview might predispose to different varieties of error in diagnostic reasoning. For example, "failure to generate hypotheses" (cognition) and "omission" (behavior) are characteristic of an interview during which the physician neglects to observe the patient carefully and

TABLE 13–2. Errors in Diagnostic Reasoning Prompted by
Errors in Interview Skills

Skill	Result of Too Much	Result of Too Little or Inadequate
Observing the patient (nonverbal communication)		Omission Failure to generate hypotheses
Open-ended questioning	Inadequate synthesis	Omission Failure to generate hypotheses Failure to demand primary data
Focused questioning	High control style Flawed database	Premature closure Inadequate synthesis

Source: Errors in reasoning derived from Platt and McMath[80] and Voytovich et al.[103]

to conduct a broad, open-ended inquiry. Platt and McMath's "failure to demand primary data" is more specific to a deficiency in the open-ended questioning part of the interview. "Inadequate synthesis" (cognition) and "premature closure" (behavior) might occur when there is too little focused questioning or when focused questioning is not skillfully used—a situation in which it would be difficult to build a robust and relevant case.

There is often, although not inevitably, a reciprocal relationship between open-ended and focused questioning, so that too little of one might be correlated with too much of the other. Platt and McMath's "high control style" and "flawed database" clearly take place when focused questioning is overemphasized and/or begins too early in the process. "Inadequate synthesis" is also favored when the interviewer lacks control or direction (e.g., too open-ended), which leads to a very nonfocused approach.

If, in fact, errors in diagnostic logic tend to be represented by deficiencies in certain interviewer behaviors, it should be possible to correlate these behaviors with inaccurate reasoning or diagnosis. Excessive premature closure or inadequate synthesis might be related to a pattern of inadequate focused questioning—perhaps because focused questioning is aborted because of time constraints or preconceived conclusions, or is simply not skillfully handled in terms of achieving a "minimal diagnostic pathway"[32] or making accurate "intermediate decisions."[47] It is possible that empirical studies of the relationship between questioning techniques and accuracy in diagnosis will reveal concrete, teachable patterns that will help us minimize such errors.

ERROR AND COMPLETENESS

Another way to categorize mistakes is to divide them into *errors of commission* and *errors of omission*. You can either *do* the wrong thing or *fail to do* the right one. These categories cut across the types of error listed previously. Factual mistakes, limitations of medical knowledge in general, breach of trust, or faulty logic can all occur, both in actions that you take or actions that you fail to take. These concepts have important ramifications when we consider the completeness of our history taking and physical examination. We often talk of doing a medical test for the sake of completeness. It is one of those pat phrases that is heard daily on rounds. We have come to think of "completeness" as something like "Big Brother" or perhaps as an unacknowledged entity that stalks our halls demanding daily sacrifices. We gaze furtively at one another, wondering what evil might befall us if we do not placate "completeness." We all do things "for completeness' sake" and, interestingly, such actions may lead to a paradoxic situation: Our job is to help sick people, but often, insofar as we do things for completeness' sake, our actions are less likely to be done for the patient's sake.

All this is another way of saying that errors of commission are generally more sanctioned in medicine than errors of omission. You rarely get into trouble with your peers if you order extra studies or make the examination more complete than necessary, unless you order a very invasive and expensive test that is obviously unnecessary. On the other hand, you are frequently asked to justify yourself if you do not order a diagnostic test that may even be only mildly relevant to a particular illness or that is relevant but unnecessary because its result will not change any therapeutic decision. We make decisions about completeness all the time when we interview patients. We may decide, for example, to forego the history of childhood diseases in the 85-year-old woman with hypertension or to skip the sexual history in a new patient who presents with acute back pain. We often feel, however, that omitting certain parts of the history is less acceptable than taking a too "invasive" history. We continually weigh the value of the information likely to be obtained against the limits of the patient's tolerance to be interviewed because he or she is too sick or too tired or would feel that certain matters are too private.

Many physicians justify completeness by a call to "defensive medicine." They claim that they have to do a computerized tomography scan in a young man who has a bump on his head and who never lost consciousness because the case may end up in court some day. The issue of malpractice suits is one we cannot consider here, except to say that such suits most often arise when bad feelings are superimposed on bad results. Many malpractice suits stem from poor communication, failure to obtain accurate and precise patient data, too little time spent explaining diagnoses or procedures, poor rapport, misunderstandings, and personality clashes. Good medical interviewing helps avoid all of those. Of course, good communication will not eliminate every threat of liability. In addition, if you are defensive and order enough tests for the sake of completeness, occasionally one of them will be truly useful. But how many errors of commission, with all their attendant costs and risks, will you have to make in order to prevent one serious error of omission? All the excessive studies and overtreatment performed in the name of completeness constitute an enormous chunk of professionally sanctioned "malpractice" that, at present, rarely ends up in court and is rarely discussed.

Defensive medicine aside, there are psychological reasons why we tend to favor errors of commission. We are action oriented, we want to help the patient, we feel ourselves under pressure to *do something* to ease suffering, and we do not like to wallow in ambiguity. We view high-technology medicine as an exciting scientific accomplishment and ourselves as applying its benefits to sick people. It is not difficult to understand why we are less sensitized to possible errors of completeness (which is a kind of muddled thinking) and overtreatment (which may lead to iatrogenic illness) than we are to possible errors of not doing enough for our patients.

HYPOTHESES AND PROBABILITY IN THE INTERVIEW

Completeness obviously does not provide a sufficient guide for making diagnoses and prescribing therapy. Facts are not enough; you have to think. It is useful to consider what is actually going on in your head as you interview your new patient and take his or her medical history. Some of your preceptors will stress completeness as if there were a certain finite body of medical facts that, once obtained, would fit together like a jigsaw puzzle. You collect nondescript volumes of data and later, when you sit down to think about it, its meaning materializes. If you collect data in this fashion during the interview, you exhaust both yourself and the patient. Diagnosis does not occur in this way. In fact, a *hypothetico-deductive* approach rather than an *inductive* one is used. In other words, you must constantly consider guesses or hypotheses, which you try to support or refute throughout the interview, physical examination, and subsequent diagnostic strategy.

Elstein and his coworkers at Michigan State University[42] showed that experienced physicians generate a variety of hypotheses about what causes the patient's problem within the first 2 minutes, and often within the first 30 seconds, of interacting with the patient. They found that data gathering is constantly changing its character based on what has gone before. They discovered that physicians have a fairly limited ability to juggle hypotheses that might explain a given problem; usually no more than five hypotheses are considered at any time. Clinicians then design their questioning and other testing to obtain data that either support one or more of the hypotheses, or tend to disprove or weigh against them. They continue this process until one hypothesis stands out sufficiently from the others. This hypothesis can then be acted on, or it can be used to generate a diagnosis. Thus, the clinical method, just like the scientific method, does not involve first gathering an enormous amount of data and then later seeing how all the parts fit together; rather, most of the data are collected for the purpose of testing hypotheses. For example, on the most elementary level, as soon as you walk into the room and see that the patient is a female of a particular race and age, you know that some diagnoses are possible while others are impossible.

The nature of this process means that *probability testing* plays a major role in the clinical judgment that is used in interviews as well as therapeutic and diagnostic decisions. We ask questions most likely to clarify the problem and use the treatment most likely to help. Ideally, probability testing requires:

1. A broad knowledge of pathophysiology and therapeutics;
2. Prior probability (or prevalence) estimates for the given disease, based upon textbook facts and, later, upon our own experience; and
3. A logical approach for estimating changes in the probability.

Good clinicians integrate these functions in making clinical judgments all the time, but the clinicians frequently find it difficult to dissect out the different elements of this process so that they can be stated clearly. Researchers in clinical judgment have discovered that we are all subject to certain psychological biases that can distort our clinical thinking. Within the interview these biases distort our hearing and understanding of the patient's symptoms and change the strategy of our deductive approach in much the same way—albeit in the opposite direction—as sound logic. These biases might make a particular diagnosis feel more probable or less probable than it really is. As human beings we are all subject to errors in judgment; however, we can minimize these errors by bringing them into the open and understanding just what they are and how they occur.

Bias

Table 13–3 lists a number of psychological biases important in medicine. The bias of *availability* means that the doctor's assessment of how probable a diagnosis is relates to how easy it is for instances or occurrences of that disease to be brought to mind. This is simply another way of saying that the things that you are more familiar with or knowledgeable about appear to be more likely than uncertain or obscure items. A diagnosis might seem more probable than it really is if, for example, you have seen a patient who proved to have a similar diagnosis last week or you

TABLE 13–3. Psychologic
Biases in Estimating
Probability

Availability
Representativeness
Sunk costs
Anchoring and adjustment
Rule in favoritism
Occam's razor

have just been reading about a certain disease in your textbook. Within the interview, you might go to a series of closed-ended or leading questions to discover what you suspect, thereby shutting out other symptoms that point to the real problem. For example, if you have just read the chapter on lymphomas, you may think that your patient with the chief complaint of "swollen glands" has Hodgkin's disease until proven otherwise. You may ask first about night sweats and weight loss, only later finding out that his 10-year-old son had a similar illness last week and that other symptoms suggest the much more likely simple streptococcal infection.

Such bias often leads to a failure within the interview to obtain data needed to make the correct diagnosis. Here is an interview of a 38-year-old patient with abdominal pain. The interviewer has been reading about peptic ulcer disease:

Dr: Tell me what brought you to the clinic today.
Pt: Well, my stomach has been acting up for the past few weeks.
Dr: Does food make it better or worse?
Pt: That's hard to say, it depends on what I eat.
Dr: How about antacids?
Pt: Antacids?
Dr: Things like Maalox or Mylanta. Have you tried anything like that?
Pt: I think that might help. It helps the gas sometimes.

Notice the poor interviewing technique here. The interviewer fails to obtain information about the location of the pain (which happened to be lower abdominal, not epigastric). Instead, the interviewer jumps into a series of closed-ended questions intended to support a diagnosis of peptic ulcer disease. Notice the patient's attempt to please the interviewer with the "correct" response ("I think that might help"). In reality this patient suffered from lactose intolerance causing lower abdominal pain, gaseousness, and diarrhea.

In a similar way, a subspecialist is likely to see diseases in his or her subspecialty as occurring more frequently than they really do in the general population or among people with the same set of symptoms who go to primary care doctors. Gastroenterologists are more likely than other doctors to diagnose GI disease, not only because their patients tend, of course, to have clear-cut GI symptom-complexes but also because gastroenterologists overvalue GI diagnoses among patients who have symptom-complexes that are also compatible with non-GI diagnoses.

Representativeness is another frequent psychologic bias, particularly among physicians who stick closely to their textbooks and clinical literature. These doctors often think a rare disease is very probable if a patient has the representative or classical symptoms of that disease. Let us say a disease has five characteristic symptoms but is extremely rare, occurring in only one out of every million people. The five symptoms might be dizziness, right upper quadrant abdominal pain, frequent headaches, difficulty sleeping, and waking up in the morning with muscle stiffness. Each of these symptoms is quite common in itself. The fact that a patient has all five at once certainly makes him considerably more likely to have the rare disease; but more prevalent, ordinary diseases are still the most probable explanation for the patient's illness. Even though the patient provides a representative picture, other common diseases are more likely to explain his or her problem than the rare disease. This does not mean that correct clinical judgment would never allow for making a very rare diagnosis, but it does mean that pursuing such a diagnosis usually has more to do with utility (see below) than it does with probability. This is a common problem early in a physician's medical career, when he or she has little practical experience with the prevalence and incidence—or probability—of diseases. Every disease seems as likely as any other, every symptom is as likely to represent a rare disease as a common one.

If a certain amount of money or effort has already been invested in pursuing a given diagnostic strategy, the outcome or yield from that strategy may appear more likely than it really is, and the doctor may continue further tests so as not to "waste" those tests already performed. This is the bias called *sunk costs*. Let us say that a patient is ill with general muscle aches, malaise, and possible intermittent fevers. He also had some nonspecific abdominal pain that, when you first took the history, you believed was suggestive of GI abnormality. You then ordered an upper GI x-ray series (normal), and on subsequent discussion with the patient you find that the GI symptoms are really not as important a part of the syndrome as you first thought. The bias of sunk costs will tend to make you feel more compelled to complete the GI workup, for example, with a barium enema and flexible sigmoidoscopy rather than to leave the GI symptoms "hanging."

In a very broad sense, the fact that you have a hypothesis, or several of them, tends to make you look more carefully at observations relevant to those hypotheses and to ignore other observations. You must have a frame of reference for your thinking. Clear thinking will necessarily lead more and more strongly in a given direction, simply because the remaining hypotheses are judged very probable or very useful or both. The bias of sunk costs is an exaggeration of this process, which leads to focusing too intently on a diagnosis simply because you are invested in it and then, perhaps, are not open to new data that may change your thinking.

Availability, representativeness, and sunk costs can be observed every day in the practice of medicine. The bias called *anchoring and adjustment* is a little more arcane. Doctors use some rough estimate of subjective probability to start with and then anchor their opinions at that level, using an adjustment factor to revise their opinion upward or downward as a result of new information. It is psychologically difficult to condense vast ranges of probability into the diagnostic problem frame, particularly since you know the patient is ill and there is a 100% probability that *something* is wrong. What can you do with a differential diagnosis in which one hypothesis has a 75% probability and another a 0.001% probability? Physicians cope with this problem by anchoring their estimates in a middle range, so that very unlikely diagnoses get overvalued and likely diagnoses often get undervalued. The adjustment factor after considering new evidence tends to be smaller in either direction than is really warranted by the facts. The net effect is that judgments hover toward the middle level of probability, and doctors often consider diseases that have vastly different likelihoods with only moderately different degrees of seriousness while pursuing their diagnostic strategy.

Since medicine demands action, there is also a bias in favor of making the diagnosis out of the array of hypotheses available. Elstein[42] and other students of clinical decision making have found that physicians often seek out and evaluate evidence to support their main hypotheses but are less aggressive in seeking out evidence that could rule out this hypothesis. This tendency might be called *rule in favoritism.* Within the interview, for example, you might actively seek symptoms such as nausea, radiation to the jaw or left arm, and sweating to support your hypothesis that the patient's chest pain is due to coronary insufficiency. You may not ask if the pain occurs upon lying down or is relieved by antacids to try to rule out esophageal reflux. The worth of an open-ended question such as "Did you notice anything else?" is its power to elicit data we simply forgot or did not think of because of this bias.

We should also mention the tendency to try to make one diagnosis rather than several. This principle of parsimony is a reasonable clinical guideline, a heuristic that all students of medicine should consider when evaluating the patient's history and physical findings. It is called *Occam's razor,* named after William of Occam, a 14th-century scholastic philosopher. In medicine this means that we should try to explain the entire illness—all the symptoms—with one diagnosis. While this is a good rule to keep in mind, it is certainly not always correct, especially in these days of multiple chronic and degenerative diseases. In particular, the concurrent occurrence of two common diseases (e.g., diabetes mellitus and peptic ulcer) is a more likely explanation of the symptom-complex of abdominal pain, vomiting, polyuria, and polydipsia than is occurrence of one rare disease (e.g., acute intermittent porphyria). Occam's razor supports the bias of representativeness when it makes us favor latching on to an uncommon diagnosis to avoid considering the less intellectually satisfying alternative of partitioning the diagnosis of the illness among several explanations.

Utility and Clinical Judgment

Clinical judgment is conditioned by utility as well as probability. Diagnoses or decisions are not ends in themselves but are tools for making the patient feel better. Thus, we want to pay particular attention to certain kinds of diagnostic hypotheses even when they are not judged to be very probable or the most probable explanation. For example, serious diseases *(seriousness)* must be considered and ruled out much more aggressively than mild or self-limited diseases. Even though a random positive test for occult blood in the stool of a healthy, asymptomatic individual most likely does *not* indicate cancer, it is medically appropriate to do a thorough evaluation of the GI tract in someone with such an unexplained finding. It would be poor judgment to ignore the results of that test (i.e., the stool guaiac), even though the risk of cancer in a person with a single positive test may only be 5%.

Treatability is another aspect of utility. There is no point in pursuing diagnosis for the sake of diagnosis unless it can have some benefit for the patient. Knowing the diagnosis and satisfying our own curiosity about the factors that led to the outcome may really have no value for the patient. Our decisions should be dictated by utility for the patient, not utility for us, unless the patient is enrolled in an experimental protocol after having given informed consent. There is no sense in doing a liver biopsy on an alcoholic patient who comes to the hospital with abnormal liver function tests once we have ascertained that the test result will have nothing to do with the patient's subsequent management. The same patient may, in the future, have recurrent episodes of abdominal problems or abnormal liver function, which would lead us to question our hypothesis of alcoholic liver disease, and at that point perhaps a biopsy would be indicated. But even then the decision must be dictated by what is best for the patient. Our "need to know" is not necessarily best for the patient, even when the risks and costs of further tests are low but particularly when they are high, as is usually the case in complex, invasive studies.

The patient's own assessment of utility should have paramount value, although physicians often have a major impact on the patient's beliefs about utility. We do not believe, as some ethical and legal commentators suggest, that all medical decisions can or should always be made entirely independently by the rational patient. In fact, sick people tend to trust their physicians and do not want to be burdened with multiple decisions, even when these patients are fully able to understand the general nature and consequences of the options. Investigators have found that informed consent, although espoused by most patients, is not so highly valued by them when faced with actual decisions about their own medical care.[68,69] Patients tend to rely on their doctors' advice, rather than on thinking through all the alternatives, expecting fidelity in their relationship. However, fidelity in this relationship depends on the physician's understanding of the patient. Within the interview a physician who helps a patient express his or her values and allows the patient to ask questions will learn what facts, from an array of many, this particular patient needs to know to make a decision. Consideration of the patient's own value system and decisions about whether to accept medical care is beyond the scope of this text but certainly has an impact on the questions of negotiation and healing that are considered in Chapter 14.

HEURISTICS FOR THE MEDICAL INTERVIEW

We have adapted a set of guidelines for improving your clinical judgment during your interview with the patient from the heuristics presented by Elstein and associates.[42] These are an attempt to give you a "handle" or set of thinking skills to use as you proceed through your patient interview and physical examination; these guidelines are also useful as you continue to judge strategies for diagnosis and management.

1. **Multiple, competing hypotheses:** Think of a number of diagnostic possibilities compatible with the chief complaint and data obtained in the early part of the medical interview. Avoid making "snap" diagnoses, as this tends to make it difficult for you to hear data that suggest other etiologies.
2. **Probability:** Consider the most common diagnoses first.
3. **Utility:** Consider more seriously those diagnoses for which effective therapies are available, for which treatment would be significantly different than that for competing diagnoses, and in which failure to treat would

hurt the patient (i.e., it would be a serious omission). Try to keep your estimates of the probability of a disease and the utility of diagnosing it separate.

4. **Branch and screen:** History taking and the physical examination should be branching procedures. You should develop screening tactics to avoid overly detailed examinations when they are unnecessary.

5. **Precision:** Strive for the degree of precision or reliability needed for the decision at hand. More than that is not necessary. For example, for many adult patients it is not necessary to know the fine details of every childhood illness. However, if a patient states that he or she had rheumatic fever as a child, you must elicit historical evidence in support of the diagnosis because that illness may have long-term consequences into adulthood.

6. **Plan:** Form a reasoned plan to test your hypotheses. There should be a reason for every piece of data you plan to gather.

7. **Disconfirmatory evidence:** Actively seek out and evaluate evidence that tends to rule out any hypothesis or action alternative as well as evidence that tends to confirm it.

8. **Multiple symptoms:** Consider the possibility that a patient with multiple symptoms or complaints may well have more than one disease.

9. **Harm versus benefit:** Consider the harm, benefit, and cost of each test you order. In addition, do not order tests whose results will not logically make a difference in your decision-making process.

10. **Revision:** Continually revise probabilities as you collect more data and alter your plan accordingly.

CHAPTER 14

Negotiation and the Healing Connection

> The free practitioner . . . treats their diseases by going into things thoroughly from the beginning in a scientific way, and takes the patient and his family into confidence. Thus he learns something from the sufferers, and at the same time instructs the invalid to the best of his powers. He does not give his prescriptions until he has won the patient's support, and when he has done so, he steadily aims at producing complete restoration of health by persuading the sufferer into compliance.
>
> Plato, *The Laws*

Most treatment in medicine requires active patient cooperation. Comatose patients receive their intravenous fluids and medications with little, if any, compliance necessary on their part, but it is difficult to imagine other medical care situations in which the behavioral component of therapy is not significant. Although "compliance" is a common term in medical parlance, it has two drawbacks. *First,* the term suggests that the physician's orders are uniquely right and that any patient who fails to be 100% compliant will have an outcome that will be less than successful. *Second,* the term suggests a passive, "plastic" patient rather than an active, participating one. To some extent, the word "adherence" does not share the second connotation, but it still contains the first. The patient must adhere, albeit actively, to the doctor's correct regimen. Rather than using these terms, we prefer to talk simply about the patient's behavior with regard to treatment and instructions and to consider how much the physician himself or herself influences that behavior.

This chapter deals with how practitioners promote patient involvement in health care. We show how the practitioner-patient interaction is a learning experience, one that can be used to encourage personal responsibility and behavioral change. The

301

interaction can, of course, also be used to teach passivity and medicalization; the interaction can teach that medicine has the answers and does the healing. Alternatively, mixed messages can be given. For example, some physicians and other practitioners recommend a treatment but do not offer explicit instructions or determine whether the patient understands the illness and treatment. In order to make these messages clear, the practitioner must know how to promote active patient involvement, and then set about creating a "healing connection" in which the patient learns such involvement.

Dozens of studies have shown that patient compliance with medications, particularly over the long term, averages around 50%.[90] This figure by itself is not very informative because it does not tell us whether 50% of the patients comply 100% of the time with their treatment (while the others stop taking their medication entirely) or whether 100% of the people actually take their medications about half the time, or which subgroups are more or less likely to be more or less compliant. The 50% figure also need not bear any direct relationship to the *success* of therapy. It could well be that a medication is effective when taken in lower doses or less frequently than prescribed, even though it may be more efficacious were it actually taken in the prescribed manner. On the other hand, lest we forget the negative side of our therapies, patients would be more likely to have side effects and to develop toxic reactions if they all took every medication prescribed in full dosage. Although complete adherence to all prescribed drugs would probably lead to somewhat better outcomes with regard to the original illnesses, it would surely also lead to more iatrogenic illness.

In reality, however, your treatment of the patient is not just the drug you prescribe. The drug is just a small part of the influence you may have on the patient and his or her healing process. Even as you complete your initial interview, history, and physical examination, you begin to bring other influences to bear in your management of the patient. You may simply be ordering further diagnostic studies while explaining your preliminary findings and expecting the patient to return to see you again. Even so, you want to do whatever you can to make sure the patient actually obtains the studies, follows your advice, and returns to your office. You also want to do what you can to make the patient feel better starting today, rather than next week or next month. You want in some way, if possible, to reduce anxiety and relieve suffering. A skillful medical interview grounded in empathy, respect, and genuineness (see Chap. 2) is the first step in creating a healing connection that will allow you to enhance your patient's active participation in health care and reduce the suffering caused by anxiety and uncertainty. In this chapter, we present three additional steps that promote the healing connection:

1. Conveying the information;
2. Understanding what the patient believes and how he or she interprets the illness; and
3. Using your knowledge about the patient's personality, psychodynamics, beliefs, and values to achieve a "best negotiated" behavioral outcome.

STEP ONE: CONVEYING THE INFORMATION

Why don't patients always follow their doctors' instructions? Ley[67] suggested four hypotheses to explain noncompliant behavior:

1. The personality hypothesis, which holds that something in the patient's basic personality structure interferes;
2. The psychodynamic hypothesis, which holds that some important defense mechanism, such as denial, prevents compliance;
3. The interpersonal hypothesis, in which affective problems arising from the doctor-patient interaction prevent full compliance; and
4. The cognitive hypothesis, which holds that the problem has to do with communication per se—words and concepts—and the simple recall of what the doctor said.

While each of these must play a part at least some of the time, Ley[67] favors the cognitive explanation and has demonstrated through his many studies that patients do not remember a good deal of what the doctor tells them. And they cannot do what the doctor recommends if they fail to remember what medication to take or how to take it.

The first step in ensuring patient involvement in the healing connection, conceptually at least, is to make sure that the patient understands what you are saying and remembers it. Investigators agree that patients, on average, remember 50% to 60% of the information doctors give them immediately and about 45% to 55% several weeks later.[59a,67] Interestingly, neither the intelligence nor age of the patient seem to be important factors in how much is remembered. Others have found that writing down the information, which on the surface would appear to be a fail-safe method, does not, in fact, necessarily lead to a better outcome in terms of better compliance or the amount of information remembered. Of note, patients who have a moderate level of anxiety about their problems are more likely to remember what the doctor tells them than if they have either very high (paralyzing and distracting) or very low (nonmotivating) anxiety levels.

It is clear that patients will be more satisfied with their care and will follow instructions better if they remember what the doctor tells them. Here is an example of the final part of a diagnostic interview in which, among other problems, the doctor appears to pay little attention to conveying understandable information in the communication:

Dr: Okay, well Mr. H., you've been having ah, these problems for some time and ah, I think they warrant ah, further investigation. I'm not quite sure right now, some of your symptoms ah, seem to be upper GI but some seem to be ah, colonic as well. It could be an ulcer problem, it could be inflammatory bowel disease. I think the first thing to do is to schedule a proctoscopy and then we'll go on from there. I can do the procto in the office here later on this week. The nurse can give you an exact time and meanwhile ah, we'll get you scheduled on the ah, x-rays. You'll need a barium enema, probably air contrast, and then an upper GI series . . .

Pt: Is that test you mentioned, is that where you insert a tube in my rectum? I had one of those about 2 years ago, I could hardly stand it . . .

Dr: Well, it's not the most comfortable thing, but it is important, it's the only way you can get the rectum,

> look at it, see the problem. It's not as bad as you think
> . . .
>
> Pt: The main problem I'm having is this bloated feeling, and the indigestion. I didn't think it was so serious. Isn't there some medicine?
>
> Dr: As you said, it's been bothering you for quite some time so I think we ought to get to the bottom of it. You can never be too careful. The problem with the GI tract is that, a lot of times, symptoms seem to blend together and it's hard to know what you're dealing with unless you look.
>
> Pt: Do you think it might be something serious, I mean like an ulcer or something . . .
>
> Dr: Well, it could be an ulcer, but it's not typical. I think we'll just have to do the workup and see. In the meantime, I'm going to give you an antispasmodic drug to take, you can take it with every meal and at bedtime. I'll give you a prescription. We'll see what happens.

Let us focus first on the doctor's initial statement in this interview segment. How might this doctor have presented the information in such a way as to facilitate understanding? *First,* the doctor could have used words and phrases more likely to be understood by the patient. The phrase "inflammatory bowel disease" and the term "proctoscopy" should not be employed unless the doctor intends to explain them, or at least check back with the patient to determine whether he knows what they mean. Medical jargon can creep into any conversation. It is almost as if English becomes the doctor's second language, and he or she must mentally translate each concept from "medicalese." You will find that some concepts (as opposed to descriptive words like "proctoscopy") are difficult to explain, but anything important to the patient that goes on in his or her body *can* be described in plain language. Often, the difficulty in translation results from our own failure to have fully mastered a particular concept.

Second, the doctor in the example could have been concrete and specific about the problems being considered, which ones that had been ruled out, what the steps in the diagnosis would entail, and why they are important. On the contrary, the doctor spoke in abstract and general terms like "further investigation" and "go on from there." What does that mean? We understand that the physician is uncertain of the actual diagnosis, but there is a failure to categorize explicitly just what the options are and, more importantly for the patient at that point, what the likely outcome will be: Will I get better? Will I probably need surgery? Is it serious? Cassell referred to this failure to be explicit by calling it *vague reference*, a technique of communicating with patients that often leads to increased anxiety about the problem,[22] because it leaves the patient room to imagine "the worst."

Third, this doctor could have stated the most important information concisely at the beginning. Patients are more likely to remember the initial chunk of information than information presented later in a discussion. You should "hook" the patient's memory by giving a succinct statement that puts the problem in a frame of reference and leads to "here's how we'll deal with it." The doctor could then employ another technique, *repetition*, to bring home the salient points during subsequent discussion with the patient.

Fourth, at the end of the segment, the doctor could have inquired about how much the patient understood and given him some feedback about that understanding. The doctor could have encouraged questions. The simple technique of requesting the patient to repeat what you have said and then giving feedback substantially increases patient satisfaction and also increases accurate recall of information.[12]

Taking the example as a whole, notice that the doctor *is* sharing uncertainty with the patient. The clinical situation is truly ambiguous and the doctor's statements accurately convey that fact. However, the *manner* in which the doctor deals with this ambiguity appears neither to be educational nor to relieve the patient's anxiety. It creates new questions and leaves the old one ("Is it something serious?") unanswered. Moreover, the doctor has really communicated no specific information or advice to the patient about his problem. While the diagnosis is admittedly still unclear, the doctor *does* have a good deal more knowledge about what the symptoms mean and what might be done about them than the patient has. Even though the doctor is uncertain, this opportunity could be used to decrease some of the patient's uncertainty while mobilizing his efforts to address the problem constructively.

In summary, communicating information need not be vague or

confusing even if the situation is uncertain. Here is an example
of how the same doctor might, on a better day, share his findings
and arrive at a plan with the patient:

Dr: Well, Mr. H., you've had a difficult time with this problem, but I believe we'll be able to get to the bottom of
it and find out what's wrong. We will have to do some
additional tests, though, before we can say for sure.
Your main symptoms, the cramps you get and the loose
bowels, are most likely caused by a problem in your
colon, one that we call irritable bowel syndrome. That
means that there's a spasm in the muscles of your large
bowel and that gives you the cramps and so on. But
your other symptoms, that bloated feeling in the stomach and pain up there, they also suggest an acid problem, like ulcer or gastritis.

Pt: Are any of those serious?

Dr: They're all medical problems that can be treated or
cured. There's nothing to suggest that you have something really serious like cancer, for example. It could be
an ulcer, but I think it's more likely that irritable bowel
syndrome can explain all of your symptoms.

Pt: I really want to get to the bottom of this, I just can't
take it anymore. I just can't get my work done feeling
like I do now.

Dr: It sounds like these attacks have really gotten to you
. . .

Pt: I'd say I'm almost paralyzed.

Dr: Okay, I understand. What I'd like to do is to schedule
some tests today. One of them is a proctoscopy; that's
a procedure in which I insert a tube into your rectum.
I can look through it and check the lining of your
bowel, like for irritation or hemorrhoids. You'll come
back to my office for that. The other two tests are x-
rays, one of the large bowel and one of the stomach and
small bowel . . .

Pt: Do you think it might be something serious, like an
ulcer or something?

Dr: What are you thinking about? Possibly it could be an
ulcer . . .

Pt: Well, ulcers can kill you, can't they?

TABLE 14–1. Step One: Maximizing Transfer of Information

Use plain English, rather than medical jargon.
Use concrete and specific language; avoid vague references.
State the important message first, then use repetition to reinforce it.
Ask the patient to restate the message, and give corrective feedback.

> Dr: It sounds like you heard something bad about ulcers.
> Pt: My uncle bled to death from one. First they said it was an ulcer, then it didn't heal, he couldn't eat anything. Finally they found out it was cancer.
> Dr: And you're worried that this could be cancer, even if the tests show something else?
> Pt: I don't know. Like I say, I can't take it anymore. My nerves are part of it, maybe.
> Dr: Let's take this a step at a time. First, your symptoms and my examination do not show any suggestion of cancer; we have no reason to suspect it. As I said, it really sounds like either an acid problem or irritable bowel. That's the most likely. Let me explain that a little more . . .

This time the doctor has done a number of things to influence the patient to have the diagnostic studies and take the medication as directed. The patient may well be more satisfied than in our first example and go home less anxious about his condition. Several of the techniques the doctor used to enhance the healing connection by better transfer of information are summarized in Table 14–1. In addition to these, the doctor also actively elicited the patient's beliefs ("It sounds like you heard something bad. . . .") and took them into account. In other words, he acknowledged that the patient's interpretation of the illness plays a role in the healing connection. We discuss this topic next in more detail.

STEP TWO: UNDERSTANDING WHAT THE PATIENT BELIEVES

Consider the following excerpt from a conversation between a doctor and a patient who has sought medical care because of epigastric pain and "heart burn."

Pt: I take shots for allergies and I take two aspirins every day for my blood pressure . . . I don't eat any sugar, any salt.

Dr: Two aspirins for . . .

Pt: Every morning.

Dr: For that, why do you take that?

Pt: Trying, trying to thin out my blood to keep my pressure down, I try to keep it around 100.

Dr: I see.

Later in the same interview the patient comes back to the issue of aspirin and blood pressure in this way:

Pt: But I always take two aspirins, I've taken two aspirins for years.

Dr: Where did you get into that habit?

Pt: Ah, when I was in the military in '68 and '69.

Dr: Um humm.

Pt: German doctor told me that ah, if you take two aspirins with milk in the morning, he says, it lowers your blood pressure and thins things out.

Dr: Um humm.

Pt: And I've always, my blood pressure is always like 100, 110, its real low.

This person *has* a perfectly logical belief regarding aspirin and blood pressure if you accept his basic premise. He assumes that high blood pressure is caused by "thick" blood. If so, and if aspirin thins the blood, it is reasonable to take aspirin to prevent hypertension. This particular belief is likely to be a simple piece of misinformation. It could easily be remedied by the doctor explaining that blood pressure and blood coagulation involve two entirely different physiological systems. It would be particularly important to address this issue if the patient were indeed found to be hypertensive and treatment is recommended, or if he had peptic ulcer disease and could not take aspirin.

This piece of "folk physiology" is reminiscent of the "high blood and low blood" beliefs in African American and rural southern white culture.[100] In these cultures, people can confuse high blood pressure with "high blood" or excessive blood volume, which is thought to cause strokes when the excess blood backs up into the brain. Anemia means "low blood" to them; too little blood puts a strain on the person's heart. It is difficult for patients with this understanding of physiology to accept the notion that they have hypertension and anemia at the same time; it just does not make sense for them to have both high and low blood.

Physicians who treat Hispanic patients may encounter similar problems prescribing a "hot" medicine for a "hot" disease. Many Puerto Ricans and Mexican-Americans subscribe to a traditional folk physiology that requires a balance of "humors" for health. Illness is believed to be an imbalance between the "hot" and "cold." Certain diseases are characterized as being cold and others hot. Medicines and other treatments are also divided in this way. You treat a cold illness with a hot medicine, to restore balance. The unsuspecting physician who prescribes hot-for-hot may well have a reluctant and noncompliant patient.[55]

Often physicians have little difficulty perceiving the health and healing beliefs of people belonging to other cultures, but they frequently fail to take into account the wide spectrum of folk physiology and healing practices presented by most ordinary people in our society regardless of age, cultural background, or education. People everywhere are concerned about the origin of their symptoms and the outcome of their illnesses, and so they formulate hypotheses about them. They learn from experience, books, television, and friends. They often seek help from a variety of sources. Sick people do not usually read medical textbooks, nor do they have the same blind faith in scientific medicine that health professionals often have. When you are sick, it is difficult to believe that the illness is a random event, a matter of probability, e.g., 22% of persons exposed to this virus become clinically ill and, of these, 14% develop jaundice. But why me? Why did I get hepatitis? Illness is not value- or meaning-free. We live in a world of symbols and interpretation. We personalize events.

The person who visits a doctor has already interpreted his or her experience and developed some beliefs about it. This is reflected in the story he or she tells and in the way he or she conceptualizes an appropriate healing response. Sick people ask themselves: What is the cause of my illness? How serious is it? What treatment do I need? Their answers may be specific to this one episode ("I was in a draft" or "I stayed up all night to study for my Serbo-Croatian final"), or they may reflect more general notions about human disease ("Disease comes from vitamin deficiencies" or "A lot of illness comes from spinal problems"). Sick people may also have beliefs about what their illness means in a larger, more personal sense. Particularly in the event of serious or chronic illness, your patient will have wondered, "What does this mean to me? Is it a punishment? Is it a challenge? Will I die like Uncle Harry whose cancer started the same way?"

Although everyone who is even a little sick has some interpretation of his or her suffering, we do not always ask about it explicitly in the medical history nor discuss it as we plan further tests or treatment. The patient has some faith in medicine or he or she would not be in the emergency room or in your office. If you are empathic and demonstrate your competence, the patient will have even more faith in you personally. You will help change (if necessary) his or her interpretation of the illness by simply doing a good job. However, in certain situations, belief factors play a more significant role, and you will not be able to optimize the healing connection unless you understand and deal with them.

How can you tell if you are dealing with a situation in which belief factors are influencing the patient's disease, illness, or behavior? *One clue* is that the acutely ill patient gets better with therapy but the sickness seems to persist, or that you successfully treat symptoms, but new symptoms keep appearing as the old ones disappear. For example, you might learn this during an initial interview when your patient tells you that ever since his bout of pneumonia 2 months ago, he has not had any energy and has developed insomnia.

A *second clue* is that the condition of a chronically ill patient is always poorly controlled despite your attempts to prescribe usually effective drugs. You suspect the patient is noncompliant but you cannot prove it and do not know why. Often, you become angry with people who do not seem to understand simple English ("I told her time and again, and explained the pills over and over") or appear to be unconcerned or, worse, self-destructive ("What is he trying to do, kill himself?").

A *third "red flag"* arises when your patient's suffering and disability are far in excess of the evident disease. A patient might bring in a disability form for you to complete because she has "high blood pressure and arthritis." Her blood pressure is mildly elevated but that, of course, is asymptomatic. She has some

Heberden's nodes (degenerative osteophytes at the distal inter-phalangeal joints), but these are usually asymptomatic. She sometimes has aching in her shoulder, but the x-rays are normal. Yet the patient believes she is disabled. She may well be, but you must address the meaning of her problems to find out why.

A *fourth and particularly problematic clue* is an extension of the third one: chronic sickliness and disability without any iden-tifiable disease. A prime example of this is "culture-bound ill-ness," a phrase anthropologists use to describe characteristic ill-nesses that originate from and are sustained entirely by sociocultural factors. An example of such a syndrome that occurs among Latin American people is "susto," or magical fright. A young woman may, for example, develop this illness shortly after she marries, enters her husband's family system, leaves her own family, and assumes new responsibilities with little support. She may become weak and dizzy, lose her appetite, and suffer from other characteristic symptoms that indicate that she is "asus-tado" (i.e., suffers from susto).[102] Such a sickness is best treated by a traditional healer, a curandero, rather than by a medical doctor. This is not an imaginary problem; it can be quite malig-nant, even fatal.[89] The physiological changes are real and uncon-trolled, even if they originate in social or psycho-emotional dys-function.[89] "Ghost sickness," suffered by American Plains Indians and "neurasthenia," a prevalent American ailment in the late 19th century, may well be other examples of culture-bound illnesses. We are likely to have such culturally defined syn-dromes in the late 20th century although they may not be so clearly visible to us as such. It is certain, however, that you will encounter many patients who are sorely disabled, who suffer greatly, and in whom you can discover no physical disease, or in whom physical disease cannot explain the symptoms (see Chap. 11).

Table 14–2 presents questions that will help you make an assessment of patients' beliefs. The questions constitute a kind of screening test to ascertain whether your patient's beliefs and expectations fall within a "normal" range, a range in which they will not seriously conflict with medical explanations or treat-ment, or whether they fall outside this range, in which case they might prevent you from effectively influencing behavior. We have adapted these questions from Kleinman and associates,[66] and arranged them to indicate three interpretive levels or types

TABLE 14–2. Step Two: Questions about the Patient's
Interpretation of His or Her Illness

Interpretive Level	Examples
Descriptive	How would you describe the problem that concerns you most?
	What are the main difficulties this problem (sickness, illness, disease, or misfortune) has caused for you?
Conceptual	What do you think is wrong, out of balance, or causing your problem?
	What does the illness do to you? How does it work? Why did it start when it did?
	What kind of treatment do you think you should receive?
	What are the results you hope for with treatment? Without treatment?
	Apart from me (a medical doctor), who else can help you get better? What else can you do?
Personal	Why did you, as opposed to somebody else, get sick? And get sick now?
	What do you fear most about your sickness?

Source: Adapted from Kleinman et al.[66]

of meaning each illness can have: descriptive, conceptual, and
personal.

The first, descriptive, level simply recaps what we discussed in
Chapter 3. You must find out what your patient identifies as the
problem for which he or she is seeking help. The "ostensible reason for coming" or chief complaint may not, in fact, be the
"actual reason for coming."[9] This is just a reminder to get the
whole story and to get it straight. Most questions on the list
address the conceptual interpretation: the concepts your patient
has about the cause, treatment, or outcome of the illness, and the
premises and logic the patient uses to work with those concepts.
The last two questions deal with personal meaning. Table 14–3
presents some general categories of personal or existential ori-
entations toward illness; often a person's attitudes about sickness
derive from more than one of these categories.

Beliefs about illness are frequently fragmented and not tightly
integrated into a coherent system. People are constantly exposed
to health information, from television, radio, magazines, and

TABLE 14-3. Step Two: Understanding the Personal Meaning of Illness and Possible Patient Responses

Personal Meaning	Patient Responses
Illness as challenge	Adapt actively
	Generate rational, task-oriented behavior
Illness as punishment	Anxious, depressed, or angry
	May see opportunity for atonement
Illness as enemy	Ready to fight, flee, or surrender
	Blame others
	Hostility or aggressiveness
Illness as weakness	Shame or loss of control
	Conceal or deny illness
Illness as relief	Reduce other obligations
Illness as strategy	Strategic ploy to manipulate
	Dependent role or clinging
Illness as loss or damage	Depression, hostility, or resistance
	Prone to suicide
Illness as value	Opportunity to reflect
	Expand personality
	Creative catalyst

Source: Adapted from Lipowski.[72]

newspapers, from which a person may garner a variety of "facts" and opinions, some of which may be inconsistent with others. A person may learn that vitamin C cures the common cold, that vitamin E relieves impotence, or that chelation therapy removes calcium deposits from the lining of arteries. Some will consider these to be unrelated bits of information, while others will see them as part of a larger value system, such as the theory that most illness is caused by nutritional imbalance and is best treated by "natural" methods.

Here is an example of an elderly woman, blind from glaucoma, who had undergone chelation therapy and was explaining it to her new physician. Chelation involves the intravenous administration of ethylenediaminetetraacetic acid (EDTA), an agent that binds calcium and other cations, thus removing them from the body when the chelator is excreted. It can be used to treat lead poisoning, for example. However, there is no sound evidence that it removes calcium from atherosclerotic plaques, and repeated intravenous treatments may be dangerous, unnecessary, and expensive. It is considered an unacceptable medical therapy. The physician has made this patient comfortable enough that she described why she did it, her feelings about it, and her evaluation of the outcome:

Dr: You had this creeping numbness, and they didn't seem to know what to do about it?

Pt: Well, no, and then after the stroke, my back actually . . . I told you about the doctor. He said that it had already happened.

Dr: That your back had already, as you said, collapsed?

Pt: Well I didn't understand, I thought that my backbones would fall down. But what really happened was I think, that the muscles that hold the bones together became like stretched out gumbands and for instance, like take an example, a car, you drive on an icy road. You want it to go one way and it goes another. I tried to go here but, I had no control over my back. No control. I was talking to Dr. Smith but he would do not a thing, didn't do a thing. I mean it didn't seem to bother him at all. And then my bitter fear for my legs. Then, it came to the point, actually where my legs were just like a couple of logs. I would try to sleep at night and turn over and I would drag my legs.

Dr: Is that what made you afraid?

Pt: I was afraid, well I explained to Dr. Smith. "Look, Dr. Smith there are people that lose the use of their legs and they go and use a wheelchair, but you got to have eyes to guide the wheelchair and I don't have that, what am I going to do?" But, like talking to the wall. Once he got very angry. "Do you think that if there would be something that would help you, I wouldn't do it for you?" Well, as if it was a sin to even be concerned about myself. So anyway, well the situation was really awful, I was really fretting my mind all the time. I just lost the use of my eyes, next I lost the use of my legs, then what to do? All right? . . . After the chelation, these things never repeated. So, then I came to Dr. Brown and he said "I'll chelate you and you'll have no more strokes." So that's when I made up my mind, I have to go to the chelation and it's better.

Dr: How often do you go now?

Pt: Well in the beginning it's good to go twice a week, but I've never been twice a week. It's not easy sitting four hours in one place. It takes three and a half to four hours.

Dr: You were afraid to tell me about this, too, weren't you?

Pt: Yes, because you're not supposed to tell nobody about it.

Dr: Who says you're not supposed to tell?

Pt: The doctors. Well you should have seen Dr. Smith. He got mad. I felt so sick that time, he got so mad actually I don't know what was the matter with him. Like he was ready to get a nervous breakdown or something. (Pauses) The thing is, it's so cruel. It's so cruel. Maybe it does do some good, and if it does then why deprive a patient, just because of politics, that's not right. Come to Dr. Brown's office and its always filled up with chelating people you know. So, I had once heard this woman telling, not to me, to others about a friend she knew. Now his legs became so bad they turned all black and his doctor advised him to have them amputated. Well that's a horrible prospect. But he, somebody told him about chelation, so he went and did it, and slowly the color came back in his legs. He started to be okay and he went back to work. This is hard to believe. So then he went to his doctor to show him and told him about the chelation, but the doctor's response was, "If it was up to me I would still amputate." It's hard to believe such extreme cruelty.

Notice how the physician has found out about the chelation, despite the patient's proviso that "you're not supposed to tell." This doctor was faced with a patient who had spent much time and money on a form of treatment orthodox medicine considers completely worthless. Earlier physicians had let her down, both by saying there was nothing to be done despite her "bitter fear for my legs," and by becoming angry if she told them about chelation. The main point for this doctor is to realize that the patient feels better, her symptoms are largely resolved, and no academic discussion of quackery will alter that fact. The questions the physician will have to ask himself during the subsequent negotiation have nothing to do with the efficacy of chelation. The important questions are these: Are the beliefs really dangerous? Do they prohibit medical care that is actually necessary? Can I work within the patient's belief system to provide good medical care? Having answered these, the doctor must take the next step and arrive at a mutually acceptable course of action through the process of negotiation, which we discuss next.

STEP THREE: NEGOTIATION

Although patients cannot follow your advice unless they understand and remember it, noncompliance may also occur if they do not agree with it. So it is necessary to learn what the patient believes needs to be done for the illness. You can use this information to help the patient get well by attempting to change the patient's beliefs, by altering your therapeutic plan to accommodate them, or by reaching some intermediate, negotiated, therapeutic alliance. *Negotiation is a process in which people use discussion and compromise to arrive at a settlement of some issue.* In practice, negotiation is a way of optimizing patient compliance and is a sign of respect for the patient's autonomy. Once you have spoken with the patient and performed a physical examination, you will have some hypotheses about the patient's illness, although you may remain uncertain about why the patient is ill or what the natural course of the patient's illness will be. You will want to influence the patient's behavior, decrease his or her anxiety, and give the patient a better sense of control over the problem. How do you do this in the clinical interview?

Let us look at what several different authors consider crucial components of *negotiation* in medical practice. Bernarde and Mayerson[11] list the following components:

1. Putting the patient at ease;
2. Having respect for the patient;
3. Having a positive attitude;
4. Communicating, which requires that you explain the information in understandable terms and provide feedback;
5. Dealing adequately with the patient's response, particularly in terms of feelings; and

6. Reaching a compromise position, when there is conflict, by a good-faith "give-and-take."

Brody[16] wrote about the mutual participation model of doctor-patient interaction and lists these components:

1. A conducive atmosphere;
2. A method of ascertaining goals and expectations of the patient;
3. Education of the patient about the problem and the treatment; and
4. Informed suggestions, preferences, and disagreements elicited from the patient.

Heaton[56] suggested that the spectrum of negotiation includes four subject areas:

1. Agreement on what the clinical information really is;
2. Consent for procedures or treatments;
3. Agreement on the nature of the problem; and
4. Agreement about what can or should be done.

Eraker and Politser[44] outlined patient characteristics, physician traits, and qualities of the doctor-patient relationship that facilitate or hinder compliance. They proposed a new way to understand and improve patient compliance that combines decision analysis, behavioral decision theory, and health beliefs. They stressed the importance of understanding the patient's "comprehension, decision-making processes, and environment," and that "acceptance of the diagnosis is particularly important because of the frequent occurrence of erroneous powerful health beliefs." These authors described certain physician tasks that influence the patient's behavior:

1. Eliciting and respecting the patient's concerns, where both the patient and physician communicate their preferences;
2. Evaluating the patient's comprehension and educating him or her in order to prevent the part of noncompliance that may be "nonvoluntary";
3. Learning about specific health beliefs, particularly those

regarding perceived susceptibility and perceived severity; and

4. Understanding the patient's perception of trade-offs between benefits and risks, and between the quality and quantity of life.

All these authors have restated in different terms the familiar themes of empathy, respect, communication skills, and acknowledgment of the patient's beliefs and expectations. You influence patients more when you respect them, communicate well with them, understand "where they're coming from," and so forth. An additional theme is that of uncertainty. The question of uncertainty is particularly important to emphasize for those just learning how to interview patients and negotiate with them. We presented elements of clinical judgment in the medical interview and discussed the problem of uncertainty in Chapter 13. The uncertainty that you experience is only partially because you are a beginner; much uncertainty is intrinsic to the doctor-patient interaction. From this perspective, you are negotiating not only to make the patient more likely to follow your suggestions or to understand your formulation but also to achieve a better healing effect than could be obtained from a unilateral decision on your part combined with 100% patient compliance. This means that negotiation requires sharing your uncertainty with the patient. Gutheil and coworkers[54] addressed this issue in the context of malpractice suit prevention. They speak of informed consent as

> an interaction between physician and patient, a dialogue intended not only to satisfy a legal requirement but to do more as well. The real clinical opportunity offered by informed consent is that of transforming uncertainty from a threat to the doctor-patient alliance into the very basis upon which an alliance can be formed. . . . Note that our approach stresses the selection of what to say to patients rather than such advice as taking more time with patients or telling them more. In practice, less time is taken and more is understood: sound efficiency of communication, not mere volume of words, is the desideratum.

We summarize the components of negotiation in Table 14–4 and end this chapter with the following case example that demonstrates the interactive nature of clinical problem solving and the negotiation that occurs as new data are added. The case illus-

TABLE 14-4. Step Three: Components of Negotiation

1. Respect the patient and deal with feelings.
2. Inform the patient, i.e., using understandable terms, present, verify, and interpret the evidence with regard to diagnosis and therapy.
3. Elicit the patient's goals (what would you like to happen? what do you think will happen?).
   Suggestions (how do you think we should handle this? what do you think is wrong?).
   Preferences (do you prefer medical therapy for this problem or do you think surgery might work better for you?).
4. Help the patient weigh risks and benefits, including trade-offs between the quality and quantity of life.
5. Formulate an agreement of the nature of the problem and a plan of action.

trates negotiation both in the "give-and-take" bargaining and the "maneuver to find a path" senses of the word. The elements of negotiation include the presentation of evidence, verification of evidence and its interpretation, weighing of risks and benefits (including how physician and patient value different outcomes), and, finally, formulation of an agreement and plan of action.

A 25-year-old woman came to her doctor's office with the complaint of a severe and persistent vaginal itch. She expressed her distress and summarized her problem in the opening statement that we encountered previously in Chapter 3:

> Pt: Well, I have a terrible vaginal itch, and I don't know whether it's from vaginitis or whether it's the urinary tract infection—you know—ah, my regular doctor treated me for vaginitis first . . .
> Dr: That was Doctor X?
> Pt: Ah, huh, then I, um, got a urinary tract infection, then the vaginitis came back, but during the whole ordeal I've never got no relief.

We learn several important things about this patient from her opening statement: she is suffering ("terrible," "ordeal," "no relief"), she is medically sophisticated ("vaginitis," "urinary tract infection"), and she is not well educated in the sense of formal schooling ("I've never got no . . .").

The physician performs an examination, then leaves the room to examine a specimen of vaginal secretions under the microscope, returning with the news that the infection is clearly caused by *Trichomonas vaginalis* and can be easily and effectively treated with a single dose of eight pills. At this point, both patient and physician agree on the nature of the problem: it is a *Trichomonas* infection. To the patient, the end of her suffering is in sight. The physician begins to write out a prescription. But, seeing the name of the drug as the physician writes it, the patient unexpectedly says:

> Pt: Flagyl. You don't have any . . . there's nothing else you can take besides Flagyl, huh?

Up until this point, it would appear as though the physician has made not only an accurate diagnosis but also a correct decision about therapy with which the patient will be happy. But the patient, instead of being appropriately grateful for the physician's expertise, is not satisfied. The negotiation begins.

> Dr: It's the *best* for it.
> Pt: Okay but I might . . . well, I'll try it.

You could imagine a scenario here in which the physician simply says "fine," and the patient is left to her own doubts about the drug, perhaps taking it, perhaps not. But the physician, listening to her hesitation, replies:

> Dr: What's the problem?
> Pt: But I think I was allergic to that.
> Dr: Why do you think that?
> Pt: Because I remember taking Flagyl before, and it did something . . . I think I broke out in hives or something.
> Dr: Really?
> Pt: But I'll try it, if I break out I'll let you know, but I think I did.
> Dr: That's a worry . . . let me look at the record . . . it says here that you were sensitive to ampicillin and sulfa . . . now could it have been . . . Oh, it does say Flagyl . . .
> Pt: I think it was just hives. Maybe I've outgrown it.
> Dr: I don't want you to take it if you had hives from it.
> Pt: Well, maybe I'll have . . . I'll have outgrown it 'cause I think it's been a while back.

> Dr: (Still looking through the chart) Yeah, it does say Flagyl.

The patient actually begins with an interpretation ("allergic") of some past event associated with the drug. Physician and patient then exchange information, together trying to verify or refute that interpretation. The patient provides supporting evidence with the descriptive term "hives," while the physician searches for other evidence by going through the patient's chart. (She is new to this physician but had previously been seen in the same clinic.) However, this is more than a simple discussion of evidence as we can see both patient ("I'll try it") and physician ("I don't want you to take it . . .") apparently on the verge of decisions, albeit opposite ones. Perhaps, seeing the physician's concern and despite her willingness to risk hives, the patient offers a new interpretation to the data ("maybe I'll have outgrown it"). The physician then offers:

> Dr: What we *could* do is we could treat your husband and we could treat you with something else but . . .
> Pt: Well, if that's the best I want that . . .
> Dr: . . . most of the "something elses" aren't as effective.
> Pt: Well, I'll take Flagyl. It can only break me out in hives a day like . . . it'll probably go away in the morning.
> Dr: I would be kind of worried about that before prescribing it for you because you *could* get an even more serious reaction to it.

Data have been exchanged ("I was allergic"), verified ("hives," written record), and now reinterpreted ("I've outgrown it"). The patient, echoing the physician's "it's the *best*," rejects the notion of "something else" by reversing the implication of concession in her earlier statement on taking Flagyl ("well, I might try it"). In the context of the physician's earlier statement, "something else" would have to be seen as decidedly inferior. We are tiptoeing on a threshold-of-risk boundary: Take Flagyl and get rid of the itch but risk an allergic reaction versus take something else and avoid the reaction but risk not curing the itch. Much of what the patient says in subsequent statements suggests that she places a higher value on getting rid of the itch than on avoiding an allergic reaction. The patient acknowledges that there is a risk involved but discounts it ("just hives"); the physician, on the other hand, stresses that the risk is more than that characterized by the patient ("you *could* get an even more serious reaction").

The decision has become problematic, and we begin to see patient and physician engage in a dialogue regarding risks and benefits. Lacking the data to successfully value or weigh the risks, the physician returns to a discussion of the evidence, by turning again to the written record to find the supporting data for the diagnosis of allergy, while the patient in turn supplies additional details pointedly aimed at discrediting her own report of an allergic reaction:

> Dr: . . . uh let me see what Dr. X said about that.
> Pt: . . . I don't even think that Dr. X was here when I had that . . .
> Dr: Dr. Y? Dr. Z? . . . because that may be why you've been treated with all this other stuff.
> Pt: But they, I remember I told them it did that to me, it might notta been that.
> Dr: But it does say you're allergic to it.
> Pt: That's cause I *told* him that.
> Dr: I've never heard anybody being allergic to it but it's . . .
> Pt: That's what I'm saying it's . . .
> Dr: . . . certainly possible . . .
> Pt: . . . Probably what happened I broke out in hives in reaction to *other* things.

It is remarkable that the patient understands that the source of the data in question—or rather the interpretation in question—is herself ("cause I *told* him that") and that she may not be the most reliable interpreter of the evidence. Perhaps, if she is the source of the original interpretation, she can also be the source of a new interpretation. In the end the physician is persuaded—to some extent. Note the ensuing discussion in which various outcomes are valued and a decision is reached:

> Dr: Well, I'll tell you what I want you to do. Since you have taken a lot of drugs because of all these urinary infections . . .
> Pt: . . . That might be why it's never left . . .

Dr: Uh hum . . .

Pt: . . . so I'd rather take the Flagyl . . .

Dr: . . . Well I'll tell you what I want you to do . . .

Pt: . . . it won't be your fault . . .

Dr: *Well*, I'm still the one that prescribes it. Let me tell you what I'd like you to do. I'd like you to take one pill out of your eight as a test dose. OK? And if you have no reaction to it, then we will hope it is safe to take the rest, though we can't know for sure.

Pt: Um hmm.

Dr: Today, just one, see what happens, and if you have no reaction to it at all, then tomorrow take the remaining seven and have your husband take his eight. OK?

Pt: OK.

Dr: OK? So if you are allergic we'll know . . .

Pt: Yeah, I'll get hives (ha ha).

Dr: Well, let's just be on the safe side, let's use a test dose . . . OK? Because *Trichomonas*, while it's uncomfortable, it can't kill you, so you know . . .

Pt: . . . It can drive you mad . . .

Dr: . . . I know, but the point is that we don't want to do anything that would be harmful to your health.

Although there was a lot of back-and-forth maneuvering, the physician takes ultimate responsibility for the decision ("I'm still the one that prescribes it"), but the decision is clearly influenced by the value the patient places on getting rid of the itch ("it can drive you mad"). The patient took the medication, had no reaction, and got rid of the itch. It is not difficult to imagine a different situation with a patient who, perhaps, had suffered more from hives. In that case, the negotiation would have resulted in a different outcome, such as the prescribing of a somewhat less effective therapy.

SUMMARY

In this chapter we have addressed the question of how you create a healing connection and influence the patient's behavior through the clinical interview. We have divided this influencing skill into three steps or components for the sake of discussion, although in practice they often flow together. *First*, the patient's understanding and recall of information must serve as a basis for any behavioral influence we might have. The patient cannot be "compliant" unless he or she knows what to do and how to do it. Moreover, the patient is not likely to be motivated to be compliant unless he or she knows why something is to be done and how it works. *Second*, the patient's own beliefs, interpretations, conceptual framework, and personal orientation must all be considered in designing an optimal therapy. Knowledge of these factors is essential for you to understand the effects of serious or chronic illnesses, as well as to promote optimal therapy for most significant illnesses. *Finally*, we discussed the role of negotiation in achieving an effective therapeutic outcome. Respect for the patient and knowledge of his or her beliefs would not necessarily help you to influence the patient unless you can use these while engaging in a process of negotiation to arrive at a mutually agreed upon plan of action.

CHAPTER 15

Ethics in Medical Interviewing

Veracity does not consist in *saying*, but in the intention of *communicating* truth.

Samuel Taylor Coleridge, *Biographia Literaria*

Medical ethics today tends to be cast in *quandaries* and *big issues*. We think of extreme cases and special situations that arise from life-sustaining technologies, transplantation, new reproductive techniques, and from the need to allocate scarce medical resources. In the last 25 years or so, the discipline of bioethics has begun to address, at least in part, the thorny moral issues created by such modern medical technology. An exclusively "high-tech" view of medical ethics limits ethical decision making to a certain kind of "expertise" (perhaps best left to "ethics" specialists) useful in certain kinds of medical situations, such as those in which questions of "pulling the plug" might arise. Such a view obscures the fact that even everyday medical practice has a moral dimension. What about day-to-day practice? What about ordinary doctor-patient interactions? There is an ethical dimension to all medical decisions, not just to some types of medical decisions. Human value questions are an integral part of everyday medicine; they are not something extra, reserved for ethicists and "experts."

In this chapter we discuss ethical aspects of common doctor-patient interactions, with a particular focus on issues that arise in the medical interview. For example, say your patient requests that you keep his sexually transmitted disease confidential, yet you believe his sexual partner would benefit from the information. What should you do? Alternatively, you meet your friend on the elevator. She tells you about the interesting patient she just saw. Is this a violation of confidentiality? How much should you tell her about your patient? Or perhaps you are interviewing an elderly person who seems a little demented; how do you evaluate his competence to consent to your suggested diagnostic procedures?

In the next section, we briefly sketch the basic ethical orientation of medical practice and two "models" of patient care based on different ethical principles. The remaining sections of the chapter present the topics of (1) confidentiality, (2) truth telling, (3) informed consent, and (4) competency, looking at the ways in which each relates to the medical interview and to ordinary doctor-patient interactions.

MORAL REASONING IN MEDICINE

We live in a pluralistic society, one in which many communities of belief with different ethical theories exist side by side. Despite this fragmentation, there is wide agreement (at least in the abstract) about the importance of certain relatively broad principles of ethical behavior (Table 15–1). A religious person might base these principles on the law of God. Others might argue that they arise from a "social contract" or that they derive from a more general theory of utility, "Do that which produces the greatest good for the greatest number of people." When applied to real clinical situations, however, two or more of these general principles often appear to conflict with one another. The "right" decision that supports beneficence is different from the "right" decision that supports autonomy. Thus, quandaries arise. How are the principles to be ranked? Does one take precedence over another?

Autonomy Model

The principle of respect for autonomy asserts personal rights and liberties. Our constitutional and political system is grounded in the notion that the state (or other people) has no authority to interfere with certain basic human rights, such as whether an individual wants to accept medical care. Numerous court decisions confirm a competent adult's right to refuse treatment and "right to die." It is only when the rights of others are at stake

TABLE 15–1. Ethical Principles in Medicine

Respect for Autonomy: Regard other persons as rightfully self-governing in their choices and actions.
Nonmaleficence: Do not harm other persons.
Beneficence: Help, or confer benefits upon, other persons.
Justice: Distribute goods and services to each person according to his or her "right" or "due."

---

that the state can readily intervene in health care decisions. For example, laws compelling childhood immunization are justified in the United States not because they protect an individual child (whose parents are perhaps objecting to the immunization on the basis of their religious beliefs) but because they protect other children from the threat of epidemics ignited by a pool of unimmunized persons. The practice of acting to benefit others without their consent is called paternalism; respect for autonomy serves to limit paternalism, both by the state and by individuals.

In medical practice, as in our larger society, respect for autonomy is prima facie the strongest principle. A model of medical care based on strong autonomy features a contract between the patient and doctor. This contract, although usually implied rather than written, defines the rights and duties of both doctor and patient. (Advocates of autonomy often fail to emphasize that patients, and not only doctors, have certain duties in the relationship.) In its most extreme form, such an autonomy model leads to the type of "provider-consumer" talk bandied about by economists, civil libertarians, and bureaucrats. The patient becomes a consumer of health care, in much the same way as he or she is a consumer of fast food or miniature golf. The doctor becomes a provider of health services, someone far removed from the ancient medical tradition of healing and philanthropy.

The autonomy model asserts respect for personal decision making, entails truthfulness and maintenance of confidentiality, and requires informed consent. In many respects, the patient should be an equal partner in the healing enterprise. However, when taken alone, the autonomy model does not tell us much about doctors or their motivations. It tells us about respecting our patients' rights but not about the virtues that drive medical practice. Physicians are not salespersons. They are professional healers with a calling grounded in philanthropy, the love of human beings. While autonomy dictates many physician obligations, it leaves out the value on which medicine itself is based.

Beneficence Model

The basis of the second model, that of beneficence, is the motivation to heal and to alleviate suffering. While we all have some moral obligation to help others in need, physicians have a special obligation to help sick people. The Hippocratic oath is a good statement of the beneficence model: "I will apply dietetic measures for the benefit of the sick according to my ability and judgment; I will keep them from harm and injustice." However, the notion of a special professional ethic tends to be ignored in much of today's writing about medical ethics. Churchill,[22a] for example, concluded that "our culture is well on its way to reducing medical ethics to legal requirements, general citizen ethics, or personal values."

Beneficence without respect for autonomy leads to paternalism. Autonomy without beneficence leads to a sterile, legalistic view of our relationships with patients. The two models complement one another, even though at times the "right" decision dictated by one model might conflict with the "right" decision demanded by the other. Both principles are required for good medical practice, whether or not lives and big issues are at stake. Ordinary doctor-patient interactions should reflect our commitment to beneficence and respect for our patients. Every medical interview is an occasion for ethical behavior. Kimball[65] summarizes this point of view well in the following:

Ethical bases for personal medicine are:

(1) awareness by the physician of his or her motivations, abilities, and competence;
(2) the physician's ability to get to know as much about the patient as a person as he or she would about the complaint;
(3) the physician's capacity for empathy;
(4) the physician's ability to maintain the confidentiality of the doctor-patient relationship;
(5) the physician's obligation to be a teacher;

(6) the physician's obligation to inform the patient about what he or she is doing and planning to do;

(7) the physician's obligation to continue care of the patient;

(8) the physician's commitment to a scientific (or analytic) approach;

(9) the physician's capacity for helping the patient reach decisions appropriate for that individual's illness and life; and

(10) the physician's awareness of his or her own humanness and limitations.

In the remainder of this chapter, we take the position that moral justification for rules of confidentiality, truthfulness, informed consent, and competency determination can be found in both models.

CONFIDENTIALITY

Bases of Confidentiality

Confidentiality is an ancient concept in medicine. The Hippocratic oath states, "What I may see or hear in the course of the treatment or even outside of the treatment in regard to the life of men, which on no account one must spread abroad, I will keep to myself holding such things shameful to be spoken about." The American Medical Association's principles of ethics[1] state that confidentiality is still an important duty in that "a physician . . . shall safeguard patient confidences within the constraints of the law." It seems natural that doctors should keep to themselves the personal information they learn about patients and that this rule of confidentiality should be asserted as a professional duty. What are the bases of this commonsense belief? What would medicine be like if there were no confidentiality?

There are four grounds on which we can justify a rule of medical confidentiality:

1. The principle of autonomy or respect for persons dictates a right to privacy that would be violated if we were to make personal information available to others.

2. The rule facilitates a trust relationship between patient and doctor.

3. The rule facilitates openness of communication. The patient feels comfortable giving more complete information because he or she knows it will not be "spread abroad." More complete information results in better diagnosis and more effective therapy.
4. The expectation of confidentiality in the patient-doctor relationship encourages persons who might not otherwise seek medical care to do so.

Limits and Exceptions

Physicians have always considered confidentiality to be a qualified duty, rather than an absolute one. The current AMA code of ethics recognizes "constraints of law" as one category of exception, but earlier AMA codes also specified that information about patients could be revealed if it was in the best interests of society or it was in the patient's own best interest. Contemporary concerns about personal rights and medical paternalism should make us circumspect about our ability to promote what we consider the patient's best interests while acting against his or her wishes. We are in a somewhat better position to identify conflicts between confidentiality and the best interests of society as a whole or of particular subsets of society like insurance companies or employers. Even so, the importance of confidentiality is such that we must give it great weight in any balancing of interests, particularly if we are not constrained by law to reveal the information.

Table 15–2 presents some standard exceptions to the rule of confidentiality. If a patient develops a seizure disorder, a physician may be required by law to report this fact to the state agency that issues driver's licenses. The patient's license might then be suspended until he or she is medically stable and certified "seizure free" for a specified period of time (e.g., 1 year). This law prevents automobile accidents by minimizing the chance that drivers will have seizure episodes while driving. However, the law also causes hardship for some individuals who, perhaps, need to drive to continue their employment. Reporting a seizure disorder can be a difficult decision for a physician, but in some states it is a course of action required by law. Similarly, reporting suspected child abuse can cause a great deal of short-term family disruption and suffering, but the physician must do so if he or she judges abuse to be probable; the doctor is supported by law

TABLE 15–2. Some Justified Exceptions to
Confidentiality

Required by law
  Gunshot wounds
  Specified communicable diseases
  Child abuse
  Dog bites
  Licensing requirements (e.g., drivers and pilots)
  Court subpoena
Significant threats of harm to the patient or to others
  Death threats
  Suicidality
  Communicable diseases
"Third-party" factors
  Doctor employed by industry
  Insurance applications
  Disability determinations

because the state has intervened to protect the interests of children who cannot protect themselves.

The tension between confidentiality and "interested third parties" is becoming more prevalent as a result of

1. New health care arrangements in which the physician is employed by a third party (e.g., health maintenance organizations or company doctors) and may have obligations other than those to his or her patients;
2. Requirements for medical information to judge disability, insurability, employability, and so forth; and
3. Computerized medical information systems to which large numbers of people might have access.

As was noted in Chapter 7, the notion of confidentiality, even as applied to "hard copy" hospital charts, is quite limited. Siegler[97] observed that between 25 and 100 persons in his hospital had legitimate access to a critically ill patient's chart. In light of this, he asked, "Is confidentiality a decrepit concept?"

Maintaining Confidentiality

A medical virtue that should be learned early and well is discretion. Discretion requires that students and physicians not share patient information with anyone who does not have a "right to know." This means that discussion of cases with friends, roommates, and spouses is generally inappropriate, even when the data in question are not strictly personal. Some people do have a right to know. Medicine is a collegial enterprise. Physicians function as members of health care teams. Consequently, we often need to discuss cases with our peers, consultants, and other health care professionals. As learners, we have a particular obligation to discuss patients with our teachers. Even here, however, discretion is important. There is rarely any justification for discussing patients on crowded elevators or in front of other patients or visitors. Presenting patients at the bedside is in many ways a good teaching technique, but it may well infringe on confidentiality if the patient has a roommate who can hear the details of his or her "case."

Another important way of maintaining confidentiality is to write only appropriate information on the chart. You should approach the chart as a document that the patient could review at any time. In fact, patients should be given the opportunity to review their own records; in some cases the record might serve as a "visual aid" to assist in teaching the person about his or her health problems. Especially with regard to sensitive information, you should always ask yourself whether writing a particular item in the chart is important to your patient's care. Some examples include: details of sexual practices, criminal record, marital conflict, and financial difficulties. Mental illness, suicide attempts, and substance abuse are also topics which, although they must be recorded, should be handled sensitively. In some cases it might be possible to write a brief "neutral" note to jog your memory, without expressing lurid details. For example, psychiatrists often keep their records in a personal file separate from the general medical record as a method of maximizing confidentiality while minimizing access.

Truthfulness and Confidentiality

When a situation arises in which you are obliged to share medical information, you should notify the patient and attempt to secure his or her permission. Failing that, you should be truthful about what is required and what you intend to do. If you diagnose a case of, for example, syphilis or tuberculosis, you must explain that the law dictates that you submit a report to the health department. While describing the public health reasons for this, you are also giving the patient crucial information about communicability and its implications for his or her behavior.

However, sometimes a patient will request explicitly that you withhold information about the patient's condition even when you have good reason to believe that others will be in danger unless the information is revealed. For example, a 35-year-old man you evaluate for fatigue and diarrhea proves to be HIV-positive. He has recently married. He indicates that, when he lived in Houston, he was an intravenous heroin abuser, but he "kicked the habit" and no longer uses drugs. He says that he will practice "safe sex" but will not tell his wife about his HIV infection because "it will just make her upset" and "she probably already has the virus by now." When pressed, he becomes angry and insists that you "bug off."

What is your responsibility in this case? After all, the patient did say he will take precautions in the future. In this case respect for autonomy must include consideration of the wife's right to know, as well as the patient's right to expect physician discretion. Likewise, an argument based on beneficence must take into account the good of other persons (wife and possible child), in addition to the patient's own good. The physician may keenly experience conflicting values in such a situation. The following guidelines may be helpful in resolving value conflicts like this one in doctor-patient interactions.

- Educate the patient by describing alternative views and possible outcomes. In this case, has the patient considered his wife's right to know? Or the risk to an infant?
- Negotiate by working within the patient's frame of reference and acknowledging his concerns. In this case, would it be easier for the physician to meet with husband and wife together to explain the situation? Granted, his wife will be distraught, but won't she be more angry and distressed to find out later, if and when the patient becomes more ill?
- Give the patient opportunity to think things over and perhaps change his mind.
- Maintain the value of confidentiality by revealing only the essential minimum of information and only to someone

who has a specific right to know if information is to be revealed against a patient's wishes. In this case, it might be the patient's wife and/or the state health department. (Some states now legally require reporting HIV positive cases. The case as described assumes that there is no legal requirement in your state.)

- Be truthful with the patient. Tell him what you must do and why you must do it.

The obligation to be truthful is discussed in the next section.

TRUTHFULNESS

Why Be Truthful?

While confidentiality and beneficence are found in ancient medical traditions, truthfulness is a rather recent addition to the medical virtues. For example, only 25 years ago most physicians did not believe it was appropriate to reveal to their patients the diagnosis of cancer. Even today in countries like Italy, Spain, and Japan such "bad news" truth telling is thought harmful to patients and, therefore, not medically indicated. Yet the requirement that we respect our patients' autonomy dictates that we be truthful, even when (or if) some possible harm might occur. It is useful in this context to review four main justifications that physicians have advanced for lying to (or not being completely honest with) their patients:

1. Some physicians have claimed that we never actually know the whole truth. All medical knowledge is probabilistic. Judgments based on probabilities and clinical judgment may well be wrong, so why do we need to confuse the issue by being too direct or too explicit? This sort of claim is in itself confused because it mixes epistemology with morality. It is important to distinguish between "truthfulness," a moral quality we should all practice, and the "truth," which is often uncertain. Truthful interactions include admitting one's uncertainty and, in the case of students, explaining one's limited role or responsibility. They also include inviting the patient's questions and answering them in understanda-

ble terms. Physicians and other clinicians should actively practice clear, simple explanations and should seek out the information needed to answer their patients' questions.

To be truthful is to express what we believe to be true. We might be wrong in a given case, but as physicians we must act by making a referral or diagnosis, or choosing a course of therapy. This means we ought to be honest in acknowledging the state of the art and the benefits and risks of a course of action. This type of disclosure is required for informed consent (see below).

2. Some physicians have generalized from the fact that sick persons often use denial as a defense mechanism to claim that patients do not want to know the truth. This is simply not the case for most persons. Studies have repeatedly shown that most people do want to know the truth about their medical condition. Sometimes patients tell their doctor, "If it's cancer, I don't want to know. Don't tell me." Such statements signal the need for a conversation in which the doctor listens attentively and sensitively explores the issues with the patient. Do you really mean you don't want to learn about your problem? Could understanding your situation allow you to live more fully and help you cope with whatever comes? A few persons have such strong denial (coupled with a heavy dose of magical thinking) that they give you an informed "waiver" from truth telling. In such cases, someone must be told. As part of the waiver process, you should discuss with the patient just who—spouse, child, parent, or friend—should be kept completely informed about the diagnosis and condition.

3. Doctors have sometimes claimed that patients cannot understand the medical facts. After all, medicine is so complex that laypersons have no way of knowing all the biochemical, pathophysiological, and pharmacological subtleties involved in a given case. While this may be true, it is irrelevant. The patient needs to know what a reasonable person would want to know, not what a physical chemist or a professor of pharmacokinetics would want to know. As was discussed in Chapter 14, explaining medical facts clearly is an important clinical skill. It

is fair to say that if you cannot explain a process in concrete "natural language," you probably do not thoroughly understand what you are talking about in abstruse "medicalese."

4. Some physicians claim that the truth will cause harm. This exemplifies the paternalistic attitude that physicians know best what is good for their patients and ought to pursue that "good" independent of (or even against) their patients' wishes. With regard to the latter, even if information is sometimes harmful, respect for personal autonomy might well dictate that, if the patient wishes, we provide the information regardless of possible consequences. Rarely, however, is the truth harmful. There is much evidence in the literature that knowing the truth generally has a positive effect on patients. To quote the Gospel of St. John, the truth does, in fact, "make you free." There are a few exceptions to this generalization. For example, some severely disturbed patients may respond to "bad news" with a decompensation of their psychiatric condition. In such cases a physician might contemplate a waiver of the truth, justifying it on the basis of potential harm. However, these situations are few and require careful consideration (and probably psychiatric consultation). The mere fact that a patient is chronically anxious, has hysterical outbursts at times, or is clinically depressed, does not take away his or her right to know the truth. The physician should be particularly cautious of family judgments: "Don't tell Aunt Clara. She won't be able to handle it. She's likely to go off the deep end." Such statements should be warnings that sensitive inquiry is necessary, but they are not waivers of responsibility to our patients.

Papers, Forms, and Clearances

Bureaucratic paperwork is the bane of modern medical practice. Enormous numbers of patient-doctor encounters are generated because people must have medical forms "filled out" for jobs, school, insurance, public assistance, nursing homes, social programs, driver's licenses, and on and on. Likewise, health insurers require the proper paperwork to justify payment for medical or laboratory services. Because of Medicare regulations, home health agencies seem to mail the doctor dozens of forms to complete on each patient with interminable regularity. It is understandable that physicians are not inclined to devote their best clinical judgment or their finest literary efforts to grinding out such administrative fodder. However, truthfulness in every-day medical practice requires honesty in the way we handle these bureaucratic headaches.

Two issues frequently arise with regard to clearances and certifications. In one case, the patient asks that information be suppressed. "Don't put down that I'm a diabetic. After all, my diabetes is in good control. And it'll cost me plenty in extra insurance premiums." Or, "Listen, that nervous breakdown was 3 years ago. It won't happen again. I'm all right now." What should you do, given the fact that telling the truth might well result in significant adverse consequences for your patient?

> *First*, you must be honest in answering any explicit questions on the form. You should explain this beforehand so the patient does not have any false expectations when they give consent for you to share their medical information.
>
> *Second*, you should take the time to write additional explanatory material if you believe that it will benefit the patient. You might indicate that the hypertension or diabetes is in excellent control or that the episode of depression has completely resolved with no residual symptoms.
>
> *Finally*, there is no need to volunteer information on such forms unless you have strong reason to believe it is relevant to the issue in question. Often, a final question will ask something like, "Any other significant medical problems or conditions?" There is no need here to detail the patient's medical history; simply put what might, in your clinical judgment, be "significant" to the insurance or job or program in question.

A different problem arises when patients ask you to make false or unsupported assertions about their illness or disability. The patient's insurance carrier or the state welfare department might ask if, in your opinion, the patient is "totally disabled." Perhaps you are unable to ascertain objective evidence of disability or the evidence is quite limited. "Yes, Mr. X does have diabetes, but there are only minor symptoms and no long-term sequelae." Or, "Yes, Mrs. Y does have some degenerative joint disease but these, in my opinion, cannot explain her chronic pain." (Of course, chronic pain is in itself a severe disability, whether or not an "objective" cause can be identified.) The important issue here is that you should never make assessments of disability that are not warranted by your clinical judgment. Your judgment, in turn, is conditioned by your level of training, area of specialization, overall practice experience, and specific knowledge of the patient's case. The point to be made here is that you must be truthful in your medical assessment. You can, of course, refuse to complete a form if you feel that your opinion is not in the patient's best interest. For generalists, it is often best to refer the patient to a specialist if you are not comfortable with the situation, remembering that there are persons who specialize in chronic pain and other "functional" disorders and in the assessment of disability.

INFORMED CONSENT

When patients answer our questions during the interview, submit to a physical examination, and allow themselves to be stuck by needles or penetrated by x-rays, they give implied consent by their actions. They came to seek help. At any time they can refuse to proceed. More invasive procedures are less "self-evident" and have sufficient potential risk that the courts have required that patients explicitly consent to them and that they do so on the basis of adequate information about benefits, risks, and alternatives. In this chapter we cannot examine fully the legal doctrine of informed consent nor the controversies about whether (and how much) true informed consent is possible in medical practice. However, medical and health care students are often required to perform procedures for which explicit informed consent is mandated, e.g., a medical student doing a thoracentesis or a nursing student inserting a Foley catheter. How do you obtain consent? What do you explain? These four guidelines should be of some help.

1. **Informed consent is a process, not a form or piece of paper:** Your clinic or hospital will have consent forms

that contain bureaucratic language and require the patient's (and a witness's) signature. You can use such a form as an outline to guide discussion, but the patient's act of signing this paper does not constitute informed consent. And, though it does serve as a piece of evidence, the signed consent form is not necessarily sufficient proof of informed consent in court. The doctrine demands four elements in the consent process (shown in Table 15–3):

a. Consent must be voluntary, i.e., there must be no evidence of coercion.
b. The patient must be competent (see discussion below) to make this medical decision at this time.

The "informed" requirement specifies:

c. That adequate information be given about the nature of the procedure, its benefits and risks, and alternative courses of action
d. That the patient understand this information

2. **Since informed consent is a process, it requires skillful patient-doctor conversation:** Katz[63] employs the metaphor of conversation to describe informed consent. Though there are ordinarily no strict rules to determine when a conversation is finished, "most people have a good intuitive grasp of what it means for a conversation to be finished, what it means to change the subject in the middle of a conversation, and what it means to later reopen a conversation one had thought was completed when something new has just arisen."[17] Brody goes on to

TABLE 15–3. Elements of Informed Consent

Informed
  Information: The patient should be provided with information that a "reasonable person" would want to know about benefits, risks, and alternatives.
  Understanding: The patient should understand the information provided.
Consent
  Voluntary: The patient's decision should be freely made, without coercion.
  Competency: The patient should be competent to make an autonomous decision in this particular setting.

---

suggest what he calls the transparency standard of consent for everyday medical practice. According to this standard,

> adequate informed consent is obtained when a reasonably informed patient is allowed to participate in the medical decision to the extent that the patient wishes. In turn, "reasonably informed" consists of two features: (1) the physician discloses the basis on which the proposed treatment, or alternative possible treatments, have been chosen; and (2) the patient is allowed to ask questions suggested by the disclosure of the physician's reasoning, and those questions are answered to the patient's satisfaction.[17]

The important issue here is that consent must be obtained in the context of a conversation during which clear explanations are given and questions are answered, and the patient's competence and understanding are assessed. Such a conversation may lead to negotiation and compromise if the patient objects to proposed procedures or treatments, and the conversation may always be reopened at a later time.

3. **The therapeutic core qualities of empathy, genuineness, and positive regard (see Chap. 2), build trust and facilitate the consent process:** Students and those in medical training should pay particular attention to the need for genuineness. This dovetails with the duty to be truthful. You might be approaching your first lumbar puncture or about to undertake your second paracentesis. (The first was unsuccessful, and your resident had to take over and complete the job.) Do you reveal your inexperience to the patient? What do you say when the patient inquires what percentage of your previous patients developed posttap headaches? Both truthfulness and genuineness dictate that you should not evade these questions, give misleading information, or play an "experienced" role. This is an awkward and sensitive situation, but it must be dealt with head-on. You are a student. This is your first attempt. Your resident should help explain your role and assure the patient that he or she will supervise every detail and be ready to step in at any time if it becomes

necessary. The patient, of course, has a right to refuse to let you do the procedure and to request that someone more experienced be called in.

4. **You should be aware of real (sometimes insurmountable) barriers to informed consent:** These barriers do not arise simply from patient ignorance and physician non-cooperation. Lidz and colleagues[68,69] studied medical inpatients and outpatients in a surgical clinic. They interviewed both patients and doctors to discover what factors inhibited strict adherence to the elements of informed consent. As shown in Table 15–4, they found a number of barriers. The two barriers most important for students to understand are:

   a. Patients often think decision making ought to be in the hands of their doctors and defer to their doctors' judgments. They opt out of the formal decision. Nonetheless, these patients desire to be thoroughly informed about what is going on. Caregivers should not confuse ready acceptance of a diagnostic test with disinterest in its purpose and characteristics. Students have an excellent opportunity to participate by listening to their patients' concerns and answering their questions.

   b. The medical care process often confuses patients because there are many decisions to be made, the

TABLE 15–4. Barriers to Informed Consent

Nature of Medical Decisions
   Treatment decisions tend to evolve over a period of time, rather than being quick and clear.
   Often numerous, related decisions must be made.
   Decision-making process often involves numerous people.
Patient Characteristics
   Patients want information but believe actual decision is the doctor's task.
   Patient does not know which doctor is responsible.
   Patient fails to "hear" because of conflict or denial.
Physician Characteristics
   Doctors do not understand rationale for patient involvement.
   Doctors do not take time to explain issues clearly to patient.

Source: Adapted from Lidz et al.[68]

decisions occur at different times, and frequently a variety of people are responsible. It is difficult to focus on one decision or one issue. Again, the student can play an important role by taking the time to explain these features in conversation with his or her patient.

COMPETENCY

Standards for Judging Competency

Competence is a legal concept, not a medical one. Formal adjudication of competence can only occur in court. The physician's role is to gather relevant information and to decide whether a patient's competence should be called into question. What clinical information is relevant to this question?

Some physicians think that a patient's refusal of needed care is in itself evidence of incompetence. This might be called an outcome standard. It means that if a patient's decision is the medically appropriate one (the right one, from our point of view), we presume the patient is competent. If the decision is medically inappropriate, we suspect incompetence. The issue of competency rarely arises if the patient agrees to the lumbar puncture or to the cardiac catheterization. It is only when the patient refuses the interventions that we wonder about his or her competence. By this definition, every elderly person who wished to refuse aggressive treatment might have his or her wishes overruled by well-meaning, paternalistic doctors. Although we should, in fact, discuss issues thoroughly and make careful observations (i.e., mental status) when patients refuse what seems to us clearly beneficial care, the fact of refusal is not in itself evidence for incompetence.

Another type of information frequently used in competency assessments is patient status. What category does this person fit into? We assume that young children are incompetent to make health care decisions. Similarly, we include those who are profoundly retarded, stuporous or delerious, and severely demented. While many cases are quite obvious, just where do we draw the boundaries? We might agree that a 6-year-old child cannot make a competent decision about whether to accept surgery, but what about a 13-year-old or 15-year-old? Neither one is legally considered an adult, yet should we not place some weight on their opinions and desires? What about a mildly retarded rather than a severely retarded patient? What about a forgetful, sometimes confused, but independent elderly man? The point here is that, while status may be suggestive, it is not the only determinant of competency.

The President's Commission on Ethical Decisions in Medical and Health Care suggested that we use information about the patient's process of decision making, rather than relying solely on information about potential outcome or patient status. Such a standard further requires that we look at the patient's decision-making process as it relates to the issue at hand, rather than relying on more global observations, such as the patient's pattern of forgetfulness or eccentricities, or the fact that the patient is sometimes incontinent or confused. What specific observations are required to apply a decision-making standard of competency?

Appelbaum and Grisso[3] suggest four criteria commonly accepted by the courts:

1. The patient must be able to communicate a choice.
2. The patient must be able to understand information about a treatment decision.
3. The patient must appreciate the medical situation and its consequences. This means awareness of illness and the relative likelihood of various outcomes, given various treatment options.
4. The patient must be able to use logical processes to evaluate information and compare options.

It is crucial here to distinguish between a logical process and a correct or reasonable conclusion. A patient's beliefs or values might be different from those of most people. However, using those beliefs as premises, that patient might reach a perfectly logical (albeit clearly wrong, from our point of view) conclusion. For example, Christian Scientists believe that illness is illusory and represents an error in thinking that can be corrected by study and prayer. A Christian Scientist could logically conclude that accepting medical treatments would be not in his or her best interest because such treatments are based on the alternate belief that sickness is real.

Competency in the Conversation

The relevant data required to apply Appelbaum and Grisso's criteria all arise from a careful and compassionate patient-doctor conversation. Inability to communicate a choice is usually obvious if it is caused by decreased consciousness or psychotic thought disorder. However, extreme ambivalence may lead a patient to switch his or her decision abruptly several times during a short period. The patient says yes, then no, then yes, then no, perhaps with increasing agitation. This should serve as a "red flag" for further evaluation. Impairments of attention span, memory, and intelligence, as well as thought disorders, may interfere with the ability to understand information and to appreciate consequences of the medical situation. These should be assessed during the routine mental status part of your interview. Assessing the capacity to reason logically is more subtle, and some courts have considered logical handling of data to be too strong a criteria to require as evidence of competency. Psychiatric consultation may be helpful to assist in this assessment. In any case, an understanding of the patient's beliefs and value system is required to see "what makes him tick."

Sometimes patient refusal of indicated tests or treatment can be very frustrating, even anger provoking. Respect for autonomy, however, demands that we be very cautious about questioning a patient's competence in order to act against his or her wishes. On the other hand, the principle of beneficence requires that we do our best to promote the patient's medical best interests. Competence is a complex topic and is ultimately, as noted above, a court determination. Here are four rules that might be helpful to you in developing your own thinking about competence in medical care decisions:

- A patient's refusal of the best medical option is not in itself evidence of incompetence; acceptance of the best medical option is not in itself evidence of competence.
- Presence of psychiatric symptoms or an identified psychiatric disorder does not in itself mean the patient is incompetent. Many severely ill patients are depressed, but depression does not necessarily impair decision-making ability (at least not to the extent that it threatens competence).

- Decisions about medical care are essentially value decisions and are determined by religious, cultural, and personal beliefs, as well as strictly biomedical factors.
- Physicians are experts about their patients' medical best interests but not necessarily about their best interests in general. Patients may have a more global view of their welfare, based on religious, cultural, or other values.

References

1. American Medical Association. Principles of Ethics (1980). In: *Current Opinions of the Council on Ethical and Judicial Affairs.* Chicago, Ill: American Medical Association; 1989.
2. American Psychiatric Association. *Diagnostic and Statistical Manual of Mental Disorders.* 3rd ed. Washington, DC, 1987.
3. Appelbaum PS, Grisso T. Assessing patients' capacities to consent to treatment. *New Engl J Med.* 1988; 319:1635–1638.
4. Balint M. *The Doctor, His Patient and the Illness.* New York, NY: International Universities Press; 1972.
5. Bankowitz RA, et al. A computer-assisted medical diagnostic consultation service: Implementation and prospective evaluation of a prototype. *Ann Intern Med.* 1989; 110:824–832.
6. Barnett GO, et al. DXplain: An evolving diagnostic decision-support system. *JAMA.* 1987; 258:67–74.
7. Baron RJ. Bridging clinical distance: An empathic rediscovery of the known. *J Med Philosophy.* 1981; 6:5.
8. Barsky AJ, Klerman GL. Overview: Hypochondriasis, bodily complaints and somatic styles. *Am J Psychiatry.* 1983; 140:273–282.
9. Bass LW, Cohen RL. Ostensible versus actual reasons for seeking pediatric attention: Another look at the parental ticket of admission. *Pediatrics.* 1982; 70:870–874.
10. Beckman HB, Frankel RM. The effect of physician behavior on the collection of data. *Ann Intern Med.* 1984; 101:692–696.
11. Bernarde MA, Mayerson EW. Patient-physician negotiation. *JAMA.* 1978; 239:1413.
12. Bertakis KD. From physician to patient: A method for increasing patient retention and satisfaction. *J Fam Pract.* 1977; 5:217.
13. Billings JA, Stoeckle JD. *The Clinical Encounter.* Chicago, Ill: Yearbook Medical Publishers; 1989.
14. Block MR, Schulberg HC, Coulehan JL, et al. Recognition and characteristics of depression in primary care practice. *J Am Board Fam Pract.* 1988; 1:91–97.
15. Broadman K, et al. Cornell medical index: Adjunct to the medical interview. *JAMA.* 1949; 140:530–534.
16. Brody DS. The patient's role in clinical decision making. *Ann Intern Med.* 1980; 93:718–722.
17. Brody H. Transparency: Informed consent in primary care. *Hastings Center Report.* 1989; 19:5–9.
18. Brownbridge G, Herzmark GA, Wall TD. Patient reactions to doctors' computer use in general practice consultations. *Soc Sci Med.* 1985; 20(1):47–52.
19. Brownbridge G, Lilford RJ, Tindale-Biscoe S. Use of a computer to take booking histories in a hospital antenatal clinic. *Medical Care.* 1988; 5(26):474–487.
20. Burnum JF. The misinformation era: The fall of the medical record. *Ann Intern Med.* 1989; 110:482–484.
21. Cassell EJ. *Talking With Patients. Vol 1: The Theory of Doctor-Patient Communication.* Cambridge, Mass: MIT Press; 1985.
22. Cassell EJ. *Talking With Patients. Vol 2: Clinical Technique.* Cambridge, Mass: MIT Press; 1985.

22a. Churchill LR. Reviving a distinctive medical ethic. *Hastings Center Rep* 1989; 19(3):28–34.

23. Churchill LR, Churchill SW. Storytelling in medical arenas: The art of self-determination. *Lit Med.* 1982; 1:73–79.

24. Colleen MF, Rubin L, Neyman J. Automatic multiphasic screening and diagnosis. *Am J Pub Health.* 1964; 54:741–750.

25. Coulehan JL. Human illness: Cases, models, and paradigms. *Pharos.* 1980; 43:2–8.

26. Coulehan JL. Adjustment, the hands, and healing. *Cult Med Psychiatry.* 1985; 9:353–382.

27. Coulehan JL, Schulberg HC, Block MR. The efficiency of depression questionnaires for case finding in primary medical care. *J Gen Intern Med.* 1989; 4:461–467.

28. Coulehan JL, Schulberg HC, Block MR, et al. Symptom patterns of depression in ambulatory medical and psychiatric patients. *J Nerv Mental Dis.* 1988; 176:284–288.

29. Coulehan JL, Schulberg HC, Block MR, et al. Medical comorbidity of major depressive disorder in primary medical practice. *Arch Intern Med.* 1990; 150:2363–2367.

30. Cutler P. *Problem Solving in Clinical Medicine.* Baltimore, Md: Williams & Wilkins; 1979.

31. Cyr MG, Wartman SA. The effectiveness of routine screening questions in the detection of alcoholism. *JAMA.* 1988; 259:51–54.

32. DeDombal FT. Medical diagnosis from a clinician's point of view. *Meth Inform Med.* 1978; 17:28–35.

33. deGruy F, Columbia L, Dickinson P. Somatization disorder in a family practice. *J Fam Pract.* 1987; 25:45–51.

34. deGruy F, Crider J, Hashimi DK, et al. Somatization disorder in a university hospital. *J Fam Pract.* 1987; 25:579–584.

35. Donnelly WJ. Medical language as symptom: Doctor talk in teaching hospitals. *Perspect Biol Med.* 1986; 30:81–94.

36. Donnelly WJ. Righting the medical record. Transforming chronicle into story. *JAMA.* 1988; 260:823–825.

37. Dudley HA. Clinical method. *Lancet.* 1971; i:35.

38. Duke University Center for the Study of Aging and Human Development. *Multidimensional Functional Assessment: The OARS Methodology.* 2nd ed. Durham, NC: Duke University; 1978.

39. Ebell MH, Heaton CJ. Development and evaluation of a computer genogram. *J Fam Prac.* 1988; 27:536–538.

40. Eisenberg L. What makes persons "patients" and patients "well"? *Am J Med.* 1980; 69:277.

41. Eisenberg L, Kleinman A. Clinical social science. In: Eisenberg L, Kleinman A, eds. *The Relevance of Social Science for Medicine.* Dordrecht, Holland: D Reidel; 1980.

42. Elstein AS, Schulman LS, Sprafka SA. *Medical Problem Solving: An Analysis of Clinical Reasoning.* Cambridge, Mass: Harvard University Press; 1978.

43. Engel GL. The need for a new medical model: A challenge for biomedicine. *Science.* 1977; 196:129–136.

44. Eraker SA, Politser P. How decisions are reached: Physician and patient. *Ann Int Med.* 1982; 97:262.

45. Escobar JI, Burnam MA, Karno M, et al. Somatization in the community. *Arch Gen Psychiatry.* 1987; 44:713–718.

46. Feinstein A. *Clinical Judgment.* Baltimore, Md: Williams & Wilkins; 1967.

47. Feinstein AR. An analysis of diagnostic reasoning. II. The strategy of intermediate decisions. *Yale J Biol Med.* 1973; 46:264–283.

48. Folstein JF, Folstein SE, McHugh PR. "Mini-mental state": A practical method for grading the cognitive state of patients for the clinician. *J Psychiatry Res.* 1975; 12:189–198.

49. Glen ES, et al. Urological history-taking and management recommendations by microcomputer. *Br J Urol.* 1989; 63:117–121.

50. Gogel EL, Terry JS. Medicine as interpretation: The uses of literary metaphors and methods. *J Med Philos.* 1987; 12:205–217.

51. Goldman RH, Peters JM. The occupational and environmental health history. *JAMA.* 1981; 246:2831–2836.

52. Greco RS, Pittenger RA. *One Man's Practice.* Philadelphia, Pa: Tavestock Publications, JB Lippincott; 1966.

53. Groves JE. Taking care of the hateful patient. *N Engl J Med.* 1978; 398:883–887.

54. Gutheil TG, Bursztajn H, Brodsky A. Malpractice prevention through the sharing of uncertainty. Informed consent and the therapeutic alliance. *N Engl J Med.* 1984; 311:49.

55. Harwood A. The hot-cold theory of disease. *JAMA.* 1971; 216:1153–1158.

55a. Haug PJ, Warner HR, Clayton PD, et al. A decision-driven system to collect the patient history. *Comput Biomed Res* 1987; 20(2):193–207.

56. Heaton PB. Negotiations as an integral part of the physician's clinical reasoning. *J Fam Pract.* 1981; 13:845.

57. Hickam DH, Sox HC, Sox CH. Systematic biases in recording the history in patients with chest pain. *J Chronic Dis.* 1985; 38:91–100.

58. Ivey AE, Authier J. *Microcounselling.* Springfield, Ill: Charles C Thomas; 1978.

59. Johnson PE, Duran AS, Hassebrock F, et al. Expertise and error in diagnostic reasoning. *Cog Sci.* 1981; 5:235–283.

59a. Joyce CRB, Caple G, Mason M, et al. Quantitative study of doctor-patient communication. *Quart J Med* 1969; 38:183–194.

60. Kahana RJ, Bibring GL. Personality types in medical management. In: Zinberg NE, ed. *Psychiatry and Medical Practice in a General Hospital.* New York, NY: International Universities Press; 1964:108–123.

61. Kassirer JP, Gorry GA. Clinical problem solving: A behavioral analysis. *Ann Intern Med.* 1978; 89:245–255.

62. Katon W, Ries RK, Kleinman A. A prospective DSM-III study of 100 consecutive somatization patients. *Compr Psychiatry.* 1984; 25:305–314.

63. Katz J. *The Silent World of Doctor and Patient.* New York, NY: The Free Press; 1984.

64. Kimball CP. Techniques of interviewing. Interviewing and the meaning of the symptom. *Ann Intern Med.* 1969; 71:147.

65. Kimball CP. *The Biopsychosocial Approach to the Patient.* Baltimore, Md: Williams & Wilkins; 1981.

66. Kleinman A, Eisenberg L, Good B. Culture, illness and care: clinical lessons from anthropological and cross-cultural research. *Ann Int Med.* 1978; 88:251.

67. Ley P. Toward better doctor-patient communication. Contributions from social and experimental psychology. In: Bennett AE, ed. *Commu-*

nication Between Doctors and Patients. Oxford, England: Nuffield Provincial Hospitals Trust, Oxford University Press; 1976:77–98.

68. Lidz CW, et al. Barriers to informed consent. *Ann Intern Med.* 1983; 99:539–543.

69. Lidz CW, et al. *Informed Consent: A Study of Psychiatric Decision Making.* New York, NY: Guilford Press; 1983.

70. Lilford RD, Glyn-Evans D, Chard T. The use of a patient interactive microcomputer system to obtain histories in an infertility and gynecologic endocrinology clinic. *Am J Obstet Gynecol.* 1983; 146:374–379.

71. Lipkin M Jr. Psychiatry and medicine. In: Kaplan H, Sadock B, eds. *Comprehensive Textbook of Psychiatry.* 5th ed. Baltimore, Md: Williams & Wilkins; 1987.

72. Lipowski ZJ. Physical illness, the individual and the coping process. *Psychiatry Med* 1970; 1:91–102.

73. Lucas RW, et al. Psychiatrists and a computer as interrogators of patients with alcohol-related illness: A comparison. *Br J Psychiatry.* 1977; 131:160–167.

74. Medical Hardware and Software Buyers' Guide Issue. *MC Computing.* 1990; 6:6.

75. Miller RA, Pople H, Myers JD. INTERNIST-II: An experimental computer-based diagnostic consultant for general internal medicine. *N Engl J Med.* 1982; 307:468–476.

76. Miller RA, et al. The INTERNIST-I/QUICK MEDICAL REFERENCE project: Status report. *West J Med.* 1986; 145:816–822.

77. Nardone DA. Differential diagnosis and heuristics. *JAMA.* 1985; 254:2890 (letter to the Editor).

78. Osler W. On the need for a radical reform in our methods of teaching senior students. *Med News (New York).* 1903; 82:49–53.

79. Pauker SG, et al. Towards the simulation of clinical cognition: Taking a present illness by computer. *Am J Med.* 1976; 60:981–996.

80. Platt FW, McMath JC. Clinical hypocompetence: The interview. *Ann Intern Med.* 1979; 91:898–902.

81. Pryor TA, et al. The HELP system. *J Med Syst.* 1983; 7:87–102.

82. Quack MJ, Westerman RF, Van Bemmel JH: Comparison between written and computerized patient histories. *Br Med J.* 1987; 295:184–190.

83. Quill TE. Recognizing and adjusting to barriers in doctor-patient communication. *Ann Intern Med.* 1989; 111:51–57.

84. Radloff L. The CES-D scale: A self-report depression scale for research in the general population. *App Psychol Meas.* 1977; 1:385–401.

85. Rakel RE. *Principles of Family Medicine.* Philadelphia, Pa: WB Saunders; 1977.

86. Reilly BM. *Practical Strategies in Outpatient Medicine.* Philadelphia, Pa: WB Saunders; 1984.

87. Rich EC, Crowson TW, Harris IB. The diagnostic value of the medical history. *Arch Intern Med.* 1987; 147:1957–1960.

88. Roter DL, Hall JA. Physicians' interviewing styles and medical information obtained from patients. *J Gen Intern Med.* 1987; 2:325–329.

89. Rubel AJ, O'Nell CW, Collado R. The folk illness called *susto.* In: Simons RC, Hughes CC, eds. *The Culture Bound Syndromes.* Dordrecht, Holland: D Reidel; 1985.

90. Sackett DL, Haynes RB. *Compliance With Therapeutic Regimens.* Baltimore, Md: Johns Hopkins University Press; 1976.

91. Schmitt BP, Kushner MS, Wiener SL. The diagnostic usefulness of the history of the patient with dyspnea. *J Gen Intern Med.* 1986; 1:386–390.

92. Schwartz WB, Patil RS, Szolovits P. Artificial intelligence in medicine: Where do we stand? *N Engl J Med.* 1988; 316:685–688.

93. Seltzer ML. The Michigan alcoholism screening test: The quest for a new diagnostic instrument. *Am J Psychiatry.* 1971; 127:1653–1658.

94. Shea SC. *Psychiatric Interviewing: The Art of Understanding.* Philadelphia, Pa: WB Saunders; 1988.

95. Shortliffe EH. Clinical decision-support systems. In: Shortliffe EH, Perreault LE, eds. *Medical Informatics: Computer Applications in Health Care.* New York, NY: Addison-Wesley; 1990.

96. Shortliffe EH. Computer programs to support clinical decision making. *JAMA.* 1987; 258:61–66.

97. Siegler M. The physician-patient accommodation. A central event in clinical medicine. *Arch Intern Med.* 1982; 142:1899–1902.

98. Skinner HA, Holt S, Schuller R, et al. Identification of alcohol abuse using laboratory tests and a history of trauma. *Ann Intern Med.* 1984; 101:847–851.

99. Slack WV, et al. A computer-based medical history system. *N Engl J Med.* 1966; 274:194–198.

100. Snow LF. Folk medical beliefs and their implications for care of patients. *Ann Intern Med.* 1974; 81:82.

101. Thomas AMC, et al. A computer-based interview system for patients with back pain: A validation study. *Spine.* 1989; 14:844–846.

102. Uzzell D. Susto revisited: Illness as strategic role. In: Landy D, ed. *Culture, Disease and Healing.* New York, NY: Macmillan; 1978.

103. Voytovich AE, Rippey RM, Suffredini A. Premature conclusions in diagnostic reasoning. *J Med Educ.* 1980; 60:302–307.

104. Warner HR, Rutherford BD, Houtchens B. A sequential Bayesian approach to history taking and diagnosis. *Comput Biomed Res.* 1972; 5:256–272.

105. Warner HR, et al. ILIAD as an expert consultant to teach differential diagnosis. In: Proceedings of the Twelfth Annual Symposium on Computer Applications in Medical Care. New York, NY: IEEE Computer Society Press; 1988:371–376.

106. Weed LL. *Medical Records, Medical Educational, and Patient Care.* Cleveland, Ohio: Case Western Reserve University Press; 1970.

107. Weiner S, Nathanson M. Physical examination. Frequently observed errors. *JAMA.* 1976; 236:852–855.

108. Wolraich ML, et al. Factors affecting physician communication and parent-physician dialogues. *J Med Educ.* 1982; 57:621–625.

109. Wright AD, et al. Patterns of acquisition of interview skills by medical students. *Lancet.* 1980; 1:964–966.

110. Wulff HR. *Rational Diagnosis and Treatment.* Oxford, England: Blackwell Scientific Publications; 1981:10.

111. Zung WK. A self-rating depression scale. *Arch Gen Psychiatry.* 1965; 12:63–70.

Additional Reading

BEAUCHAMP TL, McCULLOUGH LB. *Medical ethics: The Moral Responsibilities of Physicians.* Englewood Cliffs, NJ: Prentice-Hall; 1984.

BECKER MH, MAIMAN LA. Sociobehavioral determinants of compliance with health and medical care recommendations. *Med Care.* 1975; 70:870.

BRODY H. *Stories of Sickness.* New Haven, Conn: Yale University Press; 1987.

BURACK RC, CARPENTER RR. The predictive value of the presenting complaint. *J Fam Pract.* 1983; 16:749–754.

CASSELL EJ. *The Healer's Art.* Philadelphia, Pa: JB Lippincott; 1976.

CHARON R. To render the lives of patients. *Lit Med.* 1986; 5:58–74.

COMSTOCK LM, et al. Physician behaviors that correlate with patient satisfaction. *J Med Educ.* 1982; 57:105–112.

COULEHAN JL. Dissecting the clinical art. *Pharos.* 1984; 47(4):21.

COULEHAN JL, BLOCK M. Creating the healing connection. In: Lazes P, ed. *Handbook of Health Education.* 2nd ed. Baltimore, Md: Aspen Press; 1986.

DiMATTEO MR, PRINCE LM, TARANTA A. Patients' perceptions of physicians' behavior: Determinants of patient commitment to the therapeutic relationship. *J Community Health.* 1979; 4:280–290.

DiMATTEO MR, et al. Predicting patient satisfaction from physicians' nonverbal communcation skills. *Med Care.* 1980; 18:376–387.

DRANE JF. Competency to give an informed consent. A model for making clinical decisions. *JAMA.* 1984; 252:925–927.

DROSSMAN DA. The problem patient. Evaluation and care of medical patients with psychosocial disturbances. *Ann Intern Med.* 1978; 88:366.

DUFFY DL, HAMERMAN D, COHEN MA. Communication skills of house officers. *Ann Intern Med.* 1980; 93:354–357.

ELIOT DL, HICKAM DH. Evaluation of physical examination skills. Reliability of faculty observers and patient instructors. *JAMA.* 1987; 258:3405–3408.

ENGEL GL. The care of the patient: Art or science? *Johns Hopkins Med J.* 1977; 140:222.

ERAKER SA, KIRSHT JP, BECKER MH. Understanding and improving patient compliance. *Ann Intern Med.* 1984; 100:258–268.

FEINSTEIN AR. An additional basic science for clinical medicine: The development of clinometrics. *Ann Intern Med.* 1983; 99:843–848.

FISHER R, URY W. *Getting to Yes: Negotiating Agreement Without Giving In.* Boston, Mass: Houghton-Mifflin; 1981.

FRANK JD. The faith that heals. *Johns Hopkins Med J.* 1975; 137:127–131.

GOODWIN JS, GOODWIN JM, Vogel AV. Knowledge and use of placebos by house officers and nurses. *Ann Intern Med.* 1979; 91:106–110.

GREY G, FLYNN P. A survey of placebo use in a general hospital. *Gen Hosp Psychiatry.* 1981; 3:199–203.

HAMPTON JR, et al. Relative contributions of history taking, physical examination, and laboratory investigation to diagnosis and management of medical outpatients. *Br Med J.* 1975; 2:486–489.

HOUSTON WR. The doctor himself as therapeutic agent. *Ann Intern Med.* 1938; 11:1416.

355

HUNTER KM. "There was this one guy . . .": The uses of anecdotes in medicine. *Perspect Biol Med.* 1986; 29:619–630.

INUI TS, CARTER WB. Problems and prospects for health services research on provider-patient communication. *Medical Care.* 1985; 23:521–538.

KAPLAN C, LIPKIN M, GORDON GH. Somatization in primary care: Patients with unexplained and vexing medical complaints. *J Gen Intern Med.* 1988; 3:177–190.

KASSIRER JP, KUIPERS BJ, GORRY GA. Toward a theory of clinical expertise. *Am J Med.* 1982; 73:251–259.

KELLNER R. Hypochondriasis and somatization. *JAMA.* 1987; 258:2718–2722.

KLEINMAN A. *The Illness Narratives. Suffering, Healing and the Human Condition.* New York, NY: Basic Books; 1988.

KRAYTMAN M. *The Complete Medical History.* New York, NY: McGraw-Hill; 1979.

LAIN ENTRALGO P. *Doctor and Patient.* New York, NY: McGraw-Hill; 1969:199–205.

LARSEN KM, SMITH, CK. Assessment of nonverbal communication in the patient-physician interview. *J Fam Pract.* 1981; 12:481–488.

LAZARE A. Shame and humiliation in the medical encounter. *Arch Intern Med.* 1987; 147:1653–1658.

LAZARE A, EISENTHAL S. A negotiated approach to the clinical encounter. In: LAZARE A, ed. *Outpatient Psychiatry: Diagnosis and Treatment.* Baltimore, Md: Williams & Wilkins; 1979:141–156.

LEIGH H, REISER MF. *The Patient. Biological, Psychological and Social Dimensions of Medical Practice.* New York, NY: Plenum; 1980.

LEY P. Satisfaction, compliance and communication. *Br J Clin Psychol.* 1982; 21:241–254.

LIPKIN M JR, QUILL TE, NAPODANO RJ. The medical interview: A core curriculum for residencies in internal medicine. *Ann Intern Med.* 1984; 100:277–284.

LIPOWSKI ZJ. Somatization: The concept and its clinical application. *Am J Psychiatry.* 1988; 145:1358–1368.

MARTIN AR. Exploring patient beliefs. Steps to enhancing physician-patient interaction. *Arch Intern Med.* 1983; 143:1773–1775.

MAYFIELD D, McLEOD G, HALL P. The CAGE questionnaire: Validation of a new alcoholism screening instrument. *Am J Psychiatry.* 1974; 131:1121–1123.

MUMFORD E, SCHLESINGER HJ, GLASS GV. The effects of psychological intervention on recovery from surgery and heart attacks: An analysis of the literature. *Am J Public Health.* 1982; 72:141–151.

NOVACK DH. Therapeutic aspects of the clinical encounter. *J Gen Intern Med.* 1987; 2:346–355.

PELLEGRINO ED. The healing relationship: The architectonics of clinical medicine. In: Shelp E, ed. *The Clinical Encounter.* Dordrecht, Holland: D Reidel; 1983:153–172.

PENDLETON D, HASLER J. *Doctor-Patient Communication.* New York, NY: Academic Press; 1983.

POIRIER S, BRAUNER DJ. Ethics and the daily language of medical discourse. *Hastings Center Report.* 1988; Aug/Sept:5–9.

QUILL TE. Partnerships in patient care: A contractual approach. *Ann Intern Med.* 1983; 98:228–234.

QUILL TE. Somatization disorder. One of medicine's blind spots. *JAMA*. 1985; 254:3075–3079.

REISER DE, SCHRODER AK. *Patient Interviewing: The Human Dimension*. Baltimore, Md: Williams & Wilkins; 1980.

ROGERS C. *On Becoming a Person*. Boston, Mass: Houghton Mifflin; 1961.

SANDLER G. The importance of the history in the medical clinic and the cost of unnecessary tests. *Am Heart J*. 1980; 100:928–931.

SAPIRA JD. Why perform a routine history and physical examination? *South Med J*. 1989; 82:364–365.

SHAPIRO AK. The placebo response. In: Howells JG, ed. *Modern Perspectives in World Psychiatry: 2*. Edinburgh, England: Oliver and Boyd; 1971.

SMITH CK, POLIS E, HADAC RR. Characteristics of the initial medical interview associated with patient satisfaction and understanding. *J Fam Pract*. 1981; 12:283–288.

TVERSKY A, KAHNEMAN D. Judgment under uncertainty: Heuristics and biases. *Science*. 1974; 185:1124–1131.

WAITZKIN H, STOECKLE JD. The communication of information about illness. Clinical, sociological, and methodological considerations. *Adv Psychosom Med*. 1972; 8:180–215.

WU WC, PEARLMAN RA. Consent in medical decision-making: The role of communication. *J Gen Intern Med*. 1988; 3:9–14.

Index

Numbers in *italics* indicate figures; numbers followed by a "t" indicate tables.

359